RECENT ADVANCES IN HEMATOLOGY RESEARCH

BENIGN AND MALIGNANT DISORDERS OF LARGE GRANULAR LYMPHOCYTES

DIAGNOSTIC AND THERAPEUTIC PEARLS

RECENT ADVANCES IN HEMATOLOGY RESEARCH

Additional books in this series can be found on Nova's website under the Series tab.

Additional e-books in this series can be found on Nova's website under the eBooks tab.

RECENT ADVANCES IN HEMATOLOGY RESEARCH

BENIGN AND MALIGNANT DISORDERS OF LARGE GRANULAR LYMPHOCYTES

DIAGNOSTIC AND THERAPEUTIC PEARLS

LING ZHANG
AND
LUBOMIR SOKOL
EDITORS

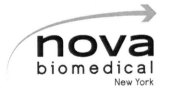

Copyright © 2018 by Nova Science Publishers, Inc.

All rights reserved. No part of this book may be reproduced, stored in a retrieval system or transmitted in any form or by any means: electronic, electrostatic, magnetic, tape, mechanical photocopying, recording or otherwise without the written permission of the Publisher.

We have partnered with Copyright Clearance Center to make it easy for you to obtain permissions to reuse content from this publication. Simply navigate to this publication's page on Nova's website and locate the "Get Permission" button below the title description. This button is linked directly to the title's permission page on copyright.com. Alternatively, you can visit copyright.com and search by title, ISBN, or ISSN.

For further questions about using the service on copyright.com, please contact:
Copyright Clearance Center
Phone: +1-(978) 750-8400   Fax: +1-(978) 750-4470   E-mail: info@copyright.com.

NOTICE TO THE READER

The Publisher has taken reasonable care in the preparation of this book, but makes no expressed or implied warranty of any kind and assumes no responsibility for any errors or omissions. No liability is assumed for incidental or consequential damages in connection with or arising out of information contained in this book. The Publisher shall not be liable for any special, consequential, or exemplary damages resulting, in whole or in part, from the readers' use of, or reliance upon, this material. Any parts of this book based on government reports are so indicated and copyright is claimed for those parts to the extent applicable to compilations of such works.

Independent verification should be sought for any data, advice or recommendations contained in this book. In addition, no responsibility is assumed by the publisher for any injury and/or damage to persons or property arising from any methods, products, instructions, ideas or otherwise contained in this publication.

This publication is designed to provide accurate and authoritative information with regard to the subject matter covered herein. It is sold with the clear understanding that the Publisher is not engaged in rendering legal or any other professional services. If legal or any other expert assistance is required, the services of a competent person should be sought. FROM A DECLARATION OF PARTICIPANTS JOINTLY ADOPTED BY A COMMITTEE OF THE AMERICAN BAR ASSOCIATION AND A COMMITTEE OF PUBLISHERS.

Additional color graphics may be available in the e-book version of this book.

Library of Congress Cataloging-in-Publication Data

ISBN: 978-1-53612-999-1
Library of Congress Control Number: 2017963333

Published by Nova Science Publishers, Inc. † New York

Contents

Preface		vii
Chapter 1	Molecular Biology and Genetics of Large Granular Lymphocytic Leukemia *T. Tiffany Wang, Jeffrey C. Xing, Thomas L. Olson, David J. Feith and Thomas P. Loughran Jr.*	1
Chapter 2	Abnormal Function of Innate and Adaptive Immune Systems in Large Granular Lymphocytic Leukemia *Lili Yang, Houfang Sun and Sheng Wei*	25
Chapter 3	NK Cell Biology and the Role of NK Cells in Hematopoietic Stem Cell Transplantation and Cellular Immunotherapy *Rawan Faramand and Asmita Mishra*	43
Chapter 4	Pathogenesis of Myelodysplastic Syndromes Harboring Clonal Large Granular Leukocytes *P. K. Epling-Burnette*	75
Chapter 5	Benign T-LGL and NK Cell Proliferations Evolved after Hematopoietic Cell Transplantation, and Anti-Neoplastic Agents *Taiga Nishihori*	101
Chapter 6	Routine Diagnostic Approaches of T-Cell Large Granular Lymphocytic Leukemia *Ling Zhang*	115
Chapter 7	Chronic Lymphoproliferative Disorder of Natual Killer Cells: An Entity Falling to a Benign or Malignant Process *Prerna Rastogi, Rawan Faramand, Lubomir Sokol and Ling Zhang*	149

Chapter 8	T-Cell Large Granular Lymphocytic Leukemia: Conventional Treatment Approaches and Novel Strategies *Magali Van den Bergh and Lubomir Sokol*	**165**
Chapter 9	Extranodal NK/T Cell Lymphoma, Nasal Type Diagnostic Approaches *Stefanie Grewe, Carolina Domiguez and Haipeng Shao*	**183**
Chapter 10	Clinical Intervention and Novel Therapeutic Strategies for Extranodal NK/T Cell Lymphoma, Nasal Type *George Yang, Daniel Grass, Kamran Ahmed and Sungjune Kim*	**225**
Chapter 11	Aggressive Natural Killer (NK) Cell Leukemia *Xiaohui Zhang*	**249**
Chapter 12	Clinical Manifestation and Management of Aggressive Natural Killer Cell Leukemia *Emilie Wang, Ling Zhang and Lubomir Sokol*	**265**
Chapter 13	Natural Killer Cell Dysfunction in Primary and Acquired Hemophagocytic Lymphohistiocytosis *Seongseok Yun and Ling Zhang*	**279**
Editors' Contact Information		**301**
Index		**303**

PREFACE

Natural killer (NK) cells are important effector cells of innate immune system implicated in many physiological processes including elimination of cancer cells and virus infected cells. NK cells comprise a majority of large granular lymphocytes circulating in peripheral blood with a minority derived from T cell lineage. Even though NK cells were first described more than 40 years ago, it was not until the 1980s when immunophenotyping was incorporated into clinical diagnostic methods and resulted in discovery of distinct disorders of large granular lymphocytes (LGLs) and NK cells. Since then, significant progress was made in our understanding of immunophenotypic and genotypic characteristics, biology, functions as well as disorders of these cells. Most recently, clinical studies using NK-cell based immunotherapy have shown promising results in treatment of some of solid tumors and hematological malignancies.

Disorders of LGLs and NK cells are rare comprising only about 1% of all lymphoid malignancies in western countries. The rarity of these conditions was a main reason that the progress in our understanding of pathogenesis and development of novel therapeutic approaches has been delayed compared to developments in more common B cell lymphoid malignancies. The low incidence of these diseases and scarcity of prospective clinical trials also limit the availability of evidence based research literature as well as comprehensive reviews about NK cell disorders. Thus, the editors decided to take on the challenging task and summarize our current knowledge about malignant and benign diseases of LGLs in this book based on the best available evidences. The editors selected topics most relevant to clinical practice in order to provide a useful guide for practicing physicians. Chapters describing four disorders (T-cell large granular lymphocytic leukemia, chronic lymphoproliferative disorder of NK cells, extranodal NK cell lymphoma and aggressive NK cell leukemia) incorporated into most recent 2016 World Health Organization (WHO) revision of classification of lymphoid malignancies are separated into diagnostic and clinical parts for easier understanding and reading. The book chapters also include experimental data for better understanding of fundamentals of

NK cell biology. Authors hope that this topic could be of interest to basic scientists who engage in the immunology and immunotherapy research.

We are aware of challenges and inherited limitations of any larger project like this one due to a rapid progress especially in the field of genomics, which may not be incorporated in this book before it is published. The editors and contributing authors would like to thank the publisher NOVA for their support.

In: Benign and Malignant Disorders …
Editors: Ling Zhang and Lubomir Sokol
ISBN: 978-1-53612-999-1
© 2018 Nova Science Publishers, Inc.

Chapter 1

MOLECULAR BIOLOGY AND GENETICS OF LARGE GRANULAR LYMPHOCYTIC LEUKEMIA

T. Tiffany Wang[1,†], Jeffrey C. Xing[2,†], Thomas L. Olson, PhD[3,4], David J. Feith, PhD[3,4] and Thomas P. Loughran Jr., MD[*,3,4]

[1]Department of Microbiology, Immunology and Cancer Biology
[2]Department of Biomedical Engineering
[3]Department of Medicine, Division of Hematology and Oncology
[4]University of Virginia Cancer Center
University of Virginia School of Medicine, Charlottesville, VA, US

ABSTRACT

Large granular lymphocyte leukemia (LGLL) is characterized by a sustained clonal proliferation of circulating large granular lymphocytes (LGL). The exact etiology and mechanisms of the development of disease are not completely understood. It is hypothesized that viral transformation, chronic antigen-driven stimulus, and somatic oncogenic mutation may each be contributing factors in a given patient and the LGLL patient population as a whole. External stimuli via certain cytokines (e.g., IL-6, IL-15, PDGF, and IL-18) could result in constitutive activation of the JAK-STAT, Ras-Raf-MEK-ERK, NFκB and PI3K/Akt pathways. Additional studies indicate a key role for the sphingolipid rheostat and FasL mediated apoptosis resistance in patients with LGLL. Together these many biochemical and genetic alterations contribute to leukemic proliferation of LGL cells. Activating somatic mutations of the *STAT3* gene occur in a subset of LGLL, leading to altered inflammatory response, autoimmunity and dysregulated apoptotic cascades. Per a clinical study cohort, LGLL patients with such mutations have favorable response to methotrexate (MTX) treatment. Notably, in the

---
[†] Authors contributed equally to this work.
[*] Corresponding author: tl7cs@virginia.edu.

proper clinical setting a positive activating *STAT3* mutation adds additional specificity to the diagnosis of T-LGLL and offers a sensitive way of tracking minimal residual disease. This chapter aims to explore the cumulative research investigating the cellular and molecular basis of LGL leukemia, with an emphasis on the more common T-cell subtype.

1. INTRODUCTION

Large granular lymphocytes (LGL) represent a morphologically distinct subset of normal circulating blood cells. They are about 2-3 times larger than red blood cells and have abundant cytoplasm with characteristic azurophilic granules [1]. Classically, this LGL subset is further divided into 85% CD3 natural killer (NK) cells and 15% CD3(+) T cells and thought to be involved in normal immune response to viruses or cancer cells. It is not uncommon to see a "reactive" lymphocytosis of LGL cells following an acute viral infection that subsides within two weeks. In contrast, LGL leukemia (LGLL) is characterized by a sustained (>6 month) clonal proliferation of circulating LGL cells, as discussed throughout this book. The majority of patients exhibit T type clones (T-LGLL) and a minority have NK type clones (NK-LGLL). Therefore, the majority of research has been conducted in T-LGLL.

2. RECAP OF LGL LEUKEMIA AND CURRENT MODEL

Currently, the World Health Organization's 2016 revised 4th edition [2] recognizes three entities: A) T-cell large granular lymphocytic leukemia (T-LGLL), B) Chronic lymphoproliferative disorder of NK cells (CLPD-NK), and C) Aggressive NK-cell leukemia (ANKL). Due to the rarity of the NK subtype, most of the following discussion focuses on research conducted in T-LGLL (A), some research on CLPD-NK (B), and only a few case reports on ANKL (C). Unless otherwise emphasized, "T-LGLL" generally refers to findings from the CD8+ T-cell subtype, and "NK-LGLL" refers to findings from the chronic lymphoproliferative NK type.

Given the sustained, chronic activation [3] of LGL cells in the leukemic condition, the question then is why are these cells accumulating in the circulation? The wide spectrum [4] of clinical presentations suggests a multi-factorial mechanism. To date, the etiology of LGLL has not been fully established. There are several hypothesized theories under investigation: viral transformation, chronic antigen-driven stimulus, and somatic oncogenic mutation. It is important to note that these mechanisms are not mutually exclusive; thus, one or more may be relevant in a given patient and the LGLL patient population as a whole.

2.1. Viral Transformation in LGLL

The etiology of viral transformation has been explored in all forms of LGLL. A documented association of Epstein-Barr virus (EBV), a known oncogenic initiator, with the aggressive form of NK-LGL leukemia was shown in several Japanese studies [5, 6]. However, this contrasts with a failure to find EBV DNA in NK-LGLL patients of Western Europe and the United States [7], which may explain the differences in clinical presentation (EBV-associated LGLL in Asia is more aggressive and invasive). In addition to EBV, human T-lymphotropic virus (HTLV), also known to be oncogenic, has been explored as a causative agent in LGLL. Retroviral infection has been only rarely documented in LGLL [8], however some studies have shown a higher prevalence of seroreactivity to human HTLV-1 envelope protein in LGLL patients [9, 10] and in patients with NK-cell variant LGLL or CLPD NK [11], compared to reference cohorts. Although not linked to disease, the HTLV *tax* protein has been successfully employed to create experimental model systems [12, 13].

2.2. Chronic Antigen Stimulation in LGLL

Chronic antigen-driven stimulus has also been explored as a cause of T- and NK cell LGL leukemia. The terminal effector memory (CD45RA+/CD62L-) phenotype of T-LGLL cells suggests the possibility of chronic antigen exposure as a driver of LGL expansion [14]. Compatible with this hypothesis, several studies examining the antigen-specific sequence of the T-cell receptor (TCR) or its combinatorial rearrangements in the variable region have found a nonrandom distribution [15, 16, 17, 18]. It is hypothesized that these restricted clonotypes may predispose an individual toward the extreme monoclonal expansions commonly found in T-LGLL [19]. However, whether the observed restricted clonotypes may be a cause (for example, a restricted repertoire that prevents clearance of antigen) or an effect (for example, the result of a chronic antigen, such as cytomegalovirus (CMV) [20] or HTLV [21]) remains inconclusive, with some studies only finding clonotype restriction in T-LGLL subtypes [18] and all studies lacking in large sample size. In the NK-LGL leukemia subtype, killer immunoglobulin-like (KIR) receptors play an analogous role to the activation of T-cell receptors in T-LGLL. Several studies [22, 23, 24, 25] have found a skewing of the ratio of activating to inhibitory KIR receptors in favor of activation. Interestingly, expansion of T cell clones has also been detected in half of a cohort of chronic NK-LGL leukemia patients, with some of these patients progressively switching to T-LGLL [26]. Activating KIRs have also been found in other autoimmune diseases, suggesting that this phenotype may contribute to the pathogenesis of the disease. Moreover, the HLA associations with HLA-

DR4 [27], HLA-DR15 [28], and HLA-B7 [19] suggest a possible autoimmune predisposition, blurring the lines between autoimmune disorders and the leukemia.

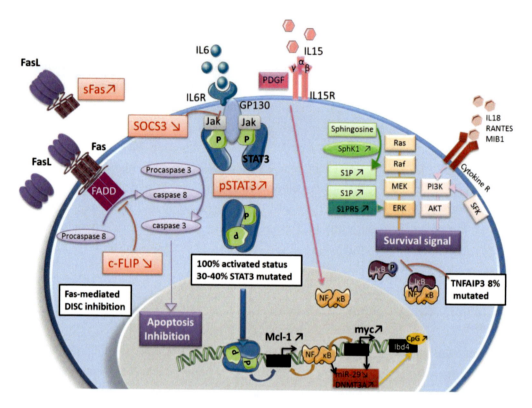

LGLL could result from alteration of several signaling pathways: inhibition of Fas-mediated death inducing signaling complex (DISC), constitutive activation of JAK/STAT pathway, stimulation of IL15/PDGF-NFκB pathway, and altered survival signals through Ras-Raf-MEK-ERK and PI3K/Akt pathway. Increased pro-survival sphingosine 1-phosphate (S1P) along with its receptor S1PR5 (sphingosine 1-phosphate receptor 5) with a consequence of activation of Raf-MEK-ERK survival signals is also observed in LGLL. Of the aforementioned pathways, the constitutive activation of *STAT3* is the main one to activate its downstream proliferative signals. Mutations of *STAT3* occur in a subset of LGLL (30-40%). Mutated TNFAIP3 is found in a minor subset of LGLL, which abrogates IκB inhibitory regulation of NFκB. Figure adapted from [97].

Figure 1. Aberrant Signaling Pathways in LGLL.

2.3. Somatic Mutation in LGLL

Aside from these "external" etiologies, a third hypothesis is that one or several somatic mutations may serve as drivers in the oncogenesis and/or progression of LGLL. Foreshadowing this possibility, clonal chromosomal abnormalities (trisomy 8 and trisomy 14) were found in several cases of LGLL in the original discovery of the disease two decades before the advent of genome-scale sequencing approaches [29]. Dysregulated apoptosis has been shown to be an important mechanism in the pathogenesis of LGLL.

Based on their expression of Fas (CD95) and Fas-Ligand (CD178) [30, 31], leukemic T cell LGLs are activated cytotoxic cells that escaped Fas-mediated activation-induced cell death (AICD) [32, 14]. In addition, soluble Fas in patient sera [33], may act as a decoy receptor that negates Fas-induced AICD. The expansion of leukemic T and NK LGL cells may result from constitutive activation of one or several survival pathways: JAK/STAT3/Mcl-1 [32], Ras/MEK/ERK [34, 35], SFK/PI3K/AKT [36, 3, 37], and sphingolipid signaling [38, 39]. The activating mutations in signal transducer and activator of transcription 3 (*STAT3*) in particular have been a major focus in recent research and will be discussed in more detail in the subsequent sections. A summary of these studied pathways is shown in Figure 1.

3. RESEARCH METHODS AND FINDINGS

To establish a better context for these interpretations, we next elaborate on some of the approaches that have been used to build our current understanding of LGLL. T-LGLL has been more extensively researched than either the chronic or the aggressive form of NK-cell leukemia as it is more common. Therefore, unless otherwise noted, this book chapter focuses on the molecular biology and genetics of T-cell LGLL.

3.1. Network Modeling

Network modeling of signaling pathways is a systems biology approach that synthesizes existing domain knowledge of signal transduction relationships into an *in silico* interaction network [40]. This is not unlike the pathway diagrams that biologists refer to when tracing the effect of one protein on the downstream pathway. The difference is that the more formalized representation as a network allows a much larger and more complex interaction of multiple, sometimes competing or even opposing, pathways to be simulated in a dynamic fashion. This enables systematic prediction of cause and effect relationships from candidate perturbations or environmental stimuli across the entire network. In the absence of quantitative kinetic measurements of enzyme rates (which is required for continuous models), discrete approximations such as Boolean models [(a classical information retrieval (IR) model]) have shown encouraging results and may provide valuable guidance for wet-bench experiments to test hypotheses related to disease pathogenesis or therapeutic targeting.

For T-LGLL, a discrete Boolean network of 60 nodes and 142 regulatory edges was curated from literature knowledge [41] and showed that signaling abnormalities in the leukemia can be reproduced with only two constitutively active external stimuli: platelet derived growth factor (PDGF) and interleukin-15 (IL-15). Experimentally, the role of

PDGF in mediating survival of T-LGLL was found to occur through an autocrine loop [42]. In addition, the pro-inflammatory role of IL-15 on both T-LGLL and NK-LGLL has been established [43, 44, 45], with a possible mechanism mediated through DNA hypermethylation in a murine disease model [46]. Moreover, systematic perturbations of the various nodes in this network identified potential therapeutic targets such as NF-κB, SPHK1, and BID, whose node reversal increases the likelihood of apoptosis. Further comprehensive dynamic and structural analysis of this network in a follow-up study [47] identified 19 potential therapeutic targets, 13 of which were experimentally corroborated and 6 are novel predictions to be validated. More recently, stable sub-network motifs [48] were analyzed to prioritize driver nodes for drug targeting in ongoing studies. These motifs represent feedback pathways that autonomously persist even upon transient activation, with some predicted to eventually direct cell fate to a steady state phenotype such as leukemia or apoptosis.

3.2. Gene Set Enrichment Analysis

Gene set enrichment analysis (GSEA) is a pathway-based approach to differential gene expression analysis between two phenotypes [49]. That is, instead of comparing each gene one by one, it compares groups of genes that are known from domain knowledge to be part of the same ontological set, such as a signaling pathway. This global approach is often applied to RNA sequencing (RNA-seq) or microarray gene expression data to identify statistically significant differences in the molecular expression profile of tumors.

Microarray gene expression data of leukemic LGLs compared with the normal activated counterpart (activated CD3+/CD8+ PBMCs) suggested that a sphingolipid metabolism and signaling-related gene set is enriched in leukemic LGLs [38]. A recent finding that sphingosine kinase 1 (SPHK1) inhibition induces apoptosis and leads to decreased phosphorylation of JAK1/JAK2/STAT3/STAT5 also in the chronic form of NK-LGLL [50] validates predictions from network modeling and gene set enrichment analysis regarding the role of sphingolipid signaling in T-LGLL.

As part of a normal physiologic response, activation of lymphocytes simultaneously increases their susceptibility to apoptosis, which is thought to help the body clear an expanded lymphocyte population after an infection subsides [51]. Interestingly, the gene expression data showed uncoupling between activation and apoptosis in leukemic LGLs. In a cohort of 30 patients [38], the gene set enrichment in T-LGLL cells showed "negative regulation of apoptosis" in contrast to phytohemagglutinin (PHA) & IL-2-activated CD8+ T-cells from normal donors, which exhibited enrichment for "induction of apoptosis."

3.3. TCR Gene Rearrangement

Both T-LGLL and CLPD-NK frequently exhibit clonal expansions of their respective cytotoxic lymphocyte populations. In T-LGLL, clonality can be tracked via the unique T-cell receptor (TCR) gene rearrangement that happens during T-cell maturation. As this is a permanent and irreversible genetic event, it may be used as a unique genetic barcode. In NK-LGLL or CLPD-NK, clonality is harder to assess since a unique receptor rearrangement is not part of the normal biology. Instead, a restricted pattern of killer immunoglobulin-like receptor (KIR) expression by immunophenotyping has been used as a surrogate of clonality, though it is difficult to say whether the same receptor expression corresponds to the same genetic clone. At present, the heterogeneous nature of T and NK cell LGLL clonality [52] calls for further refinement and substratification of disease to determine whether the current clinical categorization is too broad or that this heterogeneity is fundamental to the disease etiology itself.

The TCR is composed of two chains, either α and β or γ and δ, and its unique rearrangement is detectable by standard laboratory methods to determine the presence of a clonal expansion without necessarily yielding information about the sequence [53, 54]. However, next generation sequencing (NGS) is becoming the preferred method because it not only yields sequence data about each rearranged TCR in a sample, but also enables tracking of individual clones over time and the detection of residual disease. Clonal LGL leukemic cells typically express TCR-$\alpha\beta$ and only 1-6% of patients express TCR-$\gamma\delta$ [55].

It may be possible to find the common antigen(s) hypothesized to initiate the development of LGLL through the discovery of a common complementary determining region 3 (CDR3) sequence in LGLL patients. The CDR3 of the TCR mediates the interaction between the TCR and the presented peptide [56]. Knowing the sequences of CDR3 provides a whole repertoire of potential recognizable antigens and finding a common sequence would support the hypothesized antigen-driven model of LGLL pathogenesis. There are many levels of complexity that make finding a common antigen challenging. First, TCR repertoire is very diverse. Whereas one young adult may have as many as 100 million unique rearrangements [57] giving the opportunity for hundreds or thousands of discrete expanded clones following a single antigenic insult, the T-LGLL patient may have only one or a few persisting clone(s). In addition, large variability in HLA genotypes affects peptide binding and its recognition by CDR3 [56]. A second complication is the finding of TCR clonal drift within a patient [52, 58]. For example, Yan et al. reported a case study of a patient initially diagnosed with T-LGLL with a TCRβ9 predominant clone among smaller sub clones of TCRβ3 and TCRβ2; however, after 9 years of asymptomatic disease, he presented with increased symptoms of anemia, neutropenia and lymphocytosis. Through NGS-based deep sequencing, a switch was revealed in the clonal populations that correlated with the shift to the NK-LGLL phenotype; a loss of the TCRβ9 clone and a gain of TCRβ21 as the new predominant clone.

Common CDR3 sequences have been found among 50% of a TCR-γδ T-LGLL group of 44 patients [59], and similar CDR3 motifs were demonstrated in 42% of a separate TCR-γδ T-LGLL patient cohort [17], supporting the etiology of a common antigen as the driver of LGLL. However, similar CDR3 sequences in TCR-αβ T-LGLL patients have not been detected [18]. Compared to healthy individuals, T-LGLL patients showed a significant decrease in CDR3 repertoire diversity [19]. One illustration of the change in diversity can be seen in Figure 2, where a patient, prior to treatment, shows a low diversity score in panels A and B, indicating a monoclonal expansion, and after a complete remission, there was a restoration of T-cell diversity, shown in panel C. In addition, the leukemic clonal sequences found in LGLL patients were specific to patients and were not shared with healthy controls [19]. Deep TCR-β sequencing of patients showed that there was no homology between T-LGLL patients. However, similar TCR sequences may be found at low frequencies when analyzing the entire repertoire rather than only the large immunodominant clones [52].

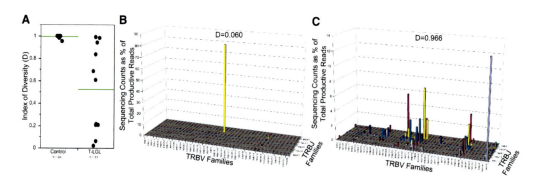

T-LGLL samples have a lower diversity score (A) compared with controls. This is further visualized in the T-cell receptor combinations of V and J regions, which show clonal combinations in a leukemic patient (B) compared with post-treatment remission in the same patient (C). In addition, note the y-axis scale difference. Figure adapted from [19].

Figure 2. Loss of TCR diversity in LGLL.

While common CDR3 motifs have not been discovered in TCR-αβ T-LGLL, this study supports the antigen-driven hypothesis for T-LGLL. Identification of specific expanded clones in the TCR repertoire may point to a "super" antigen responsible for the pathogenesis of LGLL. Future studies are clearly needed in this area and may lead to the association of specific immunodominant clonotypes with clinical characteristics and LGLL subtypes.

3.4. Genome Sequencing

Next-generation sequencing (NGS) methods such as whole-genome sequencing (WGS) and whole-exome sequencing (WES) have been shown to be more sensitive and quantitative for detection of mutations in peripheral blood samples [60] than traditional Sanger sequencing. With decreasing sequencing costs and increasing availability of bioinformatic approaches, WGS and WES have been utilized as relatively unbiased and powerful methods for high-resolution detection and quantification of genetic alterations in disease. While WGS is more expensive than WES, it has the advantage of detecting regulatory alterations such as those in enhancers and non-coding regions which may be missed by WES, gene array, and targeted studies. Among leukemias, such approaches have already been applied in examples such as acute myeloid leukemia [61, 62], chronic lymphocytic leukemia [63, 64], multiple myeloma [65] and hairy cell leukemia [66]. The findings in these cases range widely from a single, causative mutation in almost all patients [66] to multiple heterogeneous contributory mutations in a variety of pathways [61]. Although genome-wide sequencing studies in LGLL have been relatively small in scale, there is sufficient evidence from both WES and targeted studies for the role of activating *STAT* mutations in ~40% of patients. Most of the larger studies have been conducted on T-LGLL as the NK-type is much rarer. Nevertheless, existing studies in NK-LGLL have also found *STAT* mutations at a similar proportion [67, 58], which helps unify the two disease subtypes under a common molecular pathway. Even in patients without activating *STAT* mutations, the similarity of their leukemic gene expression profile, with a constitutively active *STAT3* pathway, suggests other mutations may also activate the same pathway [68], supporting the role of a more comprehensive genome-wide characterization.

Other mutations remain to be discovered in ongoing and future studies. Current directions follow the paradigm set in AML. A larger cohort of AML genomes permitted identification of recurring significant mutations [62], as well as stratification of clinical outcomes [69] to better determine which patients respond to specific therapies. Likewise, these expanded sequencing efforts in LGLL, in particular with comprehensive WGS methods, are necessary to investigate disease pathogenesis, molecular classification, and clinical stratification.

3.4.1. Mutations in STAT3

Of perhaps the most significance, *STAT3* has been found to be the most prevalent mutated gene in T and NK cell LGLL patients (reviewed in [70]). *STAT3* signaling controls the induction of downstream genes that are important for cell survival. *STAT3* is constitutively active in T-LGLL patients, regardless of *STAT3* mutation status [41]; therefore, its pathway is expected to be important in the pathogenesis of this disease. Somatic *STAT3* mutations in any human cancer were first reported in 40% of T-LGLL patients using exome sequencing of a cohort of 77 patients [71]. In a separate group of 120 T-LGLL patients, Jerez et al. found *STAT3* mutations in 27% of those patients [67]. A total of 7 mutations were found; all of which are located a few codons apart in the dimerization interface of the Src Homology 2 (SH2) domain of *STAT3* as viewed in Figure 3. These mutations include Y640F, D661V, D661Y, D661H, K658N, N674I and Y657_K658insY. Among the 31 patients with *STAT3* mutations, Y640F and D661Y were the most prevalent, found in 17% and 9% of *STAT3*-mutated patients, respectively. Using luciferase reporter constructs, all mutations were found to be activating mutations, resulting in increased *STAT3* activity [71]. *STAT3* mutations were also found in 30% of a group of 50 NK-LGLL patients, showing a similarity in the pathogenesis of T cell and NK cell derived LGLL [67].

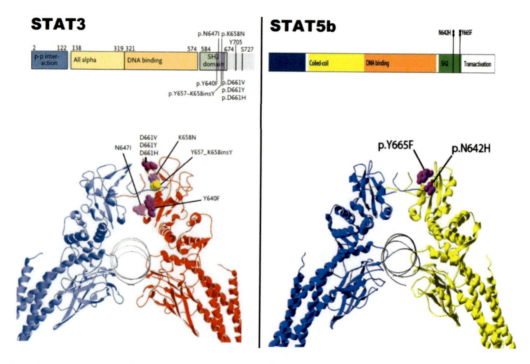

Mutations on *STAT3* (left) and *STAT5b* (right), which localize to the SH2 domain at the dimer interface. These were the first detected and most common. Figure adapted from [71, 81].

Figure 3. STAT mutations.

More recently, novel activating mutations in *STAT3* outside the SH2 domain have been found in three T-LGLL patients; two being missense mutations H410R and S381Y located in the DNA binding domain and another F174S located in the coiled-coil domain [72]. This cohort included 88 T-LGL and 18 NK-LGL leukemic patients with no *STAT3* or *STAT5* mutations in known sites within the SH2 domain. Instead, the authors found the new mutations H410R and F174S to also be activating mutations that exhibited increased *STAT3* phosphorylation and increased expression of *STAT3* responsive genes. While these studies demonstrated the occurrence of *STAT3* mutations, a subsequent study found that 22% (18 of 82) of T-LGLL patients labeled as *STAT3* mutants harbored two or up to four *STAT3* mutations [73]. These findings further support the pathogenic capabilities of *STAT3* and highlight the need to sequence the full-length *STAT3* gene.

3.4.2. Clinical Implications of STAT3 Mutation

Initial data suggest that somatic *STAT3* mutations are correlated with one large immunodominant clone, a higher association with neutropenia and the need for therapeutic treatment [67]. Not only is *STAT3* mutation associated with both T-LGLL and NK-LGLL subtypes [67], it also appears to be correlated with frequently co-occurring clinical disorders such as pure red cell aplasia (PRCA), myelodysplastic syndrome (MDS), and aplastic anemia (AA) [74, 75, 28]. The best established clinical association is with rheumatoid arthritis (RA), with up to 38% of *STAT3*-mutated patients having RA compared to 6% of patients with wild-type *STAT3* [73]. However, *STAT3* mutation comorbidity with PRCA has been controversial. The initial study of *STAT3* mutations reported no association with PRCA [67], while others such as a study of 36 patients from China showed about 50% of those with *STAT3* mutations to also have PRCA [75]. Lastly, T-LGLL patients with *STAT3* mutations have a higher probability of smaller sized leukemic LGL [76], though whether *STAT3* mutation is the causative mechanism remains unclear.

The Eastern Cooperative Oncology Group 5998 (ECOG) trial, which was the first prospective clinical trial for T-LGLL, showed that patients with the Y640F *STAT3* mutation had a more favorable response to methotrexate (MTX) treatment [77]. This highlights the potential diagnostic and therapeutic significance of *STAT3* mutations in LGLL, although additional studies in larger patient cohorts are needed to confirm these initial observations. Since the initial discovery of activating *STAT3* mutations in T-LGLL, similar mutations have been recognized in other T cell malignancies [78, 79, 80]. In the proper clinical setting a positive activating *STAT3* mutation adds additional specificity to the diagnosis of T-LGLL and offers a sensitive way of tracking minimal residual disease through methods such as ddPCR (Droplet Digital PCR) [58].

3.4.3. Mutations in STAT5b

Emphasizing the significance of STATs in the pathogenesis of LGLL, four mutations in *STAT5b* were discovered in a group of 211 *STAT3* mutation-negative T and NK cell LGLL patients, with a total frequency of 2%. This was the first evidence of mutated *STAT5b* in any human disease. Perhaps not surprisingly, just as in *STAT3*, the *STAT5b* mutations N642H and Y665F are both located in the SH2 domain (Figure 3) and increase the transcriptional activity of *STAT5b* [81]. Leukemic LGL from mutated *STAT5b* patients show increased phosphorylation of *STAT5b* in the nucleus, however, unlike with *STAT3* mutants, patients with wild-type *STAT5b* do not show increased *STAT5b* activity

[82]. Both patients with the *STAT5b* N642H mutation had a more aggressive form of LGLL, a stark contrast to the typical indolent form of LGLL [81]. Subsequent analyses (unpublished data) of two patients reported to have a previously described [83] aggressive CD3+CD56+ phenotype also demonstrated presence of the *STAT5b* N642H mutation. More recently, activating *STAT5b* mutations have been found to occur with higher frequency in the rarer CD4+ subtype of T-LGLL [84]. At the very least, these findings highlight the importance to further investigate the molecular implications and therapeutic targeting of *STAT5* mutations in LGLL.

While mutations of *STAT3* and *STAT5b* are prevalent and likely contribute to the pathogenesis of LGLL, STAT mutations alone cannot explain the entirety of this disease because the frequency of these mutations is less than 50%. Patients without *STAT3* mutations have constitutively active *STAT3* expression, along with very similar global gene expression patterns [71, 67] implying that there are other mechanisms that induce *STAT3* activation such as upstream mutations [77]. Exome sequencing of patients with both wild-type *STAT3* and *STAT5b* uncovered other somatic mutations in *PTPRT* [68], *TFNAIP3* [85], *BCL11B* [68], *TET2* [86], *DNMT3A* [86], *SLIT2* [68], and *NRP1* [101]. Selected somatic mutations detected in LGLL are summarized in Table 1.

Table 1. Summary of mutations found in LGLL

Gene	Mutation	Pathway affected	% mutated	ref
STAT3	F174S, S381Y, H410R, S614R, Y640F, N647I, Y657_K658insY, K658N, D661Y, D661V, D661H	JAK/STAT	27-43	[71, 67, 72, 73]
STAT5b	N642H, Y665F, S715F	JAK/STAT	2	[81, 84]
TFNAIP3 (A20)	F127C, E630X, A717T	NF-κB	8	[85]
DNMT3A	E907del	DNA methylation	<1	[86]
TET2	E1144K	DNA methylation	<1	[86]
PTPRT	V995M	JAK/STAT	<1	[68]
SLIT2	W647	Tumor suppressor	<1	[68]
NRP1	V391M	T-cell activation	<1	[68]
BCL11B	H126R	T-cell proliferation	<1	[68]

3.4.4. Other Mutations in the JAK/STAT Pathway

Protein tyrosine phosphatase, receptor type T (*PTPRT*) plays a role in the *STAT3* signaling cascade as a phosphatase, acting as a negative regulator of *STAT3*. *PTPRT* dephosphorylates *STAT3* at Y705 and is shown to be a tumor suppressor in several cancers [87]. A V995M mutation in the *PTPRT* gene was found in a single patient diagnosed with T-LGLL. This novel mutation occurs in the active phosphatase domain and is hypothesized to render *PTPRT* inactive [68]. Reduced phosphatase activity of *PTPRT* would allow *STAT3* to remain phosphorylated and hence activated longer, contributing to the perpetuation of oncogenesis.

Tumor necrosis factor, alpha-induced protein 3 (*TNFAIP3*) is a known tumor suppressor that encodes for A20, a negative regulator of NF-κB signaling, which is also deregulated in T-LGLL [85]. Out of 39 patients, three patients were found harboring mutations in the A20 gene, two were nonsynonymous and the third was a missense mutation. Interestingly, a correlation of *TNFAIP3* mutation and *STAT3* mutations was observed in an independent group of 34 T-LGLL patients as three out of the four patients with a *TNFAIP3* mutation also harbored a *STAT3* mutation [85]. Deregulation of both JAK/STAT and NF-κB signaling pathways are key features that contribute to the pathogenesis of T-LGLL [41], and both pathways can be constitutively activated by somatic mutation.

Most recently in a single case study, mutations in *TET2* and *DNMT3A* were found in the leukemic clone of a T-LGLL patient also harboring the Y640F *STAT3* mutation [86]. *DNMT3A* encodes for a DNA methyltransferase, and mutations in this gene have also been found in acute myeloid leukemia (AML) and result in decreased gene expression [88]. In addition, *TET2* mutations have also been detected in AML, and this gene is involved in the demethylation of DNA, which modulates chromatin structure [89]. Indeed, this may be related to a previous exploration [90] of two upstream regulators of *STAT3*: interleukin 6 (IL-6) and suppressor of cytokine signaling 3 (SOCS3), which induce and inhibit *STAT3*, respectively. In particular, the demethylating agent 5-Aza-2'-Deoxycytidine (DAC) restored SOCS3 expression and reduced *STAT3* activity, although the authors were not able to localize the causative region of demethylation in the specific SOCS3 region tested. Collectively, these findings underscore the importance of epigenetic modifiers and the need for additional studies to clarify the epigenome's role in the pathogenesis of LGLL.

3.4.5. Mutations Associated with T-Cell Activation and Proliferation

B-cell lymphoma/leukemia 11B (*BCL11B*) is a transcription factor that regulates the expression of genes important for T cell development such as IL-2 [91], NF-κB and TCRβ [92]. An H126R mutation in the *BCL11B* gene was found only in the leukemic CD8+ cells of a single T-LGLL patient [68]. In T-cell acute lymphoblastic leukemia, *BCL11B* deletions and missense mutations were found in 10-15% of patients [93]. In AML, *BCL11B* was identified as an oncogene as mutations in *BCL11B* increased expression of *BCL11B* protein, resulting in increased expression of T-cell associated genes [12]. For LGLL, it is hypothesized that increased expression of *BCL11B* may increase T-cell activation and proliferation [85].

Slit homolog 2 protein (*SLIT2*) plays a role as a tumor suppressor and can be methylated, or silenced, in chronic lymphocytic leukemia and acute lymphoblastic leukemia [94]. The mutation found in a T-LGLL patient is a W674 stop mutation, suggesting that this novel mutation may lead to loss of function and play a role in cancer development.

Lastly, neuropilin-1 (*NRP1*) is a receptor that participates in the communication between dendritic cells and T cells, which is important in initiating an immune response. A V391M *NRP1* mutation found in a single LGLL patient may affect the interaction between dendritic and T cells, which would affect their activation and proliferation [68].

These somatic mutations, while rare, are associated with either the *STAT3* pathway or T-cell activation and proliferation and may be important in the clonal expansion in T-LGLL. These findings emphasize the need to sequence a larger cohort of patients and characterize the biochemical effects of mutations on pathways vital to the survival of leukemic LGL. This will identify possible therapeutic vulnerabilities dependent on certain mutations and may facilitate personalized treatment options based upon gene mutation status.

CONCLUSION

These studies so far have been encouraging and offer many follow-up questions for subsequent investigation. Past [77] and ongoing [95] clinical trials have focused on immunosuppressive therapies, which are the mainstream of therapeutic approaches for LGLL. Despite the high frequency of activating mutations in *STAT3*, no clinical trials of rationally designed STAT inhibitors have been conducted to date in LGLL, in part due to the lack of clinical advancement and success for these molecules thus far. However, a recent study suggests that JAK/STAT pathway inhibition is at least one mechanism of action for the currently used first-line treatment, methotrexate [96]. In the absence of a curative treatment, further molecular characterization is needed to define additional targets.

The largest current limitation in understanding the molecular changes in LGLL is the lack of information regarding changes that occur in the genome outside of regions that code for proteins. Mutations in important DNA elements such as enhancers and promoters have yet to be thoroughly investigated and reported. Indeed the identification of these elements themselves in LGLL and a suitably close normal cell counterpart is also lacking. Once these regions are known, overlap with WGS comparisons of tumor and normal will provide candidate mutations in regulatory regions that may be additional drivers of this disease. These changes may explain, for example, the constitutive activation of *STAT3* in many patients despite the lack of evidence for mutation in the *STAT3* gene itself. Epigenetic changes that may lead to the same result, with the exception of a rare *TET2* and *DNMT3A* co-mutation, have similarly not been thoroughly examined and described.

A thorough cataloging of all of the mutations that occur in LGLL is also necessary to determine the temporal dynamics of clonal evolution and drift in LGLL pathogenesis and progression. Though current technology allows us to determine relative clone size through NGS of TCR sequences, we do not currently have a complete understanding of what causes clones to persist and fluctuate or how they contribute to the clinical symptoms associated with LGLL. Ideally a comprehensive mutation panel, beyond *STAT3* and other genes described here, can be performed on multiple clones from oligoclonal disease in order to determine the full mutational burden. It will be critical to our understanding of LGLL genesis to determine if clonal expansion precedes or is alternatively an end result of a mutational event. Exhaustive proof that mutations always lag behind expansion would support a continuous antigen response as the persistent driver of these expansions, with subsequent individual mutations leading to the emergence of the largest clones. In contrast, evidence for mutations that precede clonal expansion would warrant further investigation of the role of dysregulated cellular circuitry.

We do not currently have complete linkage between molecular events and the symptoms of LGLL, with cumulative studies focusing on *STAT3* mutations. It will be necessary to identify other mechanisms that may cooperate with or obviate the need for *STAT3* mutation in the transition from an indolent clonal expansion to one that causes significant pathology. Is this the result of additional mutations in the clonal expansion, the emergence of new cooperating clones, or alternatively other processes within the body that interact with the clone?

It is likely that many patients do not notice symptoms or seek a diagnosis of LGLL until the emergence of an expanded and problematic clone, which is likely to have a clear signature. In those asymptomatic patients where LGLL is more or less an incidental finding, it is important to identify the subsequent changes that cause symptoms. If this change is found to often be the expansion of an entirely new clone with a unique molecular profile it will be important to determine at what timepoint this clone appeared. Evidence of a clone with a known mutation (Table 1) at presentation, even if not dominant, may indicate the need for earlier treatment or closer clinical monitoring.

ACKNOWLEDGMENTS

LGLL research in the Loughran lab is funded by the National Cancer Institute of the National Institutes of Health under award number R01CA098472 and R01CA178393 (TPL) and T32LM012416 (JX). The content is solely the responsibility of the authors and does not necessarily represent the official views of the National Institutes of Health. Additional funding is provided by the Leukemia and Lymphoma society under award number TRP-6159-14 as well as the Bess Family Charitable Fund, the LGLL Foundation and a generous anonymous donor.

A national patient registry has been established by Dr. Loughran and current research is being pursued. Physicians are encouraged to contact Thomas Loughran at tploughran@virginia.edu for more information.

REFERENCES

[1] Lamy T, Loughran TP. How I treat LGL leukemia. *Blood.* 2011;117(10):2764-2774. doi:10.1182/blood-2010-07-296962.

[2] Swerdlow SH, Campo E, Pileri SA, et al. The 2016 revision of the World Health Organization classification of lymphoid neoplasms. *Blood.* 2016;127(20):2375-2390. doi:10.1182/blood-2016-01-643569.

[3] Kothapalli R, Nyland S, Kusmartseva I, Bailey R, McKeown T, Loughran T. Constitutive production of proinflammatory cytokines RANTES, MIP-1β and IL-18 characterizes LGL leukemia. *International Journal of Oncology.* February 2005. doi:10.3892/ijo.26.2.529.

[4] Poullot E, Zambello R, Leblanc F, et al. Chronic natural killer lymphoproliferative disorders: characteristics of an international cohort of 70 patients. *Annals of Oncology.* 2014;25(10):2030-2035. doi:10.1093/annonc/mdu369.

[5] Kawa-Ha K, Ishihara S, Ninomiya T, et al. CD3-negative lymphoproliferative disease of granular lymphocytes containing Epstein-Barr viral DNA. *J Clin Invest.* 1989;84(1):51-55. doi:10.1172/JCI114168.

[6] Suzuki R, Suzumiya J, Nakamura S, et al. Aggressive natural killer-cell leukemia revisited: large granular lymphocyte leukemia of cytotoxic NK cells. *Leukemia.* 2004;18(4):763-770. doi:10.1038/sj.leu.2403262.

[7] Loughran TP, Zambello R, Ashley R, et al. Failure to detect Epstein-Barr virus DNA in peripheral blood mononuclear cells of most patients with large granular lymphocyte leukemia. *Blood.* 1993;81(10):2723-2727.

[8] Loughran TP, Coyle T, Sherman MP, et al. Detection of human T-cell leukemia/lymphoma virus, type II, in a patient with large granular lymphocyte leukemia. *Blood.* 1992;80(5):1116-1119.

[9] Starkebaum G, Kalyanaraman VS, Kidd P, et al. Serum Reactivity to Human T-Cell Leukemia/Lymphoma Virus Type I Proteins in Patients with Large Granular Lymphocytic Leukemia. *The Lancet.* 1987;329(8533):596-599. doi:10.1016/S0140-6736(87)90236-4.

[10] Sokol L, Agrawal D, Loughran TP. Characterization of HTLV envelope seroreactivity in large granular lymphocyte leukemia. *Leukemia Research.* 2005;29(4):381-387. doi:10.1016/j.leukres.2004.08.010.

[11] Loughran TP, Hadlock KG, Yang Q, et al. Seroreactivity to an envelope protein of human T-cell leukemia/lymphoma virus in patients with CD3(-) (natural killer) lymphoproliferative disease of granular lymphocytes. *Blood.* 1997;90(5):1977-1981.

[12] Grossman WJ, Kimata JT, Wong FH, Zutter M, Ley TJ, Ratner L. Development of leukemia in mice transgenic for the tax gene of human T-cell leukemia virus type I. *Proc Natl Acad Sci USA.* 1995;92(4):1057-1061. doi:10.1073/pnas.92.4.1057.

[13] Ren T, Yang J, Broeg K, Liu X, Loughran TP, Cheng H. Developing an in vitro model of T cell type of large granular lymphocyte leukemia. *Leukemia Research.* 2013;37(12):1737-1743. doi:10.1016/j.leukres.2013.10.002.

[14] Yang J, Epling-Burnette PK, Painter JS, et al. Antigen activation and impaired Fas-induced death-inducing signaling complex formation in T-large-granular lymphocyte leukemia. *Blood.* 2007;111(3):1610-1616. doi:10.1182/blood-2007-06-093823.

[15] O'Keefe CL, Plasilova M, Wlodarski M, et al. Molecular analysis of TCR clonotypes in LGL: A clonal model for polyclonal responses. *Journal of Immunology.* 2004;172(3):1960-1969. doi:10.4049/jimmunol.172.3.1960.

[16] Wlodarski MW. Pathologic clonal cytotoxic T-cell responses: nonrandom nature of the T-cell-receptor restriction in large granular lymphocyte leukemia. *Blood.* 2005;106(8):2769-2780. doi:10.1182/blood-2004-10-4045.

[17] Garrido P, Ruiz-Cabello F, Barcena P, et al. Monoclonal TCR-Vβ13.1+/CD4+/NKa+/CD8-/+dim T-LGL lymphocytosis: evidence for an antigen-driven chronic T-cell stimulation origin. *Blood.* 2007;109(11):4890-4898. doi:10.1182/blood-2006-05-022277.

[18] Sandberg Y, Kallemeijn MJ, Dik WA, et al. Lack of common TCRA and TCRB clonotypes in CD8+/TCRαβ+ T-cell large granular lymphocyte leukemia: a review on the role of antigenic selection in the immunopathogenesis of CD8+ T-LGL. *Blood Cancer Journal.* 2014;4(1):e172. doi:10.1038/bcj.2013.70.

[19] Clemente MJ, Przychodzen B, Jerez A, et al. Deep sequencing of the T-cell receptor repertoire in CD8+ T-large granular lymphocyte leukemia identifies signature landscapes. *Blood.* 2013;122(25):4077-4085. doi:10.1182/blood-2013-05-506386.

[20] Rodriguez-Caballero A, Garcia-Montero AC, Barcena P, et al. Expanded cells in monoclonal TCRαβ+ /CD4+/NKa+/CD8-/+dim T-LGL lymphocytosis recognize hCMV antigens. *Blood.* 2008;112(12):4609-4616. doi:10.1182/blood-2008-03-146241.

[21] Nyland SB, Krissinger DJ, Clemente MJ, et al. Seroreactivity to LGL leukemia-specific epitopes in aplastic anemia, myelodysplastic syndrome and paroxysmal nocturnal hemoglobinuria: Results of a bone marrow failure consortium study. *Leukemia Research.* 2012;36(5):581-587. doi:10.1016/j.leukres.2012.02.001.

[22] Zambello R. Expression and function of KIR and natural cytotoxicity receptors in NK-type lymphoproliferative diseases of granular lymphocytes. *Blood.* 2003;102(5):1797-1805. doi:10.1182/blood-2002-12-3898.

[23] Epling-Burnette PK, Painter JS, Chaurasia P, et al. Dysregulated NK receptor expression in patients with lymphoproliferative disease of granular lymphocytes. *Blood.* 2004;103(9):3431-3439. doi:10.1182/blood-2003-02-0400.

[24] Scquizzato E, Teramo A, Miorin M, et al. Genotypic evaluation of killer immunoglobulin-like receptors in NK-type lymphoproliferative disease of granular lymphocytes. *Leukemia.* 2007;21(5):1060-1069. doi:10.1038/sj.leu.2404634.

[25] Gattazzo C, Teramo A, Miorin M, et al. Lack of expression of inhibitory KIR3DL1 receptor in patients with natural killer cell-type lymphoproliferative disease of granular lymphocytes. *Haematologica.* 2010;95(10):1722-1729. doi:10.3324/haematol.2010.023358.

[26] Gattazzo C, Teramo A, Passeri F, et al. Detection of monoclonal T populations in patients with KIR-restricted chronic lymphoproliferative disorder of NK cells. *Haematologica.* 2014;99(12):1826-1833. doi:10.3324/haematol.2014.105726.

[27] Battiwalla M, Melenhorst J, Saunthararajah Y, et al. HLA-DR4 predicts haematological response to cyclosporine in T-large granular lymphocyte lymphoproliferative disorders. *British Journal of Haematology.* 2003;123(3):449-453. doi:10.1046/j.1365-2141.2003.04613.x.

[28] Jerez A, Clemente MJ, Makishima H, et al. STAT3 mutations indicate the presence of subclinical T-cell clones in a subset of aplastic anemia and myelodysplastic syndrome patients. *Blood.* 2013;122(14):2453-2459. doi:10.1182/blood-2013-04-494930.

[29] Loughran TP, Kadin ME, Starkebaum G, et al. Leukemia of Large Granular Lymphocytes: Association with Clonal Chromosomal Abnormalities and Autoimmune Neutropenia, Thrombocytopenia, and Hemolytic Anemia. *Annals of Internal Medicine.* 1985;102(2):169. doi:10.7326/0003-4819-102-2-169.

[30] Lamy T, Liu JH, Landowski TH, Dalton WS, Loughran TP. Dysregulation of CD95/CD95 ligand-apoptotic pathway in CD3(+) large granular lymphocyte leukemia. *Blood.* 1998;92(12):4771-4777.

[31] Perzova R, Loughran TP. Constitutive expression of Fas ligand in large granular lymphocyte leukaemia. *British Journal of Haematology.* 1997;97(1):123-126. doi:10.1046/j.1365-2141.1997.d01-2113.x.

[32] Epling-Burnette PK, Liu JH, Catlett-Falcone R, et al. Inhibition of STAT3 signaling leads to apoptosis of leukemic large granular lymphocytes and decreased Mcl-1 expression. *Journal of Clinical Investigation.* 2001;107(3):351-361. doi:10.1172/jci9940.

[33] Liu JH, Wei S, Lamy T, et al. Blockade of Fas-dependent apoptosis by soluble Fas in LGL leukemia. *Blood.* 2002;100(4):1449-1453.

[34] Epling-Burnett PK, Bai FQ, Wei S, et al. ERK couples chronic survival of NK cells to constitutively activated Ras in lymphoproliferative disease of granular lymphocytes (LDGL). *Oncogene.* 2004;23(57):9220-9229. doi:10.1038/sj.onc.1208122.

[35] Liu X, Ryland L, Yang J, et al. Targeting of surviving by nanoliposomal ceramide induces complete remission in a rat model of NK-LGL leukemia. *Blood.* 2010;116(20):4192-4201. doi:10.1182/blood-2010-02-271080.

[36] Schade AE, Powers JJ, Wlodarski MW, Maciejewski JP. Phosphatidylinositol-3-phosphate kinase pathway activation protects leukemic large granular lymphocytes from undergoing homeostatic apoptosis. *Blood.* 2006;107(12):4834-4840. doi:10.1182/blood-2005-08-3076.

[37] Schade AE, Wlodarski MW, Maciejewski JP. Pathophysiology Defined by Altered Signal Transduction Pathways: The Role of JAK-STAT and PI3K Signaling in Leukemic Large Granular Lymphocytes. *Cell Cycle.* 2006;5(22):2571-2574. doi:10.4161/cc.5.22.3449.

[38] Shah MV, Zhang R, Irby R, et al. Molecular profiling of LGL leukemia reveals role of sphingolipid signaling in survival of cytotoxic lymphocytes. *Blood.* 2008;112(3):770-781. doi:10.1182/blood-2007-11-121871.

[39] Kothapalli R, Kusmartseva I, Loughran TP. Characterization of a human sphingosine-1-phosphate receptor gene (S1P5) and its differential expression in LGL leukemia. *Biochimica et Biophysica Acta (BBA) - Gene Structure and Expression.* 2002;1579(2-3):117-123. doi:10.1016/S0167-4781(02)00529-8.

[40] Saadatpour A, Albert R. Discrete Dynamic Modeling of Signal Transduction Networks. In: Liu X, Betterton MD, eds. Computational Modeling of Signaling Networks. Vol 880. Totowa, *NJ: Humana Press;* 2012:255-272. http://link.springer.com/10.1007/978-1-61779-833-7_12. Accessed November 25, 2016.

[41] Zhang R, Shah MV, Yang J, et al. Network model of survival signaling in large granular lymphocyte leukemia. *Proceedings of the National Academy of Sciences.* 2008;105(42):16308-16313. doi:10.1073/pnas.0806447105.

[42] Yang J, Liu X, Nyland SB, et al. Platelet-derived growth factor mediates survival of leukemic large granular lymphocytes via an autocrine regulatory pathway. *Blood.* 2010;115(1):51-60. doi:10.1182/blood-2009-06-223719.

[43] Zambello R, Facco M, Trentin L, et al. Interleukin-15 triggers the proliferation and cytotoxicity of granular lymphocytes in patients with lymphoproliferative disease of granular lymphocytes. *Blood.* 1997;89(1):201-211.

[44] Hodge DL, Yang J, Buschman MD, et al. Interleukin-15 Enhances Proteasomal Degradation of Bid in Normal Lymphocytes: Implications for Large Granular Lymphocyte Leukemias. *Cancer Research.* 2009;69(9):3986-3994. doi:10.1158/0008-5472.can-08-3735.

[45] Chen J, Petrus M, Bamford R, et al. Increased serum soluble IL-15R levels in T-cell large granular lymphocyte leukemia. *Blood.* 2012;119(1):137-143. doi:10.1182/blood-2011-04-346759.

[46] Mishra A, Liu S, Sams GH, et al. Aberrant Overexpression of IL-15 Initiates Large Granular Lymphocyte Leukemia through Chromosomal Instability and DNA Hypermethylation. *Cancer Cell.* 2012;22(5):645-655. doi:10.1016/j.ccr.2012.09.009.

[47] Saadatpour A, Wang R-S, Liao A, et al. Dynamical and Structural Analysis of a T Cell Survival Network Identifies Novel Candidate Therapeutic Targets for Large Granular Lymphocyte Leukemia. Ofran Y, ed. *PLoS Computational Biology.* 2011;7(11):e1002267. doi:10.1371/journal.pcbi.1002267.

[48] Zañudo JGT, Albert R. Cell Fate Reprogramming by Control of Intracellular Network Dynamics. Thieffry D, ed. *PLOS Computational Biology.* 2015;11(4):e1004193. doi:10.1371/journal.pcbi.1004193.

[49] Subramanian A, Tamayo P, Mootha VK, et al. Gene set enrichment analysis: A knowledge-based approach for interpreting genome-wide expression profiles. *Proceedings of the National Academy of Sciences.* 2005;102(43):15545-15550. doi:10.1073/pnas.0506580102.

[50] LeBlanc FR, Liu X, Hengst J, et al. Sphingosine kinase inhibitors decrease viability and induce cell death in natural killer-large granular lymphocyte leukemia. *Cancer Biology & Therapy.* 2015;16(12):1830-1840. doi:10.1080/15384047.2015.1078949.

[51] Krammer PH, Arnold R, Lavrik IN. Life and death in peripheral T cells. *Nature Reviews Immunology.* 2007;7(7):532-542. doi:10.1038/nri2115.

[52] Clemente MJ, Wlodarski MW, Makishima H, et al. Clonal drift demonstrates unexpected dynamics of the T-cell repertoire in T-large granular lymphocyte leukemia. *Blood.* 2011;118(16):4384-4393. doi:10.1182/blood-2011-02-338517.

[53] Langerak AW, Groenen PJTA, Brüggemann M, et al. EuroClonality/BIOMED-2 guidelines for interpretation and reporting of Ig/TCR clonality testing in suspected lymphoproliferations. *Leukemia.* 2012;26(10):2159-2171. doi:10.1038/leu.2012.246.

[54] van Krieken JHJM, Langerak AW, Macintyre EA, et al. Improved reliability of lymphoma diagnostics via PCR-based clonality testing: — Report of the BIOMED-2 Concerted Action BHM4-CT98-3936. *Leukemia.* 2007;21(2):201-206. doi:10.1038/sj.leu.2404467.

[55] Bourgault-Rouxel AS, Loughran TP, Zambello R, et al. Clinical spectrum of γδ+ T cell LGL leukemia: Analysis of 20 cases. *Leukemia Research.* 2008;32(1):45-48. doi:10.1016/j.leukres.2007.04.011.

[56] Borg NA, Ely LK, Beddoe T, et al. The CDR3 regions of an immunodominant T cell receptor dictate the "energetic landscape" of peptide-MHC recognition. *Nature Immunology.* 2005;6(2):171-180. doi:10.1038/ni1155.

[57] Qi Q, Liu Y, Cheng Y, et al. Diversity and clonal selection in the human T-cell repertoire. *Proceedings of the National Academy of Sciences.* 2014;111(36):13139-13144. doi:10.1073/pnas.1409155111.

[58] Yan Y, Olson TL, Nyland SB, Feith DJ, Loughran TP. Emergence of a STAT3 mutated NK clone in LGL leukemia. *Leukemia Research Reports.* 2015;4(1):4-7. doi:10.1016/j.lrr.2014.12.001.

[59] Sandberg Y, Almeida J, Gonzalez M, et al. TCRγδ+ large granular lymphocyte leukemias reflect the spectrum of normal antigen-selected TCRγδ+ T-cells. *Leukemia.* 2006;20(3):505-513. doi:10.1038/sj.leu.2404112.

[60] Kristensen T, Larsen M, Rewes A, Frederiksen H, Thomassen M, Moller MB. Clinical Relevance of Sensitive and Quantitative STAT3 Mutation Analysis Using Next-Generation Sequencing in T-Cell Large Granular Lymphocytic Leukemia. *Journal of Molecular Diagnostics.* 2014;16(4):382-392. doi:10.1016/j.jmoldx. 2014.02.005.

[61] Ley TJ, Mardis ER, Ding L, et al. DNA sequencing of a cytogenetically normal acute myeloid leukaemia genome. *Nature.* 2008;456(7218):66-72. doi:10.1038/ nature07485.

[62] The Cancer Genome Atlas Research Network. Genomic and Epigenomic Landscapes of Adult De Novo Acute Myeloid Leukemia. *New England Journal of Medicine.* 2013;368(22):2059-2074. doi:10.1056/NEJMoa1301689.

[63] Puente XS, Pinyol M, Quesada V, et al. Whole-genome sequencing identifies recurrent mutations in chronic lymphocytic leukaemia. *Nature.* 2011;475(7354): 101-105. doi:10.1038/nature10113.

[64] Wang L, Lawrence MS, Wan Y, et al. SF3B1 and Other Novel Cancer Genes in Chronic Lymphocytic Leukemia. *New England Journal of Medicine.* 2011;365(26):2497-2506. doi:10.1056/NEJMoa1109016.

[65] Chapman MA, Lawrence MS, Keats JJ, et al. Initial genome sequencing and analysis of multiple myeloma. *Nature.* 2011;471(7339):467-472. doi:10.1038/ nature09837.

[66] Tiacci E, Trifonov V, Schiavoni G, et al. BRAF Mutations in Hairy-Cell Leukemia. *New England Journal of Medicine.* 2011;364(24):2305-2315. doi:10.1056/ NEJMoa1014209.

[67] Jerez A, Clemente MJ, Makishima H, et al. STAT3 mutations unify the pathogenesis of chronic lymphoproliferative disorders of NK cells and T-cell large granular lymphocyte leukemia. *Blood.* 2012;120(15):3048-3057. doi:10.1182/ blood-2012-06-435297.

[68] Andersson EI, Rajala HLM, Eldfors S, et al. Novel somatic mutations in large granular lymphocytic leukemia affecting the STAT-pathway and T-cell activation. *Blood Cancer Journal.* 2013;3(12):e168. doi:10.1038/bcj.2013.65.

[69] Papaemmanuil E, Gerstung M, Bullinger L, et al. Genomic Classification and Prognosis in Acute Myeloid Leukemia. *New England Journal of Medicine.* 2016;374(23):2209-2221. doi:10.1056/NEJMoa1516192.

[70] Rajala HLM, Porkka K, Maciejewski JP, Loughran TP, Mustjoki S. Uncovering the pathogenesis of large granular lymphocytic leukemia—novel STAT3 and STAT5b mutations. *Annals of Medicine.* 2014;46(3):114-122. doi:10.3109/07853890.2014.882105.

[71] Koskela HLM, Eldfors S, Ellonen P, et al. Somatic STAT3 Mutations in Large Granular Lymphocytic Leukemia. *New England Journal of Medicine.* 2012;366(20):1905-1913. doi:10.1056/NEJMoa1114885.

[72] Andersson E, Kuusanmäki H, Bortoluzzi S, et al. Activating somatic mutations outside the SH2-domain of STAT3 in LGL leukemia. *Leukemia.* 2016;30(5):1204-1208. doi:10.1038/leu.2015.263.

[73] Rajala HLM, Olson T, Clemente MJ, et al. The analysis of clonal diversity and therapy responses using STAT3 mutations as a molecular marker in large granular lymphocytic leukemia. *Haematologica.* 2015;100(1):91-99. doi:10.3324/haematol.2014.113142.

[74] Ishida F, Matsuda K, Sekiguchi N, et al. STAT3 gene mutations and their association with pure red cell aplasia in large granular lymphocyte leukemia. *Cancer Science.* 2014;105(3):342-346. doi:10.1111/cas.12341.

[75] Qiu ZY, Fan L, Wang L, et al. STAT3 mutations are frequent in T-cell large granular lymphocytic leukemia with pure red cell aplasia. *Journal of Hematology & Oncology. 2013*;6. doi:10.1186/1756-8722-6-82.

[76] Tanahashi T, Sekiguchi N, Matsuda K, et al. Cell size variations of large granular lymphocyte leukemia: Implication of a small cell subtype of granular lymphocyte leukemia with STAT3 mutations. *Leukemia Research.* 2016;45:8-13. doi:10.1016/j.leukres.2016.04.001.

[77] Loughran TP, Zickl L, Olson TL, et al. Immunosuppressive therapy of LGL leukemia: prospective multicenter phase II study by the eastern cooperative oncology group (E5998). *Leukemia.* October 2014. doi:10.1038/leu.2014.298.

[78] Ohgami RS, Ma L, Merker JD, Martinez B, Zehnder JL, Arber DA. STAT3 mutations are frequent in CD30+ T-cell lymphomas and T-cell large granular lymphocytic leukemia. *Leukemia.* 2013;27(11):2244-2247. doi:10.1038/leu.2013.104.

[79] Crescenzo R, Abate F, Lasorsa E, et al. Convergent Mutations and Kinase Fusions Lead to Oncogenic STAT3 Activation in Anaplastic Large Cell Lymphoma. *Cancer Cell.* 2015;27(4):516-532. doi:10.1016/j.ccell.2015.03.006.

[80] Nicolae A, Xi L, Pham TH, et al. Mutations in the JAK/STAT and RAS signaling pathways are common in intestinal T-cell lymphomas. *Leukemia.* 2016;30(11):2245-2247. doi:10.1038/leu.2016.178.

[81] Rajala HLM, Eldfors S, Kuusanmaki H, et al. Discovery of somatic STAT5b mutations in large granular lymphocytic leukemia. *Blood.* 2013;121(22):4541-4550. doi:10.1182/blood-2012-12-474577.

[82] Rajala HLM, Mustjoki S. STAT5b in LGL leukemia – a novel therapeutic target? *Oncotarget.* 2013;4(6):808-809. doi:10.18632/oncotarget.1035.

[83] Gentile TC, Uner AH, Hutchison RE, et al. CD3+, CD56+ aggressive variant of large granular lymphocyte leukemia. *Blood.* 1994;84(7):2315-2321.

[84] Andersson EI, Tanahashi T, Sekiguchi N, et al. High incidence of activating STAT5B mutations in CD4-positive T-cell large granular lymphocyte leukemia. *Blood.* 2016;128(20):2465-2468. doi:10.1182/blood-2016-06-724856.

[85] Johansson P, Bergmann A, Rahmann S, et al. Recurrent alterations of TNFAIP3 (A20) in T-cell large granular lymphocytic leukemia: A20 mutations in T-LGL. *International Journal of Cancer.* 2016;138(1):121-124. doi:10.1002/ijc.29697.

[86] Raess PW, Cascio MJ, Fan G, et al. Concurrent STAT3, DNMT3A, and TET2 mutations in T-LGL leukemia with molecularly distinct clonal hematopoiesis of indeterminate potential: DNMT3A, TET2, and STAT3 mutations in T-LGLL. *American Journal of Hematology.* 2016;92(1):E6-E8. doi:10.1002/ajh.24586.

[87] Lee JW, Jeong EG, Lee SH, et al. Mutational analysis of PTPRT phosphatase domains in common human cancers. *APMIS.* 2007;115(1):47-51. doi:10.1111/j.1600-0463.2007.apm_554.x.

[88] Ley TJ, Ding L, Walter MJ, et al. DNMT3A Mutations in Acute Myeloid Leukemia. *New England Journal of Medicine.* 2010;363(25):2424-2433. doi:10.1056/NEJMoa1005143.

[89] Hill PWS, Amouroux R, Hajkova P. DNA demethylation, Tet proteins and 5-hydroxymethylcytosine in epigenetic reprogramming: An emerging complex story. *Genomics.* 2014;104(5):324-333. doi:10.1016/j.ygeno.2014.08.012.

[90] Teramo A, Gattazzo C, Passeri F, et al. Intrinsic and extrinsic mechanisms contribute to maintain the JAK/STAT pathway aberrantly activated in T-type large granular lymphocyte leukemia. *Blood.* 2013;121(19):3843-3854. doi:10.1182/blood-2012-07-441378.

[91] Cismasiu VB, Ghanta S, Duque J, et al. BCL11B participates in the activation of IL2 gene expression in CD4+ T lymphocytes. *Blood.* 2006;108(8):2695-2702. doi:10.1182/blood-2006-05-021790.

[92] Cismasiu VB, Adamo K, Gecewicz J, Duque J, Lin Q, Avram D. BCL11B functionally associates with the NuRD complex in T lymphocytes to repress targeted promoter. *Oncogene.* 2005;24(45):6753-6764. doi:10.1038/sj.onc.1208904.

[93] Gutierrez A, Kentsis A, Sanda T, et al. The BCL11B tumor suppressor is mutated across the major molecular subtypes of T-cell acute lymphoblastic leukemia. *Blood.* 2011;118(15):4169-4173. doi:10.1182/blood-2010-11-318873.

[94] Dunwell TL, Dickinson RE, Stankovic T, et al. Frequent epigenetic inactivation of the SLIT2 gene in chronic and acute lymphocytic leukemia. *Epigenetics*. 2009;4(4):265-269. doi:10.4161/epi.9137.

[95] Dumitriu B, Ito S, Feng XM, et al. Alemtuzumab in T-cell large granular lymphocytic leukaemia: interim results from a single-arm, open-label, phase 2 study. *Lancet Haematology*. 2016;3(1):E22-E29. doi:10.1016/s2352-3026(15)00227-6.

[96] Thomas S, Fisher KH, Snowden JA, Danson SJ, Brown S, Zeidler MP. Methotrexate Is a JAK/STAT Pathway Inhibitor. Antoniou AN, ed. *PLOS ONE*. 2015;10(7):e0130078. doi:10.1371/journal.pone.0130078.

[97] Lamy T, Moignet A, Loughran TP. LGL leukemia: from pathogenesis to treatment. *Blood*. January 2017:blood-2016-08-692590. doi:10.1182/blood-2016-08-692590.

In: Benign and Malignant Disorders …
Editors: Ling Zhang and Lubomir Sokol
ISBN: 978-1-53612-999-1
© 2018 Nova Science Publishers, Inc.

Chapter 2

ABNORMAL FUNCTION OF INNATE AND ADAPTIVE IMMUNE SYSTEMS IN LARGE GRANULAR LYMPHOCYTIC LEUKEMIA

Lili Yang[1,*], Houfang Sun[1] and Sheng Wei[2]
[1]Department of Immunology, Tianjin Medical University Cancer Institute and Hospital, Tianjin, China
[2]Department of Immunology,
H. Lee Moffitt Cancer Center, Tampa, FL, US

ABSTRACT

Large granular lymphocytes play a critical role in immunosurveillance by identifying and killing virally infected or transformed tumor cells. They function through innate and adaptive immune systems. The innate immune system is the front line barrier against virally infected cells and tumor cells, and is regulated by several biological processes. The signaling derived from the innate system can further induce cellular processes in a form of defense or to promote an adaptive immune response. Sustained abnormal proliferation of large granular lymphocytes (LGLs) post antigen stimulation can result in a spectrum of lymphoproliferative disorders. T-cell large granular lymphocytic leukemia (T-LGLL), is an excellent model of an indolent, LGL related lymphoproliferative disorders that occur due to dysregulation of both innate and adaptive immune systems. In addition to alteration of NK cell activity and dysregulation of FAS–FASL-mediated apoptosis, it is also recognized that the NKR-DAP10/DAP12 signaling pathways play critical role during T-cell activation in patients with LGLL. This chapter aims to summarize the impaired homeostasis of the immune system in LGLL with focus on autoimmunity, dysregulated immune surveillance pathways, and aberrantly activated NK and T cells bypassing normal innate and adaptive signaling.

---

[*] Corresponding Author Email: yanglili@tjmuch.com.

1. INTRODUCTION

Large granular lymphocytes (LGL) comprise 10% to 15% of normal peripheral blood mononuclear cells originating either from T cell or NK cell lineages [1-5]. Normal LGLs are cytotoxic cells with a capability to recognize and kill virally infected or transformed malignant cells. Abnormal clonal proliferation of LGLs results in a spectrum of lymphoproliferative disorders. Among those disorders the most common is indolent T-cell LGLL [3, 4]. Abnormal proliferation of LGLs is implicated in the development of disorders of the immune system such as autoimmune diseases, connective tissue diseases, as well as secondary hematologic malignancies [3, 5-8]. LGLL is an excellent model of a hematological malignancy with a dysregulated immune system. The most common hematological phenomenon associated with T-cell LGLL is neutropenia, which is observed in 70%-80% of cases. These patients can also manifest with anemia, thrombocytopenia, and hyper- or hypo-ganmmaglobuinemia etc. [1, 5]. It has been also suggested that Felty's syndrome manifesting with a triad of "rheumatoid arthritis, splenomegaly and neutropenia" shares a common pathogenesis with LGLL [5].

In the peripheral blood, the LGL cells will undergo activation and proliferation when these cells are exposed to bacterial or viral infections. After elimination of the offending stimulus activated T cells are removed via programmed cell death (apoptosis) mediated by antigen clearance; whereas, in LGLL, the LGLs are sustained despite the absence of the antigen [9, 10]. It is believed that chronic antigen stimulation can activate the survival signaling pathways and the inhibition of apoptosis pathways, including FAS–FASL, Ras–Raf-1–MEK1–ERK, PI3K–Akt, JAK–STAT, sphingolipid rheostat, NF-κB, IL-15, and PDGF signaling. A better understanding of the dysregulated signaling pathways in LGLL may provide new insights into the pathogenesis of the disease and provide novel therapeutic strategies in various clinical settings in the near future [10].

Herein, we briefly describe the normal function of innate and adaptive immune systems and subsequently discuss the impaired homeostasis of immune system in LGLL as a model to demonstrate its association with autoimmunity, dysregulated immune surveillance pathways, and aberrantly activated NK and T cells bypassing normal innate and adaptive signaling.

2. DYSFUNCTION OF INNATE IMMUNE SYSTEM IN LGL LEUKEMIA

2.1. Normal Function of Innate System

Innate immune system is the first line of immunological defense of the human body. This natural immune system is formed in the process of development and evolution after birth. The innate immune system is mainly composed of organ barriers, innate immune cells and innate immune molecules. The innate immune cells include phagocytes (neutrophils and mononuclear phagocytes), dendritic cells, nature killer (NK), cytotoxic T-cells, γδ T-cells, mast cells, eosinophils and basophilic granulocyte. Innate immune molecules include chemokines, cytokines, adhesion molecules, and regulators of the extracellular matrix, and cast important roles of activating immune mechanisms, stimulating acute phase response, upregulating adhesion molecules and recruiting immune cells. In contrast to adaptive immune system, innate immunity does not provide a longstanding protection to the host. Instead, innate cells and cellular components create an immediate physical and chemical barrier defending human body from infections. In addition to identifying foreign antigens and cells through activation of complement pathways, the functions of the innate system include releasing cytokines to recruit immune responding cells, and delivering signals via antigen presenting cells to activate adaptive immune system [11-15].

2.2. The Functions of NK Cells

NK cells account for about 15% of the total lymphocytes and 85% of the normal LGLs in peripheral blood, and play a pivotal role in immune surveillance and immune regulation [16-19]. NK cells express surface markers, such as CD56 and CD16 and lack either T or B cell receptors. NK cells have relatively large size and contain typical azurophilic granules in cytoplasm [17, 20]. Below is a simple introduction of their physiological functions.

2.2.1. Cytotoxicity of NK Cells

NK cells have spontaneous cytotoxic activity. They can directly lyse target cells that do not express self-major histocompatibility complex (MHC) antigens [16, 21, 22] through two major mechanisms 1) the perforin/granzyme pathway and 2) the Fas/FasL pathway. Granzymes and perforin are effector molecules residing in granules of cytotoxic T-cells (CTLs) and NK cells [23, 24], which can be released extracellularly upon contact with their targets [25, 26]. These enzymes can cause circular pore-like lesions in the membrane of normal cells and induce target cell death leading to acute local tissue damage and chronic cell damage. Activated NK cells can express FasL that interacts with the Fas receptor-positive target cells, and leads to the formation of the Fas-associated death domain protein (FADD), and subsequently induce the lysis of target cells via antibody-dependent cell-mediated cytotoxicity (ADCC) [19, 27]. This is also a direct pathway resulting in the destruction of target cells.

2.2.2. NK Cells and Immune Regulation

It was demonstrated elsewhere that NK cells are the main producers of cytokines, such as interferon (IFN)-γ, tumor necrosis factor (TNF), granulocyte-macrophage colony-stimulating factor (GM-CSF), interleukin 1 (IL-1), and IL-3 [27-30]. The process in which NK cells recognize target cells is nonspecific and depends on the degree of MHC I molecules expressed on the target cells rather than the specific recognition of antigen or antigen sensitization [16, 17, 30]. In the early stages of an immune response, NK cells can be stimulated to secrete these cytokines rapidly and efficiently. Thus, they are deemed to play an important role in the regulation of the immune system [30]. For example, in some viral infections, NK cells not only trigger the death of target cells, but can also be activated to secrete IFN-γ and other cytokines [28]. Furthermore, NK cells form immunological synapses with antigen-presenting cells especially with dendritic cells. Moreover, NK cells can bridge the innate immune system with the adaptive immune system [27].

2.2.3. NK Cells and Autoimmunity

NK cells have been identified in target organs of patients diagnosed with autoimmune diseases such as rheumatoid arthritis and systemic lupus erythematosus, SLE [31]. A common phenomenon in these autoimmune diseases is impaired NK cell activity, which contributes to pathogenesis of these diseases. Specifically, there were decreased levels of NK cells in peripheral blood of patients with non-organ-specific autoimmune diseases have been reported, while increased NK activity was observed in more localized autoimmune diseases [19]. These findings also indirectly suggest the importance of NK cells in maintaining the homeostasis of the immune system.

2.2.4. Other In Vitro/In Vivo Functions of NK Cells

It has been described that NK cells could kill not only circulating tumor cells, but also well-established small nodules [32]. Experimental studies showed that allogeneic and autologous fresh tumor cells were more sensitive to the lysis of NK cells. It is also shown that NK cells can destroy tumor cells effectively in vivo and play a significant role in antitumor activity. Furthermore, there are data suggesting that NK cells can react with cells from distinct histogenetic lineages in the early stages of differentiation. These cells can be immature thymocytes, bone marrow cells, or myeloid leukemic cells. It was concluded that, NK cells play an important role in hematopoietic homeostasis [29].

2.3. Neutropenia in LGL Leukemia

LGLL was first reported as a syndrome associated with the proliferation of LGL and neutropenia [1, 3-5, 7, 33]. Of note, neutropenia, the most common cytopenia, is found in approximately 80% of patients with indolent T-cell LGLL. Severe neutropenia can result in recurrent bacterial infections [3, 5, 10]. Although the mechanism of neutropenia in T-cell LGLL is not fully elucidated [1], several different hypotheses have been proposed. The two most common ones are 1) insufficient neutrophil production from the bone marrow and 2) increased neutrophil destruction [3, 5]. The latter appears more widely accepted as it is considered an immune mediated process. For instance, the presence of anti-neutrophil antibodies in LGLL suggests an antibody-mediated neutrophil destruction which most often occurs when passing the spleen. Alternatively, high levels of soluble FAS ligand in the peripheral blood, via binding to FAS receptor, can also trigger apoptosis of normal neutrophils. Given these experimental observations, the mainstream therapeutic strategy for neutropenia in LGLL is immunosuppression of LGLs. Studies have proved that stimulation of immature bone marrow myeloid cells using granulocyte-macrophage colony-stimulating factor (GM-CSF) or granulocyte colony-stimulating factor (G-CSF) does not result in durable clinical improvement of neutropenia in LGLL patients [5]. This may be due to myeloid hypoplasia which is frequently seen in bone marrow in patients with LGLL. The abnormal maturation of myeloid cells is attributed to the alterations of hematological microenvironment triggered by LGLs [5].

2.3.1. Activation of NK Cells and Signal Transduction in LGL Leukemia

As previously described, NK cells participate in the immune responses by direct lysis of transformed and allogeneic cells as well as virally-infected cells. They are part of the innate, immediate-acting arm of the immune system. Activation of NK cells is an early event during the immune response and does not require antigen-presentation in the context of MHC-peptide complex [34]. However, the function of NK cells is regulated by the net balance of the activating and inhibitory NK receptors [5, 35]. After NK-cell activation, there are two major pathways which lead to the death of target cells: granule-mediated pathway and receptor-mediated pathway.

LGLL is manifested by circulating clonal LGLs as well as tissue involvement, e.g., spleen, liver, bone marrow, by LGLs [2, 3, 10, 36]. Infiltrating LGLs are associated with endothelial damage and increased lung fibrosis in patients with LGLL [37]. In one study lung biopsies showed interstitial infiltration by LGL with extension into alveolar membranes and pneumocytes as well as increased background fibrosis. Additionally, it has been noted that some LGLL patients present with symptoms of pulmonary artery hypertension (PAH) [38]. Although the association between LGLL and PAH is not elucidated, it has been speculated that endothelial cell damage leads to lesions in the vascular wall and subsequently to vasoconstriction and ultimately PAH. In the receptor mediated pathway, the contribution of Fas was questioned in a report suggesting that despite strong expression of FAS and its ligand on vascular endothelial cells and infiltrating lymphocytes, vascular cells do not seem to undergo apoptosis. It is known that Fas-mediated target cell death accounts for only 10% of the cytotoxicity of NK cells.

Therefore, the second pathway mediated by Fas and Fas ligand does not appear to play a pivotal role in the tissue damage caused by activated NK cells. In contrast, the granule-mediated pathway by NK cells plays a more important role in the destruction of normal tissue. The identification of the signal transduction pathways and key signaling molecules that control this lytic process could lead to potential new therapeutic targets to disrupt the redistribution of granules and their exocytosis, thereby reducing the tissue damage mediated by activated NK cells.

During infection and inflammation, NK cells and cytotoxic T cells (CTLs) are recruited into peripheral tissues in human [39-42]. NK cells have been identified in target organs of patients with autoimmune disease [31, 43], numerous inflammatory diseases [44-46] and viral infections [39, 40, 47]. In addition, NK cells can destroy autologous cells in vivo such as oligodendrocytes, keratinocytes, neurons and pancreatic islet cells [48-52]. NK cell-mediated destruction of autologous cells in vivo can cause lasting cellular damage and contribute to inflammatory processes [31]. It has also been described that perforin released by activated NK cells can attack normal cells through the formation of circular pore lesions on the membrane of target cells. The pores allow the passage of large proteins such as granzyme B, which trigger apoptosis of target cells [26, 53, 54]. Several studies have shown that the pathogenesis of viral infections of heart or lungs is a direct result of viral replication [55, 56]. However, subsequent damage is dependent upon NK cells and CTL [39, 41, 45, 57].

The etiology of LGLL is not well understood. In a study of 15 patients, sera from 67% of these patients were shown to have high titers of specific antibody reactivity directed at a 34 amino acid epitope of the envelope protein of Human T Cell Leukemia Virus 1 (HTLV-I) [58]. It has been hypothesized that infection with an HTLV-like virus may be an initial trigger for activation of NK clones in such patients.

While signaling conduction thought to be play critical role in functional innate system, its impact on the development of T-LGLL is under investigated. Preliminary studies in the aspect will be discussed as following sections.

2.3.2. NK Activating Receptors

NK cells are tightly regulated by opposing signals that serve to activate or inhibit their effector functions [59]. Triggering signals can be transduced from the activating receptors into the cell via immunoreceptor tyrosine-based activation motifs (ITAMs) that propagate a signal cascade that ends in mobilization of the lytic granules [60-62]. Activating natural killer receptors (NKRs) typically recognize and bind specific molecules on target cells in the absence of MHC class I or II. Those include the killer immunoglobulin-like receptors (KIRs), NK cytotoxicity receptors (NCRs), and CD94-NKG2 families as well as NKG2D, which mediate NK-cell direct cytotoxicity and may also impart cytotoxic function to effector T cells [36]. On the other hand, the inhibitory receptors, which primarily consists of KIRs, commonly recognize classical MHC Class I molecules and dampen the ability of NK cells to kill self MHC-expressing cells, therefore, avoiding damage to normal tissue [63-65].

The binding of activating NKR ligands stimulates a cytoplasmic signaling cascade leading to NK-cell activation and cytotoxicity. Activating NKRs typically partner with and signal via membrane-bound adapter proteins that possess canonical cytoplasmic activation motifs including. DAP10 and DAP12 [36].

2.3.3. Adaptor Proteins: DAP12 and DAP10

DAP12 is an ITAM-bearing 12KDa-adaptor protein that is shared by the majority of activating NK receptors. DAP12 is expressed on the surface of NK cells as a disulfide-bonded homodimer, with each subunit expressing a single ITAM in the intracellular region [66]. Upon crosslinking of the activating receptor/DAP12 complex, the ITAMs in the adaptor proteins become phosphorylated and serve as the docking site for Syk or ZAP-70 protein tyrosine kinases [66-68]. This leads to positive signals, which trigger NK cell activation [66]. It is indicated that DAP12 signals by activating Syk protein tyrosine kinase, phosphoinositide 3-kinase (PI3K), and extracellular signal-regulated kinase (ERK/MAPK). This signaling pathway results in granule mobilization, target cell lysis, and cytokine production [36]. DAP10 is a novel 10-KD surface homodimeric adaptor that couples to a specific NK activating receptor, NKG2D, to trigger lytic function in NK cells [69]. DAP10 partners exclusively with NKG2D through interaction with a cytoplasmic PI3K binding motif (YxxM), which recruits PI3K after NKG2D recognizes its specific ligands (e.g., MICA/MICB) leading to the phosphorylation of AKT and subsequent target cell lysis and cytokine release. A large body of evidence has indicated that DAP12 and DAP10 are involved in the development and progression of various diseases, including inflammation and cancer. DAP12 and DAP10 are currently considered to be potential therapeutic targets [36]. Importantly; the cytotoxic effects in T-LGLL are increased at the same time of elevated expression of activating KIRs and their singling molecules, DAP12 and DAP10 [70].

2.3.4. Signal Cascades Associated with Lytic Function in T-LGLL

Clarification of the involved signaling mechanisms which drive effector function and cytotoxic granule movement toward target cells in activated NK cells in an area of great interest as it could provide suitable therapeutic targets for LGLL and other autoimmune diseases. Target cell lysis represents the final balance between stimulatory and inhibitory signals. It has been indicated that PI3K is pivotal for tumor cell lysis through the regulation of MAPK/ERK, which drives perforin-granzyme B movement toward the target cells [68, 71-76]. Rac1, a small GTPase, functions downstream of PI3K to regulate p21-activated kinase (PAK1), MEK, and MAPK/ERK activation. This newly defined pathway in NK cells is Ras-independent, following a specific signal sequence in the order of PI3K→ Rac1→ PAK1→ MEK→ MAPK/ERK [77, 78]. Activation of this pathway is necessary for granule release to occur. PI3K regulates a variety of cellular processes including reorganization of the actin cytoskeleton, induction of cellular survival and protection from apoptosis, antigen and IL-2 growth factor-mediated activation in T cells, membrane ruffling of T cells, and chemotaxis in neutrophils. Therefore, it is not surprising that PI3K is linked to many signaling pathways. It was also shown that the Rac1→ PAK1→ MEK→ MAPK/ERK pathway is one of the intracellular routes that PI3K employs to drive a lytic function of NK cells via granule mobilization [78]. Overall, identification of the signaling pathway during NK cell direct lysis from PI3K→ Rac1→ PAK1→ MEK→ MAPK/ERK represents important progress in the field. However, it should be noted that none of these proteins were ideal targets for drug design due to their ubiquitous expression in both immune and non-immune cells and their vital roles in many cell functions other than granule movement. Therefore, it is necessary to further define the initial activating steps mediated by DAP12 or DAP10 that are selectively and specifically required for NK-mediated lysis and granule movement after target ligation. One therapeutic strategy is to specifically target the DAP12 (or DAP10)-mediated target lysis pathway and no other signaling pathway. It is suggested that inhibitors of DAP10 and DAP12 or other proteins involved in this signaling pathway will be attractive therapeutic targets for the treatment of LGLL and other autoimmune diseases and syndromes [36].

3. THE DYSFUNCTION OF ADAPTIVE IMMUNE SYSTEM IN LGL LEUKEMIA

Adaptive immunity, also known as acquired or specific immunity, arises from antigen stimulation after birth in our body, and it has also been known as acquired immunity or specific immunity. It is mainly composed of lymphocyte, lymphoid organs and lymphoid tissue. Lymphocyte includes T cells, B cells, and NK cells. Lymphoid organs consist of two major groups; central lymphoid organs (primary lymphoid organ) and peripheral lymphoid organs (secondary lymphoid organ). Central lymphoid organs compromised of the bone marrow and thymus, are involved in the production, differentiation and maturation of immune cells. Peripheral lymphoid organs are comprised of lymph nodes, spleen, and the mucosal-associated lymphoid tissue (MALT), which is the place of mature lymphocytes to settle down [11].

3.1. Dysregulation of FAS–FASL-Mediated Apoptosis in LGL Leukemia

FAS, a member of the tumor necrosis factor (TNF) receptor family, plays an important role in CTL-mediated apoptosis of target cells [9, 33, 35]. FAS ligand is a member of the TNF family of proteins [74]. The binding of FAS and FAS ligand leads to the formation of death-inducing signaling complex (DISC), which is the complex of adaptor protein FADD and the cytosolic portion of the receptor [9, 33]. The formation of DISC causes the activation of caspase-dependent apoptosis. This is a major mechanism by which cytotoxic T cells (including LGLs) induce cell death in infected or foreign cells. It also serves as an important pathway leading to the decrease of activated T cells in vivo. The process of eliminating excess activated T cells after inflammation is called activation-induced cell death (AICD), which plays an indispensable role in maintaining T-cell homeostasis and tolerance to self-antigen in periphery. It is known that FAS-FAS ligand mediated apoptosis is one of the most important mechanisms resulting in the execution of AICD [9, 33].

However, it was suggested that malignant LGLs acquired an uncoupling of AICD and dysregulation of FAS-mediated apoptosis. LGLs express high levels of FAS and FAS ligand on their surfaces like normal activated CTLs. Unlike normal activated CTLs, leukemic LGLs are resistant to FAS-mediated apoptosis [79-81]. Nevertheless, unlike other autoimmune diseases e.g., ALPS (autoimmune lymphoproliferative syndrome) [33, 35] there are no mutations detected in the functional domain in FAS and FASL in LGLL. In addition, high levels of soluble FAS were observed in the sera of LGLL patients compared with healthy controls. Soluble FAS receptors may act as decoys for FAS ligand and then contribute to the blockade of FAS function, which eventually results in the resistance of apoptotic pathway [1, 9, 33, 35, 79]. The inhibition of FAS-dependent apoptosis leads to the dysregulation of lymphocyte homeostasis in LGLL and the T cell expansion. In fact, T-cell LGLL is an abnormal condition in which antigen-stimulated T cells expand out of homeostatic control. Although the etiology of LGLL is not elucidated [1, 3] it was proposed that antigen activation of T cells was the initiating event that led to the abnormal clonal expansion state [81]. FAS-FASL mediated apoptosis plays a pivotal role in the homeostasis of T cells through the elimination of excessive antigen-activated effector lymphocytes [10, 79, 81]. Therefore, the dysregulation of FAS-FASL mediated apoptosis pathway results in the accumulation of effector T cells. Additionally, it was demonstrated that there was a striking accumulation of CD8 terminal-effector memory T cells in LGLL [81].

As far as the treatment of the LGLL, despite elevate elevation of soluble FAS in the sera of LGLL patients, the use of specific antibodies that target the soluble FAS of tumor cells have not been extensively tested in the clinical trials due to significant risk of systemic toxicity and potential development of various hematologic malignancies. Fortunately, there are other possible therapeutic targets of this apoptosis pathway. It was hypothesized that matrix metalloproteinase (MMP) inhibitors could be used for the treatment of LGLL, since these agents could convert human FASL into a soluble FASL. One could speculate that MMP inhibitors could prevent the generation of soluble FASL and lower its levels in LGLL patients [9]. Furthermore, it was shown elsewhere, that the treatment with phytohemagglutinin (PHA) and interleukin-2 (IL-2) or treatment with ceramide can reverse FAS resistance, which provides other methods to deal with the dysregulation of FAS-mediated apoptosis pathway in LGLL [81]. In addition, the dysregulated FAS-mediated apoptosis pathway is one of the dysregulated pathway related to the abnormal immune system in LGLL. Thus, insight into activation of survival pathways and evasion of apoptosis pathways will provide new therapeutic targets of LGLL [9, 33, 80].

3.2. The Role of Abnormal CD8+ T Cells in LGL Leukemia

Recent studies in LGLL have shown that the infiltrating leukemic cells have an association with direct tissue destruction. Moreover, activated CD8+/CD28 (null) and CD4+/CD28 (null) T lymphocytes are commonly overexpressed in autoimmune diseases [36]. Autoimmune diseases, particularly rheumatoid arthritis and pulmonary arterial hypertension (PAH), are often pivotal clinical features of LGLL [5, 7, 36]. An exacerbated immune reaction against self-tissue is the key pathogenic mechanism in a variety of human diseases and is positively linked to the expansion of CD4+and/or CD8+/CD28 (null) T cells. Data presented in some studies showed that CD8+/CD28 (null) leukemic T LGL cells constitutively killed a pulmonary artery endothelial target cell line and a synovial target cell line in vitro, independently of IL-2 activation. The cytotoxicity mediated by T-LGLL cells was inherently different from that by purified CD8+CD28 (null) cells from healthy donors, suggesting that a unique cytotoxic mechanism may contribute to this disease. CD8+ CTLs share a common killing mechanism with NK cells. CD8+ T cells from LGLL patients possess higher levels of multiple NKRs on their cell surface, express higher levels of DAP10 and DAP12 mRNAs, and display activity of multiple signaling intermediates within the NKR/DAP10/DAP12 signaling cascade when compared with CD8+ T cells from healthy control subjects. These observations suggest that NKR and their associated activating adaptors must play a pivotal role in cytotoxicity by this cell population where CD8+CD28 (null) [1] T cells are normally present in the peripheral blood of healthy donors. Blockade of DAP10/DAP12 signaling pathways in CD8+ T LGLL cells with dominant-negative forms of each protein demonstrated that these pathways are directly linked to PI3K and ERK1/2 activation, granule polarization, cytotoxicity, and cytokine production. Therefore, the NKR-DAP10/DAP12 signaling pathways are essential events for NK-cell function, and also play critical roles during T-cell activation in patients with LGLL. A bridged tolerance through this NKR-generated signaling pathway may represent the key event in inflammation and tissue destruction associated with autoimmunity. It was suggested that inhibitors of DAP10 and DAP12 or other proteins involved in this signaling pathway could be attractive therapeutic targets for the treatment of LGLL and autoimmune diseases and syndromes [36].

CONCLUSION

Abnormal proliferation of LGLs can results in malignancies such as LGLL, which is tightly associated with the impaired homeostasis of the immune system in vivo. Alterations of the innate immune systems are observed in LGLL Hematological and/or autoimmune disorders are often present simultaneously in those with LGLL and frequently associated with neutropenia. The coexistence of activated NK cells is seen in LGLL. The increased adaptor proteins DAP10 and DAP12 result in the upregulation of the signal transduction pathway PI3K→ Rac1→ PAK1→ MEK→ MAPK/ERK. Therefore, the inhibition of DAP10 and DAP12 serves as an attractive therapeutic strategy in the treatment of LGLL. Such therapeutic approach could alleviate the lysis function of activated NK cells to target cells and reduce CD8+ T-cell mediated tissue damage [36]. In addition, there are also several other dysregulated signaling pathways in LGLL such as ineffective FAS-mediated apoptosis, which leads to significant accumulation of CD8+ terminal-effector memory T cells in LGLL. Reactivation of FAS mediated apoptotic pathway would be is an alternative option for the treatment of LGLL.

LGLL is a lymphoproliferative disorder associated with ineffective hematopoiesis [82]. Immunosuppressive therapies using methotrexate or cyclophosphamide were shown to be effective in about a half of patients [83]. Thus, a novel therapy is needed [9]. In the era of genomic and molecular medicine, novel insight into dysregulated signaling pathways and abnormal immune system by whole genomic sequencing, exome sequencing or RNA sequencing will help us discover immunogenic profiles and develop more specific therapeutic targets for the treatment of LGLL.

REFERENCES

[1] Lamy T, Loughran TP, Jr. Current concepts: large granular lymphocyte leukemia. *Blood Rev.* 1999;13(4):230-240.

[2] Sokol L, Loughran TP, Jr. Large granular lymphocyte leukemia. *Curr Hematol Malig Rep.* 2007;2(4):278-282.

[3] Sokol L, Loughran TP, Jr. Large granular lymphocyte leukemia. *Oncologist.* 2006;11(3):263-273.

[4] Loughran TP. Large granular lymphocytic leukemia: an overview. *Hosp Pract (1995).* 1998;33(5):133-138.

[5] Zhang R, Shah MV, Loughran TP, Jr. The root of many evils: indolent large granular lymphocyte leukaemia and associated disorders. *Hematol Oncol.* 2010;28(3):105-117.

[6] Mailloux AW, Zhang L, Moscinski L, et al. Fibrosis and subsequent cytopenias are associated with basic fibroblast growth factor-deficient pluripotent mesenchymal stromal cells in large granular lymphocyte leukemia. *J Immunol.* 2013;191(7):3578-3593.

[7] Gentile TC, Wener MH, Starkebaum G, Loughran TP, Jr. Humoral immune abnormalities in T-cell large granular lymphocyte leukemia. *Leuk Lymphoma.* 1996;23(3-4):365-370.

[8] Prochorec-Sobieszek M, Rymkiewicz G, Makuch-Lasica H, et al. Characteristics of T-cell large granular lymphocyte proliferations associated with neutropenia and inflammatory arthropathy. *Arthritis Res Ther.* 2008;10(3):R55.

[9] Leblanc F, Zhang D, Liu X, Loughran TP. Large granular lymphocyte leukemia: from dysregulated pathways to therapeutic targets. *Future Oncol.* 2012;8(7):787-801.

[10] Steinway SN, LeBlanc F, Loughran TP, Jr. The pathogenesis and treatment of large granular lymphocyte leukemia. *Blood Rev.* 2014;28(3):87-94.

[11] Janeway C, Travers P, Walport M, Shlomchik M. *Immunology.* 5th ed. New York and London2001.

[12] Janeway CA, Jr., Medzhitov R. Innate immune recognition. *Annu Rev Immunol.* 2002;20:197-216.

[13] Newton K, Dixit VM. Signaling in innate immunity and inflammation. *Cold Spring Harb Perspect Biol.* 2012;4(3).

[14] Brubaker SW, Bonham KS, Zanoni I, Kagan JC. Innate immune pattern recognition: a cell biological perspective. *Annu Rev Immunol.* 2015;33:257-290.

[15] Turvey SE, Broide DH. Innate immunity. *J Allergy Clin Immunol.* 2010;125(2 Suppl 2):S24-32.

[16] Alam R. A brief review of the immune system. *Prim Care.* 1998;25(4):727-738.

[17] Moretta L, Ciccone E, Mingari MC, Biassoni R, Moretta A. Human natural killer cells: origin, clonality, specificity, and receptors. *Adv Immunol.* 1994;55:341-380.

[18] Cooper MA, Fehniger TA, Caligiuri MA. The biology of human natural killer-cell subsets. *Trends Immunol.* 2001;22(11):633-640.

[19] Grunebaum E, Malatzky-Goshen E, Shoenfeld Y. Natural killer cells and autoimmunity. *Immunol Res.* 1989;8(4):292-304.

[20] Roder JC, Pross HF. The biology of the human natural killer cell. *J Clin Immunol.* 1982;2(4):249-263.

[21] Ortaldo JR, Mathieson BJ, Wiltrout RH. Characterization and functions of natural killer cells. *Ann Inst Pasteur Immunol.* 1988;139(4):444-450.

[22] Reyburn H, Mandelboim O, Vales-Gomez M, et al. Human NK cells: their ligands, receptors and functions. *Immunol Rev.* 1997;155:119-125.

[23] Smyth MJ, Trapani JA. Granzymes: exogenous proteinases that induce target cell apoptosis. *Immunol Today.* 1995;16(4):202-206.

[24] Trapani JA, Sutton VR, Smyth MJ. CTL granules: evolution of vesicles essential for combating virus infections. *Immunol Today.* 1999;20(8):351-356.

[25] Trinchieri G. Biology of natural killer cells. *Adv Immunol.* 1989;47:187-376.

[26] Smyth MJ, Thia KY, Street SE, MacGregor D, Godfrey DI, Trapani JA. Perforin-mediated cytotoxicity is critical for surveillance of spontaneous lymphoma. *J Exp Med.* 2000;192(5):755-760.

[27] Sinkovics JG, Horvath JC. Human natural killer cells: a comprehensive review. *Int J Oncol.* 2005;27(1):5-47.

[28] Biron CA. Activation and function of natural killer cell responses during viral infections. *Curr Opin Immunol.* 1997;9(1):24-34.

[29] Trinchieri G, Perussia B. Human natural killer cells: biologic and pathologic aspects. *Lab Invest.* 1984;50(5):489-513.

[30] See DM, Khemka P, Sahl L, Bui T, Tilles JG. The role of natural killer cells in viral infections. *Scand J Immunol.* 1997;46(3):217-224.

[31] Flodstrom M, Shi FD, Sarvetnick N, Ljunggren HG. The natural killer cell -- friend or foe in autoimmune disease? *Scand J Immunol.* 2002;55(5):432-441.

[32] Yang Q, Goding SR, Hokland ME, Basse PH. Antitumor activity of NK cells. *Immunol Res.* 2006;36(1-3):13-25.

[33] Shah MV, Zhang R, Loughran TP, Jr. Never say die: survival signaling in large granular lymphocyte leukemia. *Clin Lymphoma Myeloma.* 2009;9 Suppl 3:S244-253.

[34] Lanier LL. Turning on natural killer cells. *J Exp Med.* 2000;191(8):1259-1262.

[35] Epling-Burnette PK, Loughran TP, Jr. Survival signals in leukemic large granular lymphocytes. *Semin Hematol.* 2003;40(3):213-220.

[36] Chen X, Bai F, Sokol L, et al. A critical role for DAP10 and DAP12 in CD8+ T cell-mediated tissue damage in large granular lymphocyte leukemia. *Blood.* 2009;113(14):3226-3234.

[37] Lamy T, Bauer FA, Liu JH, et al. Clinicopathological features of aggressive large granular lymphocyte leukaemia resemble Fas ligand transgenic mice. *Br J Haematol.* 2000;108(4):717-723.

[38] Rossoff LJ, Genovese J, Coleman M, Dantzker DR. Primary pulmonary hypertension in a patient with CD8/T-cell large granulocyte leukemia: amelioration by cladribine therapy. *Chest.* 1997;112(2):551-553.

[39] Hussell T, Openshaw PJ. Intracellular IFN-gamma expression in natural killer cells precedes lung CD8+ T cell recruitment during respiratory syncytial virus infection. *J Gen Virol.* 1998;79 (Pt 11):2593-2601.

[40] Spender LC, Hussell T, Openshaw PJ. Abundant IFN-gamma production by local T cells in respiratory syncytial virus-induced eosinophilic lung disease. *J Gen Virol.* 1998;79 (Pt 7):1751-1758.

[41] Kambayashi T, Assarsson E, Chambers BJ, Ljunggren HG. Expression of the DX5 antigen on CD8+ T cells is associated with activation and subsequent cell death or memory during influenza virus infection. *Eur J Immunol.* 2001;31(5):1523-1530.

[42] Glas R, Franksson L, Une C, et al. Recruitment and activation of natural killer (NK) cells in vivo determined by the target cell phenotype. An adaptive component of NK cell-mediated responses. *J Exp Med.* 2000;191(1):129-138.

[43] Reinitz E, Neighbour PA, Grayzel AI. Natural killer cell activity of mononuclear cells from rheumatoid patients measured by a conjugate-binding cytotoxicity assay. *Arthritis Rheum.* 1982;25(12):1440-1444.

[44] Zeng X, Moore TA, Newstead MW, Hernandez-Alcoceba R, Tsai WC, Standiford TJ. Intrapulmonary expression of macrophage inflammatory protein 1alpha (CCL3) induces neutrophil and NK cell accumulation and stimulates innate immunity in murine bacterial pneumonia. *Infect Immun.* 2003;71(3):1306-1315.

[45] Andrews DM, Farrell HE, Densley EH, Scalzo AA, Shellam GR, Degli-Esposti MA. NK1.1+ cells and murine cytomegalovirus infection: what happens in situ? *J Immunol.* 2001;166(3):1796-1802.

[46] Saunders BM, Cheers C. Intranasal infection of beige mice with Mycobacterium avium complex: role of neutrophils and natural killer cells. *Infect Immun.* 1996;64(10):4236-4241.

[47] Kearney MT, Cotton JM, Richardson PJ, Shah AM. Viral myocarditis and dilated cardiomyopathy: mechanisms, manifestations, and management. *Postgrad Med J.* 2001;77(903):4-10.

[48] Antel JP, McCrea E, Ladiwala U, Qin YF, Becher B. Non-MHC-restricted cell-mediated lysis of human oligodendrocytes in vitro: relation with CD56 expression. *J Immunol.* 1998;160(4):1606-1611.

[49] Morse RH, Seguin R, McCrea EL, Antel JP. NK cell-mediated lysis of autologous human oligodendrocytes. *J Neuroimmunol.* 2001;116(1):107-115.

[50] Molinero LL, Gruber M, Leoni J, Woscoff A, Zwirner NW. Up-regulated expression of MICA and proinflammatory cytokines in skin biopsies from patients with seborrhoeic dermatitis. *Clin Immunol.* 2003;106(1):50-54.

[51] Backstrom E, Chambers BJ, Kristensson K, Ljunggren HG. Direct NK cell-mediated lysis of syngenic dorsal root ganglia neurons in vitro. *J Immunol.* 2000;165(9):4895-4900.

[52] Nakamura N, Woda BA, Tafuri A, et al. Intrinsic cytotoxicity of natural killer cells to pancreatic islets in vitro. *Diabetes.* 1990;39(7):836-843.

[53] Yoneda O, Imai T, Goda S, et al. Fractalkine-mediated endothelial cell injury by NK cells. *J Immunol.* 2000;164(8):4055-4062.

[54] Sutton VR, Davis JE, Cancilla M, et al. Initiation of apoptosis by granzyme B requires direct cleavage of bid, but not direct granzyme B-mediated caspase activation. *J Exp Med.* 2000;192(10):1403-1414.

[55] Shioi T, Matsumori A, Sasayama S. Persistent expression of cytokine in the chronic stage of viral myocarditis in mice. *Circulation.* 1996;94(11):2930-2937.

[56] Matsumori A. Molecular and immune mechanisms in the pathogenesis of cardiomyopathy--role of viruses, cytokines, and nitric oxide. *Jpn Circ J.* 1997;61(4):275-291.

[57] Watters RJ, Liu X, Loughran TP, Jr. T-cell and natural killer-cell large granular lymphocyte leukemia neoplasias. *Leuk Lymphoma.* 2011;52(12):2217-2225.

[58] Loughran TP, Jr., Hadlock KG, Yang Q, et al. Seroreactivity to an envelope protein of human T-cell leukemia/lymphoma virus in patients with CD3- (natural killer) lymphoproliferative disease of granular lymphocytes. *Blood.* 1997;90(5):1977-1981.

[59] Lanier LL. On guard--activating NK cell receptors. *Nat Immunol.* 2001;2(1):23-27.

[60] Tomasello E, Blery M, Vely F, Vivier E. Signaling pathways engaged by NK cell receptors: double concerto for activating receptors, inhibitory receptors and NK cells. *Semin Immunol.* 2000;12(2):139-147.

[61] Djeu JY, Jiang K, Wei S. A view to a kill: signals triggering cytotoxicity. *Clin Cancer Res.* 2002;8(3):636-640.

[62] Cerwenka A, Lanier LL. Ligands for natural killer cell receptors: redundancy or specificity. *Immunol Rev.* 2001;181:158-169.

[63] Colonna M, Samaridis J. Cloning of immunoglobulin-superfamily members associated with HLA-C and HLA-B recognition by human natural killer cells. *Science.* 1995;268(5209):405-408.

[64] Olcese L, Lang P, Vely F, et al. Human and mouse killer-cell inhibitory receptors recruit PTP1C and PTP1D protein tyrosine phosphatases. *J Immunol.* 1996;156(12):4531-4534.

[65] Campbell KS, Dessing M, Lopez-Botet M, Cella M, Colonna M. Tyrosine phosphorylation of a human killer inhibitory receptor recruits protein tyrosine phosphatase 1C. *J Exp Med.* 1996;184(1):93-100.

[66] Lanier LL, Corliss BC, Wu J, Leong C, Phillips JH. Immunoreceptor DAP12 bearing a tyrosine-based activation motif is involved in activating NK cells. *Nature.* 1998;391(6668):703-707.

[67] McVicar DW, Taylor LS, Gosselin P, et al. DAP12-mediated signal transduction in natural killer cells. A dominant role for the Syk protein-tyrosine kinase. *J Biol Chem.* 1998;273(49):32934-32942.

[68] Jiang K, Zhong B, Gilvary DL, et al. Syk regulation of phosphoinositide 3-kinase-dependent NK cell function. *J Immunol.* 2002;168(7):3155-3164.

[69] Wu J, Song Y, Bakker AB, et al. An activating immunoreceptor complex formed by NKG2D and DAP10. *Science.* 1999;285(5428):730-732.

[70] Kirchhoff S, Muller WW, Krueger A, Schmitz I, Krammer PH. TCR-mediated up-regulation of c-FLIPshort correlates with resistance toward CD95-mediated apoptosis by blocking death-inducing signaling complex activity. *J Immunol.* 2000;165(11):6293-6300.

[71] Wei S, Gamero AM, Liu JH, et al. Control of lytic function by mitogen-activated protein kinase/extracellular regulatory kinase 2 (ERK2) in a human natural killer cell line: identification of perforin and granzyme B mobilization by functional ERK2. *J Exp Med.* 1998;187(11):1753-1765.

[72] Trotta R, Puorro KA, Paroli M, et al. Dependence of both spontaneous and antibody-dependent, granule exocytosis-mediated NK cell cytotoxicity on extracellular signal-regulated kinases. *J Immunol.* 1998;161(12):6648-6656.

[73] Trotta R, Fettucciari K, Azzoni L, et al. Differential role of p38 and c-Jun N-terminal kinase 1 mitogen-activated protein kinases in NK cell cytotoxicity. *J Immunol.* 2000;165(4):1782-1789.

[74] Brumbaugh KM, Binstadt BA, Billadeau DD, et al. Functional role for Syk tyrosine kinase in natural killer cell-mediated natural cytotoxicity. *J Exp Med.* 1997;186(12):1965-1974.

[75] Billadeau DD, Brumbaugh KM, Dick CJ, Schoon RA, Bustelo XR, Leibson PJ. The Vav-Rac1 pathway in cytotoxic lymphocytes regulates the generation of cell-mediated killing. *J Exp Med.* 1998;188(3):549-559.

[76] Gismondi A, Jacobelli J, Mainiero F, et al. Cutting edge: functional role for proline-rich tyrosine kinase 2 in NK cell-mediated natural cytotoxicity. *J Immunol.* 2000;164(5):2272-2276.

[77] Wei S, Gilvary DL, Corliss BC, et al. Direct tumor lysis by NK cells uses a Ras-independent mitogen-activated protein kinase signal pathway. *J Immunol.* 2000;165(7):3811-3819.

[78] Jiang K, Zhong B, Gilvary DL, et al. Pivotal role of phosphoinositide-3 kinase in regulation of cytotoxicity in natural killer cells. *Nat Immunol.* 2000;1(5):419-425.

[79] Liu JH, Wei S, Lamy T, et al. Blockade of Fas-dependent apoptosis by soluble Fas in LGL leukemia. *Blood.* 2002;100(4):1449-1453.

[80] Zhang R, Shah MV, Yang J, et al. Network model of survival signaling in large granular lymphocyte leukemia. *Proc Natl Acad Sci U S A.* 2008;105(42):16308-16313.

[81] Yang J, Epling-Burnette PK, Painter JS, et al. Antigen activation and impaired Fas-induced death-inducing signaling complex formation in T-large-granular lymphocyte leukemia. *Blood.* 2008;111(3):1610-1616.

[82] Epling-Burnette PK, Sokol L, Chen X, et al. Clinical improvement by farnesyltransferase inhibition in NK large granular lymphocyte leukemia associated with imbalanced NK receptor signaling. *Blood.* 2008;112(12):4694-4698.

[83] Burks EJ, Loughran TP, Jr. Perspectives in the treatment of LGL leukemia. *Leuk Res.* 2005;29(2):123-125.

In: Benign and Malignant Disorders …
Editors: Ling Zhang and Lubomir Sokol
ISBN: 978-1-53612-999-1
© 2018 Nova Science Publishers, Inc.

Chapter 3

NK Cell Biology and the Role of NK Cells in Hematopoietic Stem Cell Transplantation and Cellular Immunotherapy

Rawan Faramand[1] and Asmita Mishra[2],*

[1]University of South Florida, H. Lee Moffitt Cancer Center
and Research Institute, Tampa, FL, US
[2]Department of Blood and Marrow Transplantation and Cellular Immunotherapy,
H. Lee Moffitt Cancer Center and Research Institute, Tampa, FL, US

Abstract

Natural Killer (NK) cells are an important part of the innate immune system that are implicated in immune-surveillance, transplantation alloreactivity, and tolerance. A critical function of NK cells in immune response to cancer cells and viralinfections has been attracting increased attention for their potential clinical use via immune-based therapies. However, when compared with our progress in understanding B- and T-Cell functions in the biology of allogeneic hematopoietic stem cell transplantation (alloHSCT), the comprehension of the role of NK cells in alloHSCT and in adoptive immunotherapy is limited. Numerous studies have proposed several models of NK cell alloreactivity including ligand incompatibility, receptor-ligand interaction, missing ligand and killer-immunoglobuline-like receptor (KIR) mismatch. These studies facilitated improved understanding of the role of NK cells in mediating immune reconstitution, graft-versus host disease (GVHD), disease relapse, and infection control during the process of alloHSCT. The selection of donors based on KIR genotyping is an ongoing focus of several clinical trials and identifying the hematopoietic stem cell setting in which KIR matching has the most impact remains an area to be explored. Similarly, the role of NK cells on GVHD remains controversial and is dependent on several parameters

---

* Corresponding Author Email: asmita.mishra@moffitt.org.

including the degree of T cell depletion and mode of NK cell stimulation. Future studies are necessary to identify predictive factors of GVHD development in NK cellular therapy to maximize graft-versus leukemia (GvL) and minimize the risk of GVHD. Emerging data supports the exploitation of NK cell alloreactivity for patients with hematologic malignancies. In addition, the potential clinical applications of *ex-vivo* manipulated chimeric antigen receptor NK cells in clinical trials as well as other mechanisms of adoptive immunotherapy will lead a greater success in the alloHSCT setting.

1. INTRODUCTION

The role of immunotherapy in cancer management has recently demonstrated tremendous growth. Progress in the methods of gene engineering, development of effective and safe cellular delivery systems, utilization of immune checkpoint blockade in the treatment of hematopoietic or non-hematopoietic neoplasms and most recently the federal drug administration (FDA) approval of CD19 expressing chimeric antigen receptor T cells (CAR-T) for children and young adults with relapsed/refractory B cell acute lymphoblastic leukemia contributed to the growth in this field [1-3]. Adaptive immunotherapy with monoclonal antibodies has now become standard of care for the management of many malignancies [4]. While our understanding of B cells and T cells and our ability to manipulate their activity has significantly improved, the role of natural killer (NK) cells specifically in allogeneic hematopoietic stem cell transplantation (alloHSCT) is limited by comparison.

Allogeneic hematopoietic stem cell transplantation (alloHSCT) is a potentially curative therapy for many hematologic malignancies such as leukemia and lymphoma, as well as congenital or acquired bone marrow disorders. What was once perceived to have insurmountable mortality burden, alloHSCT has now become a standard of care therapy for many hematologic disorders due to improvements in donor selection and transplant-directed supportive care [5]. Advances in immunotherapy have improved our understanding of the role of donor derived T-cells in the allograft setting including promoting engraftment and attacking residual leukemia cells, i.e., graft- versus- leukemia effect (GvL). Additionally, donor derived T-cells can mediate adverse reactions such as acute and chronic graft- versus- host disease (GVHD), a multisystem disorder associated with high morbidity and mortality after receiving alloHSCT [6].

While our understanding of the B- and T-Cell function and biology in the alloHSCT setting is robust, the role of NK cells is limited despite being discovered more than 40 years ago [7]. This may be in part due to the lack of familiarity and understanding with their basic biology and function, and subsequently the clinical applicability. The key role of NK cells in various aspects of immune response is now being recognized and has been attracting increased attention for its potential clinical use as a part of immune-based therapies [7]. NK cells are an important member of the innate immune system that can recognize and kill target cells without previous exposure [8]. This is particularly important when evaluating biologic studies of NK cells and factors that influence NK-cell effect in cancer immune-surveillance, viral immunity, and transplantation alloreactivity. In this chapter, we will review NK cell biology, discuss their role in the alloHSCT setting, and review advances in incorporating NK cells as therapeutic options for the treatment of hematologic malignancies.

2. NK Cell Biology and Function

Normal large granular lymphocytes (LGL) are derived from two major lineages based on immunophenotype; T cell and NK cells. Immunophenotypically, NK cells are characterized as lymphocytes with the absence of expression of surface CD3 (sCD3-) but positive expression of the CD56 (CD56+) antigen. Thus, NK cells do not express the CD3/T-cell receptor (TCR) complex or undergo TCR gene rearrangement during maturation. NK cells can be further divided into two distinct subsets identified as the mature CD16+CD56^{dim} population and less mature CD16+CD56^{bright} population [7, 9, 10]. These cells play an integral role within the innate immune system that can mediate non-major histocompatibility complex (MHC)-restricted cytotoxicity. Granules within the mature NK cells contain perforin (membrane-disrupting protein) and granzymes (family of proteolytic enzymes) that facilitate NK cell mediated killing [11]. NK cells also secrete pro-inflammatory cytokines and chemokines that bridge the innate and adaptive immune responses [8]. These features allow NK cells to spontaneously kill cells that express dangerous signals that are deemed harmful to the host. Furthermore, NK cells are activated quickly and require a short duration of time to generate a cytolytic response, in comparison to other immune mechanisms [10].

2.1. NK Cell Biology: A Complex Interplay of Activating and Inhibitory Ligands

To prevent killing of healthy host cells, NK cells are regulated by a complex mechanism that prevents them from attacking autologous cells, while ensuring that stressed (virally infected or cancer cells) MHC Class I absent cells are eliminated (Figure 1a) [10]. These unique features underscore the importance of NK cells and their vital role in viral immunity, cancer immune-surveillance, immune reconstitution, and transplantation alloreactivity [10]. In humans, T-cell activation and subsequent cytotoxicity are highly restricted to an antigen peptide presented in the groove of MHC class of proteins which is recognized by the T-cell receptor (TCR) [10]. NK cell activation is not antigen-specific and thus requires mechanisms to ensure that autoreactivity is avoided against normal host cells [7, 10]. By employing different receptors, NK cells exhibit an elegant and complex interplay between cytotoxic activation (activating receptors) against harmful stimuli and self-tolerance (inhibitory receptors) to ensure healthy functioning of the immune system (Figure 2) [7]. Compromised cells can activate NK cell cytolytic activity by either the loss of self identifying inhibitory receptors (Figure 1b), or by overexpression of stress ligands (Figure 1c) which are recognized by the NK cell activating receptors [10].

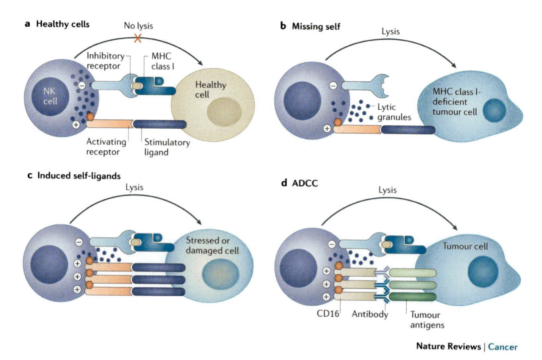

A) A balance of signals delivered by activating and inhibitory receptors regulates the recognition of healthy cells by natural killer (NK) cells. B) Tumor cells that downregulate major histocompatibility complex (MHC) class I molecules are detected as 'missing self' and are lysed by NK cells. C) Tumor cells can overexpress induced stress ligands recognized by activating NK cell receptors, which override the inhibitory signals and elicit target cell lysis. D) Tumor antigen-specific antibodies bind to CD16 and elicit antibody-dependent NK cell-mediated cytotoxicity.

Figure 1. Function of Natural Killer Cells [10].

The main receptor families expressed on NK cells that maintain this immune balance are killer immunoglobulin-like receptors (KIRs), C-type lectin receptors, and natural cytotoxicity receptors (NCRs). NCRs are activating receptors mediating cytotoxic killing and include constituently expressed receptors such as NKp30 and NKp46 as well as receptors expressed only after activation of the NK cell such as NKp44 [10]. KIRs and C-type lectin receptors have both activating and inhibitory properties that facilitate recognition of self to prevent attack of healthy autologous cells and additionally promote

NK cell activation in the presence of danger on a target cell (Figure 2) [7, 9]. C-type lectin receptors are expressed predominantly on the surface of NK cells and a subset of T-lymphocytes. One of the members of this family of receptors is the CD94 (also known as KLRD1-NKG2 system). By forming a disulfide-linked heterodimer with theNKG2A receptor the CD94/NKG2A complex recognizes a relatively non-polymorphic MHC class I ligand named Human Leukocyte Antigen- (HLA) E, thereby providing one mechanism to identify normal host cells as "self" [12].

2.2. Function of Killer Immunoglobulin-Like Receptors (KIRs)

KIRs are encoded by a diverse family of 17 genes on chromosome 19q13.4 and segregate independently from HLA genes [7,9]. The naming convention for these receptors is based on the number of immunoglobulin-like domains in the molecule, and the length of the cytoplasmic tail, integrating both structure and function [13]. A short-tailed cytoplasmic tail (S) indicates an activating tail, whereas a long-tailed cytoplasmic tail (L) indicates an inhibitory KIR. The number prefaced before the letter "D" (i.e., "2D") references the number of extracellular immunoglobulin domains [9, 14]. For example, KIR2DL1 signifies 2 immunoglobulin domains and a long cytoplasmic tail with inhibitory functionality [7]. The last number of the name refers to the number of that protein in the family [9]. In the example given above, the #1 denotes being the first member of the inhibitory KIRs containing two immunoglobulin domains.

KIRs demonstrate ligand specificity recognizing the HLA family including the polymorphic HLA-A, -B, and –C; however not all ligands have been identified yet [12]. Similar to HLA genes, each person expresses a unique KIR pattern, which has varying frequencies of KIR alleles amongst different ethnicities [9]. Despite their heterogeneity, there are patterns of conserved genomic regions within different populations. Two distinct KIR haplotypes have been recognized and are classified according to distinct centromeric and teloremic gene regions and activity [7, 15]. The group A haplotype has a set number of genes encoding mostly inhibitory receptors [7, 15]. The B haplotype group has variable gene content which includes both activating and inhibitory receptors containing at least one of the following B specific genes; KIR2DS1, KIR2DS2, KIR2DS3, KIR2DS5, KIR2DL2, and KIR2DL5 [15]. This becomes particularly important when considering translational models that utilize KIRs for direct immune checkpoint blockage of NK cells. For example, the fully human, first-in-class, anti-KIR, monoclonal antibody, Lirilumab (IPH2102/BMS-986015), blocks three inhibitory KIRs, KIR2DL1, KIR2DL2, and KIR2DL3 [16]. By targeting these specific KIR regions, the usage of Lirilumab facilitates NK cell activation by blocking their inhibitory receptors and is being tested against several malignancies in Phase I and II trials [16, 17].

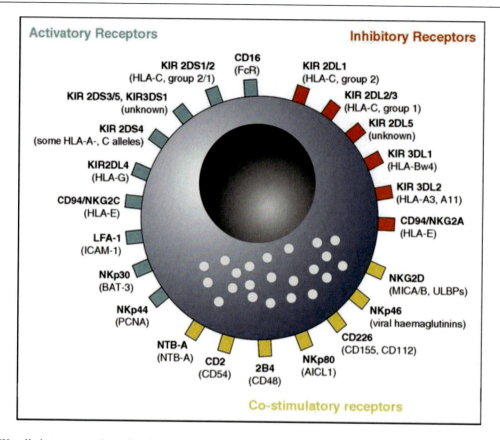

NK cells integrate various signals in response to leukemic cells. The precise function of some of the receptors is not yet well known, and some activatory receptors might be costimulatory, and vice versa. Note that recent evidence suggests that NKG2D and NKp46 are co-stimulatory receptors because they are not able to induce NK cell activity on their own [18]. In addition, KIR2DL4 is, to date, considered to convey activatory rather than inhibitory signals [18]. Many other receptors, including cytokine, chemotactic, and adhesion molecule receptors, as well as other costimulatory receptors, are not shown. Ligands are shown in parentheses. AICL; activation-induced C-type lectin; BAT-3, HLA-B-associated transcript 3; CD16, FcRIII receptor; LFA-1, leukocyte functional antigen 1; MICA/B, MHC class I–related chain A/B; NTB, natural killer T- and B-cell antigen; PCNA, proliferating cell nuclear antigen; ULBPs, UL-16 binding proteins [7].

Figure 2. Overview of activating, inhibitory, and costimulatory NK cell receptors [7].

3. ADOPTIVE IMMUNOTHERAPY WITH NK CELLS

Utilizing the antitumor effects of NK cells, several groups have explored the adoptive transfer of NK cells to treat hematologic malignancies. The beneficial utilization of Interleukin 2 (IL2) stimulated lymphokine-activated killer cells for metastatic cancer was first reported in 1985 by the Rosenberg group [19, 20]. Building upon early therapeutic successesin the refractory setting, the Miller group conducted a phase I study using low dose IL-2 after autologous transplant to evaluate the cytolytic tumor activity by IL-2 activated autologous NK cells [21]. While the study did demonstrate IL-2-mediated augmented *in vivo* NK cell activity, it did not lead to clinically significant antitumor effect. This was hypothesized to be secondary to NK cell recognition of "self" MHC molecules of autologous cells thereby resulting in suppressive NKcell function [22].

To overcome suppression of autologous NK cells, several groups have evaluated adoptive immunotherapy utilizing donor derived allogeneic NK cells [23-26]. The importance of NK cells in alloHSCT can be characterized by their role in mediating immune reconstitution, GVHD, disease relapse, and infection control [27]. As such, the importance of NK cells is underscored by the fact that they are the first lymphoid cells to appear in peripheral blood after alloHSCT engraftment [9, 28, 29]. One of the critical features of NK cell cytotoxic activity is dependent on the interaction and recognition of self-HLA molecules, thereby "educating" or "licensing" the NK cell [7, 30]. Licensed NK cells are defined as having an inhibitory KIR (iKIR) for self HLA class I ligands [7]. These "licensed" NK cells become activated upon recognition of the paucity of self-HLA expression, as observed in tumor cells or virally infected cells [31]. Various murine models, human *in vitro* studies, and clinical trials have studied the impact of NK alloreactivity of such "educated cells" and the impact of ligand matching on GvL, GVHD and allo-tolerance [23, 24, 32-36].

The "missing-self" hypothesis was first proposed by Ljunggren and Karre in 1985 based on the observation that tumor cells with absent MHC class I molecules are susceptible to killing by NK cells (Figure 3b) [7, 31]. In the setting of alloHSCT, donor NK cells can be activated by "sensing" the absence of HLA class I ligands in the recipient that would interact with the donor iKIR [37]. Thus, engrafted stem cells are activated by the "missing self" on recipient targets leading to donor versus recipient alloreactivity (Figure 3b) [7, 32]. In the absence of HLA class I ligand interaction with recipient leukemic cells, NK cell cytotoxicity is activated against the tumor cells (Figure 3c) [7].

Emerging data demonstrates that the interactions between KIR and HLA can play an important role on the clinical outcomes of alloHSCT. Given that the location of the KIR locus is on chromosome 19q13.4 whereas the HLA locus is located on chromosome 6p21.3, chromosomal segregation occurs independently [14, 38]. Thus, donor recipient pairs can be KIR-ligand mismatched even in HLA matched allogeneic transplants. KIR-ligand mismatches in the graft versus host direction may occur when the recipient lacks one or more major KIR ligands [39]. Several NK cell alloreactivity models with varying efficacy have been proposed to predict post-alloHSCT outcomes. These models include the ligand-ligand model, receptor-ligand model, and KIR gene-gene model (Figure 4) and are described in the following sections [37]. Selecting a HSC (hematopoietic stem cell) donor based on KIR genotyping is currently under investigation and no guidelines have been established yet.

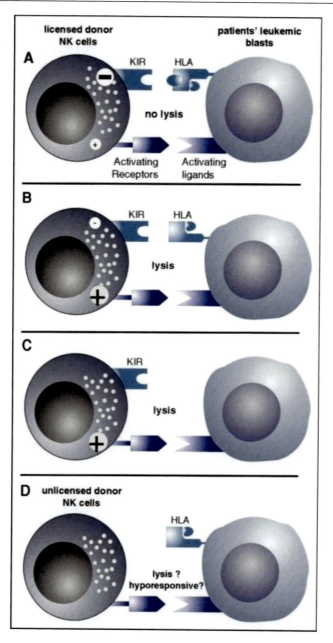

(A) Licensed donor NK cells (i.e., NK cells that have iKIRs for self–HLA class I) are inhibited via engagement of the iKIR by the recipients' ligands (HLA class I), which exert a strong inhibitory signal; thus, these donor NK cells cannot lyse recipients' leukemic blasts (NK cell non-alloreactivity). (B) iKIRs of licensed NK cells are not engaged by the KIRLs, and the donor NK cells are activated and lyse recipients' leukemic blasts (NK cell alloreactivity). (C) Recipients' blasts lack HLA class I expression and, therefore, cannot inhibit donor NK cells, resulting in activation of donor NK cells. (D) NK cells do not express KIRs and, therefore, have not been licensed. KIR-negative NK cells are one of the earliest lymphocyte populations that reconstitute after T cell–depleted HSCT. These NK cells are hyporesponsive but might become responsive upon cytokine stimulation.

Figure 3. NK cell Alloreactivity [7].

3.1. The KIR Ligand Incompatibility Model

The KIR ligand incompatibility model, also known as the "ligand-ligand" model was first suggested by the Perugia group, and predicts NK cell alloreactivity in the GVHD direction when the recipient lacks expression of an iKIR ligand (Figure 4a) [23, 24, 36, 37]. This seminal study demonstrated the first clinical evidence of the efficacy of adoptive immunotherapy via NK alloreactivity [23, 24]. Utilizing HLA-mismatched haploidentical donors, Ruggeri and colleagues evaluated ninety two patients with high risk leukemia; 57 with acute myeloid leukemia (AML) and 35 with acute lymphoblastic leukemia (ALL) using T- cell depleted graft to further investigate the role of NK cell alloreactivity based on the principles described by the "missing-self" hypothesis [23, 24, 40]. To predict NK cell alloreactivity after alloHSCT, high resolution HLA typing of the donor and recipient pair was utilized to describe KIR-KIR Ligand (KIRL) mismatch. KIR incompatibility was defined as the absence of one donor KIR ligand class I allele in the recipient. Patients received a conditioning regimen which included total body irradiation, thiotepa, fludarabine and anti-thymocyte globulin (ATG) and no additional GVHD prophylaxis [23, 24]. Patients were stratified based on KIR phenotypes expressing recognition of HLA-C alleles; the first with KIR ligand incompatibility in the GvHdirection (donor-versus-recipient NK cell alloreactivity), and the second without it [24]. In the presence of alloreactive NK cells in prior studies, this group demonstrated disease control by eradication of leukemia cells *in vivo* that resulted in marked improvement of survival in AML patients, with 65% event-free survival (EFS) at five years in KIR ligand mismatched cohort compared to 5% in non-alloreactive group. These results were particularly notable given advanced stage disease (3rd complete remission or relapse) with 85% of patients with KIR-ligand incompatibility (KIRL) [24]. Furthermore, none of the patients with KIR mismatch experienced graft rejection or GVHD [23, 24]. In a multivariate analysis, KIR ligand incompatibility was the only predictor of survival in AML. While substantial survival benefit was seen in patients with AML, KIR incompatibility did not benefit patients with ALL suggesting the role of NK cells may be disease specific and requiring further evaluation [24].

To determine if improved survival with KIRL incompatibility as demonstrated in haploidentical transplants was applicable for other donor types, Giebel and colleagues subsequently evaluated NK alloreactivity using unmanipulated, unrelated donor HSCs [38]. One hundred and thirty patients with hematologic malignancies had high resolution HLA typing and were stratified by KIRL compatibility (n=20) and incompatibility (n=100) [38]. With a follow up period of 4.5 years, those with KIRL incompatibility had a higher probability of overall survival(OS) (87% vs. 48%, P = 0.006), and disease free survival (87% vs. 39%, P=0.0007) in comparison to KIRL compatible group, respectively [38] Results of a prospective multicenter trial using unrelated donors were unable to replicate these findings as the two year survival and leukemia free survival did not differ based on KIRL mismatch [41]. Variations in patient population between the studies may have in part contributed to the different outcomes.

3.2. The Receptor-Ligand Model

The "receptor-ligand" model defines alloreactivity as the presence of at least one iKIR with the absence of the corresponding KIR ligand in the recipient's HLA repertoire (figure 4b) [7, 37, 42]. Leung et al. evaluated the impact of receptor-ligand modeling in thirty six pediatric patients with myeloid and lymphoid hematologic malignancies who underwent a haploidentical HSCT [42]. The recipient's KIR repertoire was derived from highly purified, HLA disparate CD^{34+} cells [42]. Thirteen patients were classified as having high risk disease based on having KIR ligands for all KIRs in the donor repertoire. In multivariate analysis, the receptor-ligand model remained the only significant prognostic factor (p<0.042) after accounting for factors such as age, disease, and remission status [42]. The accuracy of this model has been noted when applied in T cell depleted HLA-identical sibling HSCT and unrelated donor HSCT [43, 44]. Unlike the ligand-ligand model, the receptor-ligand model has also been accurately used as a prognostic tool in both myeloid and lymphoid malignancies [42].

3.3. The Gene-Gene Model

Although less commonly used, the "gene-gene" model relies on mismatched gene content between the donor and the recipient (Figure 4d) [7, 37]. This method requires KIR genotyping of both donor and recipient, and evaluates the differences in the expression of either inhibitory or activating receptors between the donor and the recipient. Using this method, Symons and colleague evaluated KIR genes using polymerase chain reaction (PCR) of eighty six patients with poor risk hematologic malignancies [37]. They observed that 30 patients had KIR haplotype mismatches while the other 55 donor-recipient pairs had a compatible KIR haplotype. Using the KIR "gene-gene" model, the donor-recipient pairs with mismatched inhibitory KIR genes had improved OS, EFS and lower rates of relapse in T-cell replete haploidentical HSCT [37]. The selection of donors based on KIR gene content, such as haplotype B, is currently being investigated in a clinical trial from the University of Minnesota (Clinicaltrials.gov NCT01288222). In this prospective trial, the role of the donor KIR genotype on outcomes will be evaluated in patients with AML undergoing match unrelated transplant (MUD).

NK Cell Biology and the Role of NK Cells in Hematopoietic Stem Cell ...

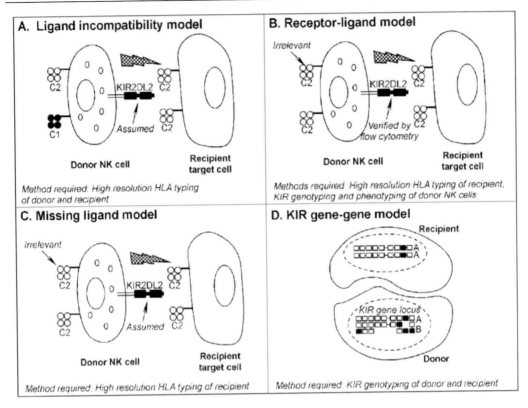

"Models of natural killer cell alloreactivity after allogeneic cell transplantation. A) The KIR ligand incompatibility, or ligand-ligand model predicts NK cell alloreactivity in the GVH direction (depicted by jagged arrow) when the recipient lacks expression of an inhibitory KIR ligand, in this case a member of the HLA-C1 group, that is present in the donor. This model assumes the presence of functional donor NK cells expressing KIR2DL2, the receptor for HLA-C1 molecules, as their inhibitory receptor. B) The receptor-ligand model predicts NK cell alloreactivity in the GVH direction when the recipient lacks the expression of an HLA ligand for a verified donor inhibitory KIR. The HLA type of donor cells is not considered in this model. C) The missing ligand model predicts NK cell alloreactivity in the GVH direction when recipient cells lacks expression of at least one of the HLA ligands (C1, C2, or –Bw4) for a verified donor inhibitory KIR. As in B., the HLA type of the donor is not considered in this model. D) The KIR gene-gene model predicts NK alloreactivity when the donor and recipient are mismatched for KIR gene content. This model characterizes the KIR genotype of both donor and recipient and asks whether differences in the expression of individual inhibitory or stimulatory genes between the donor and the recipient KIR (i.e., donor includes inhibitory KIR genes that the recipient is missing or vice versa) have any effect on the outcome of allogeneic SCT. Inhibitory KIR genes are shown here as unshaded boxes, whereas black boxes represent activating KIR genes. In the example shown, the donor has several activating and inhibitory genes that the recipient lacks. This example also illustrates the KIR haplotype characterization. In this case, the donor is haplotype group B, based on the presence of several activating KIR genes, while the recipient is haplotype group A based on the presence of inhibitory genes and only one activating gene" [37].

Figure 4. Models of NK cell alloreactivity following alloHSCT [37].

4. THE ROLE OF NK CELLS IN HEMATOPOIETIC STEM CELL TRANSPLANTATION

4.1. The Role of NK Cells in Match Related Donor Transplants

Survival outcomes of alloHSCT depend on numerous factors including underlying disease, transplant chemotherapy conditioning regimen, HLA match between the donor and the recipient, presence or absence of GVHD development, and infectious complications [43]. More recently, the role of donor derived alloreactive NK cells has also been recognized as an important consideration when considering disease free survival (DFS) after alloHSCT [24]. Earlier studies highlighting the importance of KIR ligand incompatibility in haploidentical transplants, demonstrate reduction of GVHD and disease-free survival in patients with myeloid malignancies [24, 36, 38]. Since HLA genes segregate independently from KIR genes, NK alloreactivity may still occur in the setting of alloHSCT using an HLA identical sibling. In a single institution study by Hsu and colleagues, 178 patients with AML, ALL, chronic myelogenous leukemia (CML), or myelodysplastic syndrome (MDS) receiving T-cell-depleted HSCT from HLA-identical siblings were evaluated for the impact of donor KIR genotyping on survival [43]. While there was no benefit seen in CML or ALL patients, those with AML and MDS had improved DFS and OS if they lacked HLA ligand for the donor KIR [43]. Additionally, AML and MDS patients lacking 2 HLA ligands (HLA-B and –C) for donor-inhibitory KIR, resulting in increased NK activation, had the greatest DFS and OS benefit [43]. Verheyden et al. further evaluated the potential impact of donor KIR genotypeon GvL effect in HLA-identical HSCT in AML, CML, and ALL using a myeloablative regimen [45]. Similar to the analysis by Hsu et al. the impact of donor KIR genotyping was most pronounced in the subset of AML patients. In these patients, the combined presence of activating donor KIRs, 2DS1 & 2DS2, had significant decreased relapse rates with 5-year relapse of patients with donor 2DS1(+)2DS2(+) genotype found to be 17% in comparison to patients without this donor genotype demonstrating nearly 4-fold increase in leukemia relapse rate [45].

Despite the beneficial effect demonstrated by the above mentioned studies, NK alloreactivity remains a complex issue. Several studies have reported a deleterious outcome in relation to iKIRLs T-cell-replete donor grafts, in direct contrast to outcomes in T-cell depleted grafts [26]. In a large single center retrospective analysis by Sun and colleagues, 378 patients with ALL, AML, MDS and CML who underwent HLA mismatched alloHSCT were subdivided into three cohorts based on KIR genotyping [26]. Group 1 were HLA class 1 antigen and iKIR matched, Group 2 included HLA class 1 antigen mismatches, and Group 3 included HLA class 1 antigen and iKIR mismatches [26]. Transplant related factors were evenly distributed amongst the three groups including diagnosis, disease status at time of transplantation, and conditioning intensity. One-year OS was 59%, 49% and 30% amongst group 1, group 2, and group 3, respectively [26]. Furthermore, relapse rates were highest among patients who were mismatched at both HLA class 1 antigens as well iKIRs. The authors postulated that one potential reason to explain the differences between studies is likely related to definitions of mismatching, as Sun et al. used the presence of iKIR ligand in the corresponding KIR gene to define mismatches as opposed to HLA typing [24, 38].

4.2. The Role of NK Cells in Match Unrelated Donor Transplants

While the role of donor and recipient HLA matching on morbidity and mortality in unrelated donor transplants is well established, the impact of KIR ligand mismatching and degree of disparate loci in matched unrelated donors (MUDs) remains an active area of research. The KIR study group sought to evaluate the complex issue of KIR ligand mismatching in unrelated donor transplants using large registry datasets from the National Marrow Donor Program, the European Bone Marrow Transplant, and Dutch registries [46]. The study population included 1571 MUD recipients with a diagnosis of AML, MDS or CML using amyeloablative conditioning regimen followed by bone marrow graft [46]. KIR ligand mismatches in donor-recipient pairs were defined by HLA typing of HLA-B and/or -C. In contrast to the studies in haploidentical transplants, there were no statistically significant differences in GVHD, non-relapse mortality, or incidence of relapse[46]. While these results are consistent with other groups that have demonstrated lack of benefit in KIR ligand mismatching, one limitation of this analysis includes a lack of KIR genotyping. Rather, HLA typing was used to determine KIR ligand incompatibility based on previous studies by the Perugia group [46]. Furthermore, KIR ligand incompatibility affect may be masked by the effect of T-cell alloreactivity and post-transplant immunosuppression.

While the majority of analyses have focused on inhibitory KIRs, little was known about the effect of activating KIR genes in the match unrelated setting. Using 1700 patients with AML (75%) or ALL (25%) who received a match unrelated alloHSCT, the Center for International Blood and Marrow Transplant Research group designed a retrospective study to evaluate this issue [47]. Using the gene-gene model, patients whose donors were homozygous or heterozygous for HLA-C1 antigens (KIR2DS1 positive allografts) had lower relapse rates than recipients of KIR2S1 negative allografts [47]. This study highlighted the importance of KIR haplotypes and activating genes in determining clinical outcomes in alloHSCT.

The conflicting data between various studies is multifactorial due to differences in degree of T-cell depletion in the graft, differences in immunosuppressive regiments for GVHD prophylaxis, methods of determining KIR ligand incompatibility, and underlying malignancies. The key factor appears to the balance between T cell and NK cell reactivity. In minimally T-cell depleted grafts, T-cell alloreactivity dominates over NK cell alloreactivity and impairs their function *in vivo* [10]. In the majority of the studies, the beneficial role of NK cell alloreactivity was only observed in adult patients with AML, suggesting that myeloid blasts may have increased sensitivity to NK mediated cytotoxicity.

Table 1. Studies evaluating the role of KIR ligand mismatch in match unrelated transplants

Study	Giebel [38]	Bornhauser [48]	Schaffer [49]	Farag [46]	Miller [22]
No. of patients	130	118	190	1571	2062
Disease	ALL, AML, MDS, CML, NHL, HL, MM	AML, CML, MDS	ALL, AML, CML, MDS, NHL, HL, MM	AML, MDS, CML	AML, CML, MDS
TCD	ATG (100%)	TCD (20) + ATG (100)	TCD (17) + ATG (100)	20	
Relapse (p)	NS	Higher in KIR-ligand mismatch (0.02)	NS	Higher in KIR- ligand mismatch (0.04)	Lower in KIR-ligand mismatches (only myeloid early disease)
OS (p)	Higher in KIR ligand mismatch (0.006)	NS	Lower in KIR-ligand mismatch (0.01)	Lower in KIR-ligand mismatch (<0.001)	NS

ATG, anti-thymocyte globulin; CML, chronic myeloid leukemia; HL, Hodgkin lymphoma; MDS, myelodysplastic syndrome; MM, multiple myeloma; NHL, non-Hodgkin lymphoma; NS, nonsignificant; TCD, T-cell depletion. (Table adapted from Mehta et al.) [9].

4.3. The Role of NK Cells in Haploidentical Transplants

The role of NK cells in haploidentical transplants was pioneered by the Perugia group as discussed earlier in this chapter [23, 24, 36]. A follow up study published in 2007 included the 57 patients with AML whose outcomes were reported in the seminal 2002 study, in addition to 52 patients who received a transplant after the original publication [36]. All patients evaluated received a myeloablative T cell depleted haploidentical transplant [36]. Alloreactions in the graft versus host direction were identified in 51 patients [36]. In contrast to the initial study, transplantation from alloreactive NK cells did not significantly reduce graft rejection or incidence of GVHD. Despite no increased protection from GVHD, there was a marked improvement in EFS in patients who had alloreactions in the GVHD direction (67% vs. 18%, P=0.02) irrespective of whichever of the 3 KIR ligand were mismatched [36]. Furthermore, there was a 52% reduction in the risk of relapse or death in the mismatched group compared to the group of patients who were KIR-ligand matched (P <0.001) [36]. This survival advantage is mediated by a marked GVL effect in which alloreactive NK cells kill recipient leukemic cells [36]. It is notable that these studies from the Perugia group used intensive myeloablative regimens without post-transplant GVHD prophylaxis [36]. The absence of post-transplant immunosuppression is thought to provide a favorable environment for NK cell expansion and alloreactions leading to improved survival in this setting.

To further evaluate the role of NK cells of non-myeloablative haploidentical HSCT outcomes, Symons et al. retrospectively studied 86 patients with high-risk hematologic malignancies who were transplanted between 1999 and 2007 [37]. This study differs from the Perugia group in that all patients had a non-myeloablative conditioning regimen, which included post-transplant cyclophosphamide. No significant difference in cumulative incidence of GVHD or engraftment among patients with inhibitory KIR gene mismatches and those with identical iKIR gene content were noted [37]. However, there was a significantly improved OS (HR=0.37; CI: 0.21-0.63; p=0.0003) and EFS (HR=0.51; CI: 0.31-0.84; p=0.01) in patients who were mismatched when compared to those patient-donor pairs with identical iKIR gene content [37]. Unlike previously described studies that only showed a benefit in myeloid malignancies, this study showed favorable outcomes in both myeloid and lymphoid malignancies. Since T-cell depleted transplants offer a favorable environment for NK cell expansion, it is hypothesized that the elimination of host reactive T cells by post-transplant cyclophosphamide unmasked the benefit of the NK cell alloreactivity [37].

While the role of inhibitory KIRs has been extensively studied in both *in vitro* and clinical studies, the role of activating KIRs and their ligands is less understood. The only well-established interaction is between KIR2DS1 and the HLA-C2 ligand [9]. While all populations have both group A and B KIR haplotypes, their frequency varies depending on ethnic group. As discussed previously, the group B KIR haplotype contains combinations of activating and while the group A haplotype contains 5 inhibitory genes and a single activating gene KIR2DS4 [50]. Oeverman and coworkers studied the outcomes of 85 pediatric patients who received a T-cell depleted haploidentical HSCT for ALL [51]. The majority (74%) had a KIR haplotype B which is consistent with previous reports in the Caucasian population (www.allelefrequencies.net). Incidence of relapse was significantly reduced among patients who had a KIR haplotype B donor rather than a KIR haplotype A (33% vs. 64%) [51]. The five-year EFS of patients transplanted from KIR haplotype B or KIR haplotype A donor was 50.6% vs. 29.5% respectively (P=0.033) [51]. While this study was limited by a small number of patients, it highlights the potential importance of identifying KIR haplotypes in the haploidentical setting. It is also noteworthy that this study only included patients with ALL as prior studied adult alloHCT studies overwhelmingly reported impact in myeloid malignancies. Activating KIR ligand expression may be varied in pediatric versus adult ALL blasts in their susceptibility to lysis by activating haplotype B donor NK cells [52].

The role of donor activating KIR genotypes in haploidentical T-cell depleted HSCT was also studied in an adult population of 161 patients with acute leukemias (121 with AML and 40 with ALL) [35]. Sixty nine patients received transplants from NK alloreactive donors and did not receive subsequent GVHD prophylaxis. In consensus with previous studies by the same group, multivariate analysis showed that donor-vs-recipient NK cell alloreactivity was associated with reduced relapse and improved EFS in patients with AML (HR 0.60; 95% CI, 0.37-0.96, P= 0.034) [35]. In the subset of patients with NK cell alloreactivity, transplantation from B haplotype donors who possess KIR2DS1 and/or KIR3DS1 activating genes was an independent factor predicting lower NRM (nonreplapse mortality), improved EFS, and lower infectious mortality [35]. There were no differences in GVHD or relapse rates. Since the majority of NRM was accounted for by infectious mortality, it appears that transplantation from NK-alloreactivity donors who possess activating genes may improve EFS by potentially reducing infectious mortality. *In vitro* analysis by the same group found that KIR2DS1 triggered NK cells to release IFN-γ which has known antiviral effects and enhances antigen-presenting cell functions [35]. The above data highlights the promise of donor selection based on KIR ligand matching for allogeneic transplant recipients.

4.4. The Role of NK Cells in Cord Blood Transplants

In those patients from whom a suitably matched hematopoietic stem cell donor is unavailable, umbilical cord blood (UCB) is a potential alternative in the of treatment patients with hematologic malignancies [53, 54]. The major advantages of HLA-mismatched transplantation using UCB include rapid availability of the donor product and decreased risk of developing severe GVHD [55]. Several studies have evaluated the role of NK alloreactivity using UCB given the paucity of T-cells within the UCB graft and potential NK ligand mismatches between the two UCB units to compose a complete graft in adult patients [55-58]. As noted above, the majority of donor-recipient pairs are HLA-mismatched either at the antigen level (low resolution HLA-A and –B) or at the allelic level (HLA-DRB1), with HLA-C not routinely considered for matching. These studies have had conflicting and varying results with some studies demonstrating beneficial survival results with KIR-mismatched and others showing none to negative impact [56-60].

One of the first reports of the positive clinical impact of KIR-ligand mismatching in single unit UCB transplant (UCBT) was demonstrated by the Eurocord group, in concordance with findings of the Perugia group in related haploidentical transplants. In the retrospective registry analysis, 218 patients in remission from acute leukemia (AML n=94, ALL n=124) received a single unit UCBT after receiving a myeloablative regimen [58]. KIR-ligand mismatch between the patient and the cord blood unit (CBU) was associated with improved 2-year leukemia-free survival (LFS) (55% vs. 31%, $P= 0.005$) and OS (57% vs. 40%, $P= 0.02$) in comparison to KIR-ligand matched, respectively [58]. In multivariate analysis, KIR-ligand incompatibility was found to be an independent predictive factor on improved LFS and OS [58].

Contrary to the positive outcomes noted by the Eurocord group, the detrimental impact of KIR-ligand mismatching in UCBT patients who received reduced intensity conditioning has been also been reported. Patients with KIR-ligand mismatch between the CBU and the transplant recipient who received one of several reduced intensity transplant preparatory regimens were reported to have higher rates of grade III-IV acute GVHD (42% vs. 13%, P <0.01), increased NRM (27 vs 12%, $P=0.03$) and inferior survival (32% vs. 52%, P =0.03) [61]. In patients who received a myeloablative regimen (n=155), there was no significant difference on NRM, OS, relapse, and incidence of acute and chronic GVHD based on KIR-ligand mismatching versus matching status [61].

The largest series evaluating the effect of KIR-ligand matching on outcomes after UCBT used registry data obtained from both the Center for International Blood and Marrow Transplant Research and the European Group for Blood and Marrow Transplantation. Rocha et al. studied 461 patients with AML from whom transplant was performed between 2000-2010 and received a single UCB unit after conditioning chemotherapy with a myeloablative regimen [56]. In contrast to prior studies, high resolution donor and recipient HLA typing was completed using molecular techniques [56]. KIR-ligand matching and mismatching was based on donor and recipient KIR-ligand expression for HLA C group 1, 2, or Bw4. For patients with 6-/8 HLA matched transplants, KIR ligand matching status was not associated with overall mortality, NRM, or rates of acute or chronic GVHD [56]. This study differed from an earlier Eurocord report in which there was significant leukemia-free and OS benefit for AML patients with KIR-ligand mismatch [57]. The prior Eurocord study was conducted using low resolution HLA-matching typing between recipient and the UCB unit in comparison to the subsequent analysis. Additionally, Rocha and colleagues analyzed transplants mismatched at 1 to2 HLA loci separately to those with >3 HLA mismatches to control for confounding effect of HLA disparity [56, 57].

In summary, current studies evaluating the role of NK cells show that UCBT are limited to retrospective data with heterogeneous patient populations, conditioning regimens, and usage of single and double UCB units. The studies also differ in the methods in which KIR-Ligand mismatches are determined and the role of activating

KIRs was not considered. Additionally, variances in matching definitions for HLA-A, -B, -C, and –DRB1 and typing resolution including both low and high resolution typing are notable amongst the studies. At this time, while large series data suggest KIR-ligand matching does not impact survival outcomes in this setting, the effect of KIR-ligand mismatching in the UCBT setting remains controversial and further studies are needed to elucidate predictive NK-cell alloreactivity models.

5. THE ROLE NK CELLS IN GVHD PATHOGENESIS

The role of NK cells in GVHD induction or exacerbation remains controversial. The well-established model of GVHD pathogenesis includes activation of donor-derived T cells with evidence from murine and human models showing both promotion and prevention of this post-HSCT complication by NK cells [6, 62]. The association of NK cells in GVHD was first reported in 1979 by investigators at Memorial Sloan Kettering Cancer Center [63]. This group documented the association between pre-transplant levels of NK cell activity and the development of GVHD in a pilot cohort of thirteen patients undergoing myeloablative allo HSCT [63]. This seminal report opened the field for further evaluation of the relationship between NK cells and pathogenesis of GVHD. Early studies focused on the presence of NK cells in GVHD target organs such as the skin in both murine and human models [64-66]. To confirm the donor origins of the NK cells in patients manifesting with cutaneous acute GVHD, Horn and Haskel studied 35 skin biopsies of women transplanted with bone marrow grafts from male donors [67]. They noted that patients with grade 1 cutaneous GVHD had minimal infiltration of Y chromosome containing cells identified in the dermis. However, for those specimens with features of grade 2 GVHD, the majority of lymphocytes were donor-derived Y chromosome containing cells with increased relative infiltration of NK cells confirming the presence of donor NK cells during evidence of acute GVHD in target organs [67].

Several murine models were developed to evaluate the relationship between NK cells and the development of GVHD, given NK cell infiltration in GVHD target organs [68, 69-71]. Experiments using NK cell depleting antibodies directed against either the cell surface glycolipid asialo GM1 or cell surface NKR-P1receptor in murine minor mismatch models had inconsistent reduction of GVHD and failed to clarify the impact of NK cell on GVHD [68, 69-71]. Discrepancies in these studies were hypothesized to be due to the presence of activated T-cells which expressed epitopes recognized by the anti-asialo GM1 and NKR-P1 receptor NK1.1, making it difficult to distinguish the impact of one cell line versus the other [62, 72]. Ghayur and colleagues employed a new approach using a murine model containing beige mice that carried a homozygous mutation resulting in severe NK cell deficiency. In this model, adoptive transfer of heterozygous mutant splenocytes induced hepatic GVHD, while transfer of homozygous mutant splenocytes (i.e., NK cell deficient) did not induce GVHD [70]. While encouraging, deficit in adaptive T cells remained a confounding feature in determining GVHD pathogenesis in these studies [73, 74].

While early observations suggested that NK cells mediate GVHD, subsequent studies using adoptive transfer of NK cells painted a different picture. Murphy and colleagues examined the adoptive transfer of NK cells from purified severe combined immunodeficiency (SCID) mice into lethally irradiated mice along with T-cell-replete bone marrow graft [75]. Surprisingly, despite the transfer of mismatched NK cells, there were no observations of GVHD induction similar to human haploidentical models [75]. Similar results were confirmed by several other groups including the Peguria group in which adoptive transfer of alloreactive Ly49 ligand mismatched NK cells in a mismatched murine model prevented the development of GVHD [24]. The mechanism by which GVHD was prevented was thought to be secondary to inhibition of T-cell proliferation. It is well established that donor T cell activation, proliferation, and differentiation play an important role in the pathophysiology of acute GVHD [6]. Decrease in T-cell activity as a consequence of antigen presenting cell (APC) depletion by the alloreactive NK cells is thought to mitigate induction of GVHD [24, 76]. Furthermore, in alloreactive NK cell responses, the activating ligand KIR2DS1 has been observed to play an important role in reducing GVHD and promoting engraftment by contributing to APCs' killing of dendritic cells and T-cells blasts [77].

In addition to depleting APCs, NK cells have the ability to directly kill activated T-cells and thereby suppress the development of GVHD [78]. Upregulation of the activating receptor NKG2D during T-cell activation *in vitro* renders these cells susceptible to lysis by NK cell [78]. This finding has been corroborated by Olson and colleagues using an *in vivo* major mismatch HSCT model and demonstrating NKG2D mediated NK cell lysis among animals treated with allogeneic NK cells [79]. Notably, an increase in the ratio of regulatory T cells was also found, which has been previously demonstrated to reduce GVHD [79, 80].

Most clinical studies do not observe an increased incidence of GVHD when using adoptive NK cellular therapy; however a recent study by Shah and colleagues reports the potential role of NK cell cytokine production on the development of acute GVHD [81]. In a phase I dose escalation trial, nine pediatric patients with high risk solid tumors were infused with donor derived IL-15/4-1BBL-activated NK cells, following T-cell depleted, HLA-matched alloHSCT [81]. Five of the nine recipients developed acute GVHD with severe grade 4 disease reported in three of the patients [81]. Given the limited population reported, no overt clinically relevant factors were identified as contributing to the clinical manifestation of GVHD. While NK cells can enhance clinically undetectable T cells by producing cytokines such as IFN-γ and TNF-α, it is unclear if this mechanism contributed to the development of GVHD [62]. The role of NK cell cytokine productive on the development of GVHD has been demonstrated in a xenogeneic model with detectable production of both IFN-γ and TNF-α in IL-2 activated human NK cells. Irradiated, severe combined immunodeficiency (SCID) mice infused with these activated NK cells subsequently went on to develop findings suggestive of acute GVHD [82]. Increased NK cell IFN-γ production has been correlated with increased GVHD, but the exact mechanism has not been fully elucidated [83].

These observations led to further investigation into the relationship between regeneration of mature NK cells and the development of acute GVHD following alloHSCT [84]. In a single center study, blood samples were collected from 107 patients prior to and following alloHSCT at regular intervals up to 200 days after transplant [84]. An inverse correlation between the development and severity of acute GVHD and the early expansion of the immature NK cell subset expressing CD56^{bright} was identified [84]. Patients who did not develop acute GVHD had a higher number of NK cells, specifically the CD56^{bright} subset, than patients who developed acute GVHD [84]. Furthermore, there was a significant correlation between the degree of acute GVHD and the disturbance of the CD56^{bright} NK subset, which suggests a negative impact of acute GVHD on NK cell maturation [84]. Bunting and colleagues recently demonstrated that acute GVHD prevents NK cell maturation following alloHSCT through competition for IL-15 by donor T cells [85]. These alterations in NK cell reconstitution resulted in defective *in vivo* cytotoxicity with subsequent reduction in the GvL effect [62, 85]. However, it remains unclear if the reduced number of CD56^{bright} NK cells is a consequence or a cause of acute GVHD.

While our understanding of the role of NK cells in HSCT has improved, the complex role of NK cells in mediating or protecting against GVHD remains elusive. Early observational studies and mouse models suggested that NK cells can induce an exacerbation of GVHD. However, subsequent studies in humans revealed that NK cells can promote GvL while protecting against GVHD. Nonetheless, more recent data has challenged the concept and showed that NK cells can promote GVHD in some cases. Further research is needed to clarify the impact of the pleiotropic NK cells on GVHD induction so that the role of adoptive NK cells can be maximized in the treatment of hematologic malignancies.

6. THE USE OF ADOPTIVE NK CELLS IN THE TREATMENT OF HEMATOLOGIC MALIGNANCIES

6.1. Chimeric Antigen Receptor-Modified NK cells

Chimeric antigen receptors (CARs) are genetically modified constructs of engineered receptors typically composed of a binding domain such as a specific monoclonal antibody or receptor that binds to tumor antigen target, linked to an intracellular signaling domain [1, 9]. Genes that encode for these receptors are inserted most commonly into recipient T-cells to generate autologous tumor-specific reactive T-cells that are infused back into patients. CAR-T cells have been extensively investigated using constructs predominantly targeting CD19+ B cells for lymphoid malignancies demonstrating their efficacy with favorable clinical outcomes [1]. Since the development of CD19+CAR T-cells, there have been efforts to develop additional CAR-T cell against surface antigen targets found on many malignancies [86]. One of the main challenges is the expression of target antigens on healthy tissues, thereby increasing potential risk of off-target/off-cancer toxicity by CAR-T cells. NK cells are an attractive cell lineage for development CAR-based therapy and offer an alternative source of cellular immunotherapy that mediates direct cytotoxicity against various types of solid and hematological malignancies, facilitates activation of macrophages and myeloid cells within the tumormicro-environment, and harbors an anti-cancer memory response for long-term surveillance [87-89]. Thus, CAR-engineered NK cells can be a complementary treatment option to CAR-T cells.

One of the potential barriers related to the infusion of activated T cells when considering an allogeneic source is the likelihood and increased risk of developing GVHD. Given prior results on treatment using haploidentical NK cells outlined earlier in this chapter, the risk of GVHD, when using T-cell deplete NK cells, can potentially be minimized [33, 90]. As such, the feasibility and safety of adoptive NK cell therapies has already been demonstrated in numerous phase I/II trials in the non-transplant and the post-transplantation settings [25, 91].

In comparison to CAR-T cells, experience with engineered CAR-NK cells remains limited. Despite encouraging preclinical studies, clinical data on the safety and efficacy of CAR modified NK cells continues to be an area of active research and is currently being investigated in clinical trials. In addition to the large number of clinical trials utilizing CAR T cells for treatment, several studies evaluating the efficacy of CAR-NK cells are also now available for patient accrual. As noted above, the ability to specifically redirect NK cells towards CD19+ presents a novel strategy against aggressive leukemias such as B-cell acute lymphoblastic leukemia (ALL). This concept is being evaluated in two clinical trials (Clinicaltrials.gov NCT00995137 and NCT01974479) using haploidentical retrovirally transduced anti CD19-BB-ζ CAR. In the study led by the St. Jude Children's Research Hospital (clinialtrials.gov NCT00995137), donor NK cells are expanded by co-culture with irradiated K562 cell line modified to express membrane bound IL-15 and 41BB ligand, and then transduced with a signaling receptor that binds to CD19. In 2014, this study completed enrollment of eligible children with relapsed/refractory ALL who were otherwise not candidates for HSCT and final results are currently pending. Another study sponsored by the National University Health System in Singapore is currently recruiting both pediatric and adult patients to a phase II trial that uses the same construct as the St. Jude trial in patients with persistent residual disease who have been treated for ALL (clinialtrials.gov NCT01974479).

In an effort to expand target-antigen recognition beyond B-cell malignancies expressing CD19, several alternative approaches for CAR-modified NK cells have been developed including targeting of NKG2D ligands [92]. NKG2D is a key receptor for NK cell activation which is expressed on NK cells as well as tumor cell surface of a variety of malignancies. Development of a NKG2D-DAP10-CD3ζ receptor, composed of the extracellular domain of NKG2D for recognition of NKG2D ligand on tumor surfaces in addition 2 key signaling molecules, DAP10 and CD3ζ results in enhanced cytotoxicity against leukemia and solid tumor cell lines, particularly in the presence of increased NKG2D surface expression [92]. The safety of the CAR using human NKG2D was first evaluated in a phase I dose-escalation trial by Nikiforow et al. in patients with AML/MDS-refractory anemia with excess blasts or relapsed/refractory multiple myeloma (MM) for whom standard conventional treatment options were not available (clinicaltrials.gov NCT02203825) [93]. Eleven patients were infused with a single dosage of the CAR NK product (CM-CS1) without evidence of infusion reaction. The first 10 patients had no dose-limiting toxicities and no cases of cytokine release syndrome, neurotoxicity, or CAR-T related deaths. While there was no objective tumor response with the initial infusion at 28 days, there were some surprisingly unexpected outcomes in patients with aggressive disease. For example, an AML patient harboring a p53 mutation survived 4 months after infusion despite significant disease burden at time of infusion [93]. While no data is yet available on prior treatment of these patients, this phase I trial established that a single dose of the CAR NK product was safe with warrants further investigation into efficacy.

Based on the safety profile and feasibility demonstrated by the Dana Farber group, NKR-2, the autologous transduced T cells product with chimeric NKG2D receptor construct is currently being evaluated in the "THINK" trial (clinicaltrials.gov NCT030118405), a multinational, open-label phase I dose escalation study. This multiple infusion trial is currently actively recruiting patients to evaluate the safety and clinical activity. While CAR immunotherapy has been encouraging in the treatment of hematologic malignancies, this study will also evaluate the efficacy of NKR-2 in five solid tumors (colorectal cancer, ovarian cancer, urothelial cancer, triple negative breast cancer, and pancreatic cancer) in addition to two hematologic tumors (AML and MM). Primary aims of the study include incidence of treatment specific adverse events of NKR-2 administration and subsequent potential adverse events during study treatment. Secondary aim includes the determination of the efficacy of NK CAR-T in each of the tumor types. Table 2 provides a summary of ongoing clinical trials investigating the use of modified CAR-NK cells.

Table 2. Ongoing clinical trials investigating CAR-NK immunotherapy for the treatment of hematologic malignancies and solid tumors

Trial	Condition	Investigation	Phase
NCT03018405	CRC, Ovarian Cancer, Urothelial Cancer, TNBC, Pancreatic cancer, AML, MDS, MM	NKR-2 cells	I
NCT02203825	AML, MDS, MM	CM-CS1 T-cell infusion	I
NCT03050216	AML	Haploidentical Donor NK Cells Infusion with Subcutaneous ALT-803	II
NCT02944162	AML	anti-CD33 CAR-NK cells	I/II
NCT03056339	B-lymphoid malignancies, ALL, CLL, NHL	19/IL15-Transduced CB NK cells	
NCT02892695	ALL, CLL, Follicular lymphoma, MCL, DLCL, B-cell prolymphocytic leukemia	anti-CD19 CAR-NK cells	I/II
NCT02742727	AML, T-Cell acute Lymphoblastic Leukemia/Lymphoma, T-cell prolymphocytic leukemia, T-cell large granular Lymphocytic leukemia, Peripheral T-cell Lymphoma, Angioimmunoblastic T-cellLymphoma, Extranodal NK /T-cell lymphoma, Enteropathy-type intestinal T-cell lymphoma, Hepatosplenic T-cell lymphoma	anti-CD7CAR-pNK cells	I/II

AML: Acute myeloid leukemia; CRC: colorectal cancer; MCL: mantle cell lymphoma; MM: multiple myeloma; ALL: acute lymphoblastic leukemia/lymphoma; TNBC: triple negative breast cancer.

CONCLUSION

Recent scientific advances have significantly improved our understanding of the role of NK cell as a critical part of the innate immune system that participates in immune-surveillance, transplantation alloreactivity, and tolerance in the alloHSCT setting. While several models exist to define NK cell alloreactivity, the selection of donors based on KIR genotyping is an ongoing focus of several clinical trials in the HCT setting. Additionally, the setting in which KIR matching has the most impact remains an area to be addressed. Similarly, the role of NK cells in GVHD remains controversial and is dependent on several factors such as degree of T cell depletion and mode of NK cell stimulation [7]. Further research is warranted to identify predictive factors of GVHD development in NK cellular therapy to minimize risk of GVHD while maximizing GvL. There is encouraging evidence to support the exploitation of NK cell alloreactivity for patients with hematologic malignancies. Furthermore, the introduction of *ex-vivo* manipulated CAR NK cells in clinical trials as well as other mechanisms of adoptive immunotherapy may lead to future clinical applications with promising results.

REFERENCES

[1] Lee DW, Kochenderfer JN, Stetler-Stevenson M, et al. T cells expressing CD19 chimeric antigen receptors for acute lymphoblastic leukaemia in children and young adults: a phase 1 dose-escalation trial. *Lancet.* 2015;385(9967):517-528.

[2] Maude SL, Frey N, Shaw PA, et al. Chimeric antigen receptor T cells for sustained remissions in leukemia. *N Engl J Med.* 2014;371(16):1507-1517.

[3] Postow MA, Chesney J, Pavlick AC, et al. Nivolumab and ipilimumab versus ipilimumab in untreated melanoma. *N Engl J Med.* 2015;372(21):2006-2017.

[4] Davila ML, Brentjens RJ. CD19-Targeted CAR T cells as novel cancer immunotherapy for relapsed or refractory B-cell acute lymphoblastic leukemia. *Clin Adv Hematol Oncol.* 2016;14(10):802-808.

[5] Little MT, Storb R. History of haematopoietic stem-cell transplantation. *Nat Rev Cancer.* 2002;2(3):231-238.

[6] Ferrara JL, Levine JE, Reddy P, Holler E. Graft-versus-host disease. *Lancet.* 2009;373(9674):1550-1561.

[7] Handgretinger R, Lang P, André MC. Exploitation of natural killer cells for the treatment of acute leukemia. *Blood.* 2016;127(26):3341-3349.

[8] Guillerey C, Huntington ND, Smyth MJ. Targeting natural killer cells in cancer immunotherapy. *Nat Immunol.* 2016;17(9):1025-1036.

[9] Mehta RS, Rezvani K. Can we make a better match or mismatch with KIR genotyping? *Hematology Am Soc Hematol Educ Program.* 2016;2016(1):106-118.

[10] Morvan MG, Lanier LL. NK cells and cancer: you can teach innate cells new tricks. *Nature reviews. Cancer.* 2016;16(1):7-19.

[11] Voskoboinik I, Whisstock JC, Trapani JA. Perforin and granzymes: function, dysfunction and human pathology. *Nature reviews. Immunology.* 2015;15(6):388-400.

[12] Thielens A, Vivier E, Romagné F. NK cell MHC class I specific receptors (KIR): from biology to clinical intervention. *Curr Opin Immunol.* 2012;24(2):239-245.

[13] Marsh SG, Parham P, Dupont B, et al. Killer-cell immunoglobulin-like receptor (KIR) nomenclature report, 2002. *Hum Immunol.* 2003;64(6):648-654.

[14] Bashirova AA, Martin MP, McVicar DW, Carrington M. The killer immunoglobulin-like receptor gene cluster: tuning the genome for defense. *Annu Rev Genomics Hum Genet.* 2006;7:277-300.

[15] Hsu KC, Liu XR, Selvakumar A, Mickelson E, O'Reilly RJ, Dupont B. Killer Ig-like receptor haplotype analysis by gene content: evidence for genomic diversity with a minimum of six basic framework haplotypes, each with multiple subsets. *J Immunol.* 2002;169(9):5118-5129.

[16] Vey N, Bourhis JH, Boissel N, et al. A phase 1 trial of the anti-inhibitory KIR mAb IPH2101 for AML in complete remission. *Blood.* 2012;120(22):4317-4323.

[17] Kohrt HE, Thielens A, Marabelle A, et al. Anti-KIR antibody enhancement of anti-lymphoma activity of natural killer cells as monotherapy and in combination with anti-CD20 antibodies. *Blood.* 2014;123(5):678-686.

[18] Long EO, Kim HS, Liu D, Peterson ME, Rajagopalan S. Controlling natural killer cell responses: integration of signals for activation and inhibition. *Annu Rev Immunol.* 2013;31:227-258.

[19] Rosenberg SA, Lotze MT, Muul LM, et al. Observations on the systemic administration of autologous lymphokine-activated killer cells and recombinant interleukin-2 to patients with metastatic cancer. *N Engl J Med.* 1985;313(23):1485-1492.

[20] Rosenberg SA, Lotze MT, Muul LM, et al. A progress report on the treatment of 157 patients with advanced cancer using lymphokine-activated killer cells and interleukin-2 or high-dose interleukin-2 alone. *N Engl J Med.* 1987;316(15):889-897.

[21] Miller JS, Tessmer-Tuck J, Pierson BA, et al. Low dose subcutaneous interleukin-2 after autologous transplantation generates sustained in vivo natural killer cell activity. *Biol Blood Marrow Transplant.* 1997;3(1):34-44.

[22] Miller JS, Cooley S, Parham P, et al. Missing KIR ligands are associated with less relapse and increased graft-versus-host disease (GVHD) following unrelated donor allogeneic HCT. *Blood.* 2007;109(11):5058-5061.

[23] Ruggeri L, Capanni M, Casucci M, et al. Role of natural killer cell alloreactivity in HLA-mismatched hematopoietic stem cell transplantation. *Blood.* 1999;94(1):333-339.

[24] Ruggeri L, Capanni M, Urbani E, et al. Effectiveness of donor natural killer cell alloreactivity in mismatched hematopoietic transplants. *Science.* 2002;295 (5562):2097-2100.

[25] Miller JS, Soignier Y, Panoskaltsis-Mortari A, et al. Successful adoptive transfer and in vivo expansion of human haploidentical NK cells in patients with cancer. *Blood.* 2005;105(8):3051-3057.

[26] Sun JY, Dagis A, Gaidulis L, et al. Detrimental effect of natural killer cell alloreactivity in T-replete hematopoietic cell transplantation (HCT) for leukemia patients. *Biol Blood Marrow Transplant.* 2007;13(2):197-205.

[27] Farhan S, Lee DA, Champlin RE, Ciurea SO. NK cell therapy: targeting disease relapse after hematopoietic stem cell transplantation. *Immunotherapy.* 2012;4(3):305-313.

[28] Almeida-Oliveira A, Smith-Carvalho M, Porto LC, et al. Age-related changes in natural killer cell receptors from childhood through old age. *Human immunology.* 2011;72(4):319-329.

[29] Small TN, Papadopoulos EB, Boulad F, et al. Comparison of immune reconstitution after unrelated and related T-cell-depleted bone marrow transplantation: effect of patient age and donor leukocyte infusions. *Blood.* 1999;93(2):467-480.

[30] Kim S, Poursine-Laurent J, Truscott SM, et al. Licensing of natural killer cells by host major histocompatibility complex class I molecules. *Nature.* 2005;436(7051):709-713.

[31] Ljunggren HG, Kärre K. In search of the 'missing self': MHC molecules and NK cell recognition. *Immunol Today.* 1990;11(7):237-244.

[32] Haas P, Loiseau P, Tamouza R, et al. NK-cell education is shaped by donor HLA genotype after unrelated allogeneic hematopoietic stem cell transplantation. *Blood.* 2011;117(3):1021-1029.

[33] Curti A, Ruggeri L, D'Addio A, et al. Successful transfer of alloreactive haploidentical KIR ligand-mismatched natural killer cells after infusion in elderly high risk acute myeloid leukemia patients. *Blood.* 2011;118(12):3273-3279.

[34] Eapen M, Rocha V, Sanz G, et al. Effect of graft source on unrelated donor haemopoietic stem-cell transplantation in adults with acute leukaemia: a retrospective analysis. *Lancet Oncol.* 2010;11(7):653-660.

[35] Mancusi A, Ruggeri L, Urbani E, et al. Haploidentical hematopoietic transplantation from KIR ligand-mismatched donors with activating KIRs reduces nonrelapse mortality. *Blood.* 2015;125(20):3173-3182.

[36] Ruggeri L, Mancusi A, Capanni M, et al. Donor natural killer cell allorecognition of missing self in haploidentical hematopoietic transplantation for acute myeloid leukemia: challenging its predictive value. *Blood.* 2007;110(1):433-440.

[37] Symons HJ, Leffell MS, Rossiter ND, Zahurak M, Jones RJ, Fuchs EJ. Improved survival with inhibitory killer immunoglobulin receptor (KIR) gene mismatches and KIR haplotype B donors after nonmyeloablative, HLA-haploidentical bone marrow transplantation. *Biol Blood Marrow Transplant.* 2010;16(4):533-542.

[38] Giebel S, Locatelli F, Lamparelli T, et al. Survival advantage with KIR ligand incompatibility in hematopoietic stem cell transplantation from unrelated donors. *Blood.* 2003;102(3):814-819.

[39] Moretta A, Bottino C, Pende D, et al. Identification of four subsets of human CD3-CD16+ natural killer (NK) cells by the expression of clonally distributed functional surface molecules: correlation between subset assignment of NK clones and ability to mediate specific alloantigen recognition. *J Exp Med.* 1990;172(6):1589-1598.

[40] Kärre K. Immunology. A perfect mismatch. *Science.* 2002;295(5562):2029-2031.

[41] Weisdorf D, Cooley S, Devine S, et al. T cell-depleted partial matched unrelated donor transplant for advanced myeloid malignancy: KIR ligand mismatch and outcome. *Biology of blood and marrow transplantation: journal of the American Society for Blood and Marrow Transplantation.* 2012;18(6):937-943.

[42] Leung W, Iyengar R, Turner V, et al. Determinants of antileukemia effects of allogeneic NK cells. *J Immunol.* 2004;172(1):644-650.

[43] Hsu KC, Keever-Taylor CA, Wilton A, et al. Improved outcome in HLA-identical sibling hematopoietic stem-cell transplantation for acute myelogenous leukemia predicted by KIR and HLA genotypes. *Blood.* 2005;105(12):4878-4884.

[44] Arima N, Nakamura F, Yabe T, et al. Influence of Differently Licensed KIR2DL1-Positive Natural Killer Cells in Transplant Recipients with Acute Leukemia: A Japanese National Registry Study. *Biol Blood Marrow Transplant.* 2016;22(3):423-431.

[45] Verheyden S, Schots R, Duquet W, Demanet C. A defined donor activating natural killer cell receptor genotype protects against leukemic relapse after related HLA-identical hematopoietic stem cell transplantation. *Leukemia.* 2005;19(8):1446-1451.

[46] Farag SS, Bacigalupo A, Eapen M, et al. The effect of KIR ligand incompatibility on the outcome of unrelated donor transplantation: a report from the center for international blood and marrow transplant research, the European blood and marrow transplant registry, and the Dutch registry. *Biol Blood Marrow Transplant.* 2006;12(8):876-884.

[47] Venstrom JM, Dupont B, Hsu KC, et al. Donor activating KIR2DS1 in leukemia. *N Engl J Med.* 2014;371(21):2042.

[48] Bornhäuser M, Schwerdtfeger R, Martin H, Frank KH, Theuser C, Ehninger G. Role of KIR ligand incompatibility in hematopoietic stem cell transplantation using unrelated donors. *Blood.* 2004;103(7):2860-2861; author reply 2862.

[49] Schaffer M, Malmberg KJ, Ringdén O, Ljunggren HG, Remberger M. Increased infection-related mortality in KIR-ligand-mismatched unrelated allogeneic hematopoietic stem-cell transplantation. *Transplantation.* 2004;78(7):1081-1085.

[50] Parham P. MHC class I molecules and KIRs in human history, health and survival. *Nat Rev Immunol.* 2005;5(3):201-214.

[51] Oevermann L, Michaelis SU, Mezger M, et al. KIR B haplotype donors confer a reduced risk for relapse after haploidentical transplantation in children with ALL. *Blood.* 2014;124(17):2744-2747.

[52] Torelli GF, Peragine N, Raponi S, et al. Recognition of adult and pediatric acute lymphoblastic leukemia blasts by natural killer cells. *Haematologica.* 2014;99(7):1248-1254.

[53] Barker JN, Weisdorf DJ, DeFor TE, et al. Transplantation of 2 partially HLA-matched umbilical cord blood units to enhance engraftment in adults with hematologic malignancy. *Blood.* 2005;105(3):1343-1347.

[54] Brunstein CG, Barker JN, Weisdorf DJ, et al. Umbilical cord blood transplantation after nonmyeloablative conditioning: impact on transplantation outcomes in 110 adults with hematologic disease. *Blood.* 2007;110(8):3064-3070.

[55] Rocha V, Labopin M, Sanz G, et al. Transplants of umbilical-cord blood or bone marrow from unrelated donors in adults with acute leukemia. *The New England journal of medicine.* 2004;351(22):2276-2285.

[56] Rocha V, Ruggeri A, Spellman S, et al. Killer Cell Immunoglobulin-Like Receptor-Ligand Matching and Outcomes after Unrelated Cord Blood Transplantation in Acute Myeloid Leukemia. *Biol Blood Marrow Transplant.* 2016;22(7):1284-1289.

[57] Willemze R, Rodrigues CA, Labopin M, et al. KIR-ligand incompatibility in the graft-versus-host direction improves outcomes after umbilical cord blood transplantation for acute leukemia. *Leukemia.* 2009;23(3):492-500.

[58] Willemze R, Ruggeri A, Purtill D, et al. Is there an impact of killer cell immunoglobulin-like receptors and KIR-ligand incompatibilities on outcomes after unrelated cord blood stem cell transplantation? *Best Pract Res Clin Haematol.* 2010;23(2):283-290.

[59] Brunstein CG, Wagner JE, Weisdorf DJ, et al. Negative effect of KIR alloreactivity in recipients of umbilical cord blood transplant depends on transplantation conditioning intensity. *Blood.* 2009;113(22):5628-5634.

[60] Garfall A, Kim HT, Sun L, et al. KIR ligand incompatibility is not associated with relapse reduction after double umbilical cord blood transplantation. *Bone marrow transplantation.* 2013;48(7):1000-1002.

[61] Brunstein CG, Wagner JE, Weisdorf DJ, et al. Negative effect of KIR alloreactivity in recipients of umbilical cord blood transplant depends on transplantation conditioning intensity. *Blood.* 2009;113(22):5628-5634.

[62] Simonetta F, Alvarez M, Negrin RS. Natural Killer Cells in Graft-versus-Host-Disease after Allogeneic Hematopoietic Cell Transplantation. *Front Immunol.* 2017;8:465.

[63] Lopez C, Kirkpatrick D, Sorell M, O'Reilly RJ, Ching C. Association between pre-transplant natural kill and graft-versus-host disease after stem-cell transplantation. *Lancet.* 1979;2(8152):1103-1107.

[64] Guillén FJ, Ferrara J, Hancock WW, et al. Acute cutaneous graft-versus-host disease to minor histocompatibility antigens in a murine model. Evidence that large

granular lymphocytes are effector cells in the immune response. *Lab Invest.* 1986;55(1):35-42.

[65] Ferrara JL, Guillen FJ, van Dijken PJ, Marion A, Murphy GF, Burakoff SJ. Evidence that large granular lymphocytes of donor origin mediate acute graft-versus-host disease. *Transplantation.* 1989;47(1):50-54.

[66] Acevedo A, Aramburu J, López J, Fernández-Herrera J, Fernández-Rañada JM, López-Botet M. Identification of natural killer (NK) cells in lesions of human cutaneous graft-versus-host disease: expression of a novel NK-associated surface antigen (Kp43) in mononuclear infiltrates. *J Invest Dermatol.* 1991;97(4):659-666.

[67] Horn TD, Haskell J. The lymphocytic infiltrate in acute cutaneous allogeneic graft-versus-host reactions lacks evidence for phenotypic restriction in donor-derived cells. *J Cutan Pathol.* 1998;25(4):210-214.

[68] Charley MR, Mikhael A, Bennett M, Gilliam JN, Sontheimer RD. Prevention of lethal, minor-determinate graft-host disease in mice by the in vivo administration of anti-asialo GM1. *J Immunol.* 1983;131(5):2101-2103.

[69] Blazar BR, Widmer MB, Soderling CC, Gillis S, Vallera DA. Enhanced survival but reduced engraftment in murine recipients of recombinant granulocyte/macrophage colony-stimulating factor following transplantation of T-cell-depleted histoincompatible bone marrow. *Blood.* 1988;72(4):1148-1154.

[70] Ghayur T, Seemayer TA, Kongshavn PA, Gartner JG, Lapp WS. Graft-versus-host reactions in the beige mouse. An investigation of the role of host and donor natural killer cells in the pathogenesis of graft-versus-host disease. *Transplantation.* 1987;44(2):261-267.

[71] Varkila K. Depletion of asialo-GM1+ cells from the F1 recipient mice prior to irradiation and transfusion of parental spleen cells prevents mortality to acute graft-versus-host disease and induction of anti-host specific cytotoxic T cells. *Clin Exp Immunol.* 1987;69(3):652-659.

[72] Charley MR, Mikhael A, Hoot G, Hackett J, Bennett M. Studies addressing the mechanism of anti-asialo GM1 prevention of graft-versus-host disease due to minor histocompatibility antigenic differences. *J Invest Dermatol.* 1985;85(1 Suppl):121s-123s.

[73] Carlson GA, Marshall ST, Truesdale AT. Adaptive immune defects and delayed rejection of allogeneic tumor cells in beige mice. *Cell Immunol.* 1984;87(2):348-356.

[74] Halle-Pannenko O, Bruley-Rosset M. Decreased graft-versus-host reaction and T cell cytolytic potential of beige mice. *Transplantation.* 1985;39(1):85-87.

[75] Murphy WJ, Bennett M, Kumar V, Longo DL. Donor-type activated natural killer cells promote marrow engraftment and B cell development during allogeneic bone marrow transplantation. *J Immunol.* 1992;148(9):2953-2960.

[76] Meinhardt K, Kroeger I, Bauer R, et al. Identification and characterization of the specific murine NK cell subset supporting graft-versus-leukemia- and reducing graft-versus-host-effects. *Oncoimmunology.* 2015;4(1):e981483.

[77] Sivori S, Carlomagno S, Falco M, Romeo E, Moretta L, Moretta A. Natural killer cells expressing the KIR2DS1-activating receptor efficiently kill T-cell blasts and dendritic cells: implications in haploidentical HSCT. *Blood.* 2011;117(16):4284-4292.

[78] Rabinovich BA, Li J, Shannon J, et al. Activated, but not resting, T cells can be recognized and killed by syngeneic NK cells. *J Immunol.* 2003;170(7):3572-3576.

[79] Olson JA, Leveson-Gower DB, Gill S, Baker J, Beilhack A, Negrin RS. NK cells mediate reduction of GVHD by inhibiting activated, alloreactive T cells while retaining GVT effects. *Blood.* 2010;115(21):4293-4301.

[80] Edinger M, Hoffmann P, Ermann J, et al. CD4+CD25+ regulatory T cells preserve graft-versus-tumor activity while inhibiting graft-versus-host disease after bone marrow transplantation. *Nat Med.* 2003;9(9):1144-1150.

[81] Shah NN, Baird K, Delbrook CP, et al. Acute GVHD in patients receiving IL-15/4-1BBL activated NK cells following T-cell-depleted stem cell transplantation. *Blood.* 2015;125(5):784-792.

[82] Xun C, Brown SA, Jennings CD, Henslee-Downey PJ, Thompson JS. Acute graft-versus-host-like disease induced by transplantation of human activated natural killer cells into SCID mice. *Transplantation.* 1993;56(2):409-417.

[83] Cooley S, McCullar V, Wangen R, et al. KIR reconstitution is altered by T cells in the graft and correlates with clinical outcomes after unrelated donor transplantation. *Blood.* 2005;106(13):4370-4376.

[84] Ullrich E, Salzmann-Manrique E, Bakhtiar S, et al. Relation between Acute GVHD and NK Cell Subset Reconstitution Following Allogeneic Stem Cell Transplantation. *Front Immunol.* 2016;7:595.

[85] Bunting MD, Varelias A, Souza-Fonseca-Guimaraes F, et al. GVHD prevents NK-cell-dependent leukemia and virus-specific innate immunity. *Blood.* 2017;129(5):630-642.

[86] Adoptive therapy with CAR redirected T cells: the challenges in targeting solid tumors. *Immunotherapy.* 2015;7(5):535-544.

[87] Barber A, Rynda A, Sentman CL. Chimeric NKG2D expressing T cells eliminate immunosuppression and activate immunity within the ovarian tumor microenvironment. *Journal of immunology* (Baltimore, Md.: 1950). 2009;183 (11):6939-6947.

[88] Zhang T, Barber A, Sentman CL. Generation of antitumor responses by genetic modification of primary human T cells with a chimeric NKG2D receptor. *Cancer research.* 2006;66(11):5927-5933.

[89] Spear P, Barber A, Sentman CL. Collaboration of chimeric antigen receptor (CAR)-expressing T cells and host T cells for optimal elimination of established ovarian tumors. *Oncoimmunology*. 2013;2(4):e23564.

[90] Rubnitz JE, Inaba H, Ribeiro RC, et al. NKAML: a pilot study to determine the safety and feasibility of haploidentical natural killer cell transplantation in childhood acute myeloid leukemia. *Journal of clinical oncology: official journal of the American Society of Clinical Oncology*. 2010;28(6):955-959.

[91] Stern M, Passweg JR, Meyer-Monard S, et al. Pre-emptive immunotherapy with purified natural killer cells after haploidentical SCT: a prospective phase II study in two centers. *Bone marrow transplantation*. 2013;48(3):433-438.

[92] Chang YH, Connolly J, Shimasaki N, Mimura K, Kono K, Campana D. A chimeric receptor with NKG2D specificity enhances natural killer cell activation and killing of tumor cells. *Cancer Res*. 2013;73(6):1777-1786.

[93] Nikiforow S, Murad J, Daley H, et al. A first-in-human phase I trial of NKG2D chimeric antigen receptor-T cells in *AML/MDS and multiple myeloma*. Vol 34: 15_suppl, TPS3102-TPS3102 2016.

In: Benign and Malignant Disorders …
Editors: Ling Zhang and Lubomir Sokol

ISBN: 978-1-53612-999-1
© 2018 Nova Science Publishers, Inc.

Chapter 4

PATHOGENESIS OF MYELODYSPLASTIC SYNDROMES HARBORING CLONAL LARGE GRANULAR LEUKOCYTES

P. K. Epling-Burnette
Department of Immunology and Affiliate of the Malignant Hematology Division, Moffitt Cancer Center and Research Institute, Tampa, FL, US

ABSTRACT

Large Granular Lymphocyte (LGL) leukemia is a defined clinical entity associated with the clonal expansion of differentiated $CD3^+$ T cells or $CD3^-$ NK cell clonal expansion. A spectrum of clonal myeloid diseases including myelodysplastic syndromes (MDS), aplastic anemia and paroxysmal nocturnal hemoglobinuria (PNH) also exhibit clonal T cell expansion with cells of a similar LGL phenotype. Understanding the emerging patterns of clinical overlap across these hematological diseases may aide in the identification of shared genetic loci or etiological events that will inform the development of new diagnostic or therapeutics in these diseases. While the debate still rages about the immune system's ability to identify and destroy abnormal bone marrow cells, the primary function of T cells and NK cells is to act as a barrier to cancer development. MDS, in particular, develops along a spectrum leading to clonal evolution and transformation to acute myeloid leukemia (AML). The presence of clonal T cells may indicate active immune surveillance that protects against the expanding malignant clone. Therefore, distinguishing between immune surveillance and oncogenic events will alter the clinical actions and understanding of the mechanistic convergence points that will likely have a clinical impact. Both intrinsic genetic factors and extrinsic parameters may foster the clonal selection and persistence of T cells in MDS and other related myeloid diseases. In this chapter, the concepts of immune surveillance, autoimmunity, and oncogenic events are discussed as it relates to MDS and clonal LGLs.

Keywords: large granular lymphocytes, large granular lymphocytic leukemia, myelodysplastic syndrome, aplastic anemia, paroxysmal nocturnal hemoglobinuria, autoimmunity

1. INTRODUCTION

LGLL represents a spectrum of clonal lymphoid malignancies that are originally classified into two major groups based on affected lineages: CD3-positive T cell LGLL and CD3-negative natural killer (NK) LGLL [1-5]. The latter is now categorized as clonal lymphoproliferative disorder of NK cells (CLPD- NK) according to 2008 WHO classification of hematopoietic and lymphoid neoplasms. The term LGLL was proposed in 1985 based on the demonstration of clonality and tissue invasion by LGLs in the marrow, spleen and liver [1]. Sequence restriction in the complementarity-determining region (CDR3) of the T cell receptor (TCR) gene was used to define the clonal nature of the expanded lymphocyte population [6]. Based on the action of the recombination-activating genes (RAG), the TCR contains distinct regions that recombine to form the mature receptor [7]. Somatic recombination of the variable (V), diversity (D), and joining (J) regions (VDJ) facilitates the diversification of the TCR gene sequence and enables the interactions between a vast array of unique antigenic peptides presented in the context of major histocompatibility complex (MHC) expressed on antigen-presenting cells (APCs) [7]. The TCR CDR3 is assembled with highly varying lengths due to this process of random gene rearrangements. Clonality of the T cell population is characterized by enrichment of T cells with common CDR3-variable β (CDR3-Vβ) chain size distribution that is known as TCR-CDR3-Vβ skewing. In LGLL, the TCR clonality appears to be driven by oncogenic drivers in some cases, but remains idiopathic in most cases [8-10].

2. TCR CLONAL DOMINANCE IN LGL LEUKEMIA, MDS AND RELATED DISEASES

An exaggerated clonal expansion of T and NK cells may occur in response to specific antigen stimulation, to aberrant retraction caused by apoptosis resistance, or in some cases, to driver mutations [10, 11]. In immune-mediated bone marrow failure syndromes and myeloid neoplasms such as myelodysplastic syndromes (MDS), aplastic anemia, and PNH the expansion of clonal T cells has been long considered a result of sustained aberrant autoantigen stimulation induced by pre-malignant bone marrow progenitors [10-16]. MDS is an age-associated disease characterized by dysplastic bone marrow morphology [17, 18]. It is now appreciated that the causes of MDS relate to the acquisition of diverse somatic driver mutations that alter signaling and epigenetic pathways, genome stability, splicing, or immune responses that contribute to ineffective hematopoiesis (Table 1) [19-28].

Table 1. Frequency and clinical consequences of recurrent gene mutations in patients with MDS

Gene	Chromosome	Frequency (%) MDS	Frequency (%) in sAML	Survival Impact
Epigenetic Pathways				
ASXL1	20q	11-15	23	Unknown
DNMT3A	2p	8	NA	Decrease
EZH2	7p	2-6	NA	Decrease
IDH1/IDH2	2q/15q	4-11	8-10	Decrease
TET2	4q	11-26	11-24	Favorable
Signaling				
FLT3ITD	13q	0-2	12-13	Decrease
JAK2	9p	2	<1	Unknown
N/KRas	1p/12p	2-6	0-12	Unknown
RUNX1	21q	4-14	8-28	Decrease
cCBL	11q	1	8	Unknown
Genome Stability				
NPM1	5q	2	9	Unknown
TP53	17p	10-18	21-42	Decrease
Spliceosome				
SF3B1	2q	7-75* (RS)	3-9	Unknown
U2AF1	21q	16	1-10	Unknown

In the United States, the incidence of MDS was first established from 2001 to 2003 using data from US population-based cancer registries including the National Cancer Institute's Surveillance, Epidemiology, and End Results (SEER) Program and North American Association of Central Cancer Registries (NAACCR) databases. From 2001-2003, the overall incidence was 3.3 per 100,000 (4.5 in men and 2.7 in women) per year. Recent analysis based on 2007-2011 reporting showed the age-adjusted incidence of MDS to be 4.9 per year [29]. This increase may reflect changes in reporting and awareness of the disease. The median age at diagnosis is 76 years, with 86% of cases over 60 years of age [30, 31]. Among racial groups in the US, white individuals had the highest incidence rate (3.5/100,000 in Whites) followed by African Americans (3.0/100,000), native Americans (1.3/100,000) and Asians and Pacific Islanders (2.6/100,000). The occurrence of large granular lymphocytosis or LGLL concurrent with MDS, and other blood malignancies, was first reported in 1988 by Bassan [32]. At that time, LGLL cells were thought to have emerged from a malignant hematopoietic stem cell population with both myeloid and lymphoid differentiation potential. Of 100 patients referred to the National Institutes of Health for immunosuppressive treatment, nine presented characteristics of both T-LGLL and MDS overlap syndrome [33]. Matsutani [34] then later reported the clonal expansion of $CD8^+$ T cells in three of four MDS patients suggesting that there may be a more common co-occurrence of these two disease entities. TCR sequencing and flow cytometry of a larger cohort identified the presence of immunodominant T cell clones in 50% (n = 52 cases) with MDS compared to 5% of age-matched healthy controls (n = 20) [9, 11]. Depending on the sensitivity of the molecular technique, MDS and LGLL overlapping syndromes appear to be common. Saunthararajah [35] and Zhang [36] defined the clinicopathological features of T-LGL proliferation in MDS patients. Both described higher lymphocyte counts in the coincident cases compared to MDS alone and the former showed improved responses to immunosuppressive therapy. In the study by Zhang, an impact on lineage dysplasia was identified with more frequent hypoplasia, and particularly erythroid hypoplasia in MDS cases with T-LGLs, but no difference in overall survival.

3. Classification of MDS

Understanding the overlapping LGLL and MDS syndrome requires analysis of disease diversity. MDS classification, first described in 1976 by the French-American-British (FAB) classification system [37], has rapidly evolved to describe the impact of various factors on transformation to AML evaluation and overall survival [38]. After the French-American-British (FAB) system was established, the classification was refined by the World Health Organization (WHO) [39]. Major classification systems are based, primarily, on the characterization of pathological features that includes: (1) refractory cytopenia with unilineage dysplasia (RCUD) that includes refractory anemia (RA), refractory neutropenia (RN), and refractory thrombocytopenia (RT); (2) refractory anemia with ring sideroblasts (RARS); (3) refractory anemia with multilineage dysplasia (RCMD); (4) refractory anemia with excess blasts-1 (RAEB-1); (5) refractory anemia with excess blasts-2 (RAEB-2); (6) myelodysplastic syndrome, unclassified (MDS-U); (7) MDS associated with isolated del(5q); and (8) refractory cytopenia of childhood (RCC) as a group of provisional entities [40, 41]. The aforementioned terminology and subclassification has recently modified in accordance with the 2016 revision of WHO classification [17]. Other classification systems are designed for survival prognostication. The International Prognostic Scoring System (IPSS) [42] considers the percentage of marrow blasts, the number of cytopenias, and bone marrow cytogenetics. Patients with untreated MDS were first classified into one of four IPSS prognostic risk groups; low, intermediate-1 (Int-1), intermediate-2 (Int-2), and high-risk with median survival estimates of 5.7, 3.5, 1.2, and 0.4 years, respectively. The risk of AML evolution of 25% of patients was determined to be 9.4 (low-risk), 3.3 (Int-1), 1.1 (Int-2), and 0.2 (high-risk) years, respectively. Since this system was validated at diagnosis in patients with *de novo* MDS, recent classification systems including the MD Anderson classification and IPSS-revised (IPSS-R) have assessed the prognostic models using multiple time points during the natural course of MDS and further stratified patients into very low (score = 0), low (1), intermediate (2), high (3–4), or very high [43-45]. Significant differences can be seen among these five groups in overall survival (*p<0.0001*) and risk of AML transformation (*p<0.0001*). T cell clonality has not associated with World Health Organization (WHO) diagnostic category, karyotype, marrow cellularity, sex, age or other known prognostic features [9], but larger case studies are needed to clarify the association between LGLL and MDS prognosis.

4. DEREGULATED IMMUNITY IN TRISOMY 8 MYELODYSPLASTIC SYNDROME

LGLs have been definitely linked to other myeloid diseases such as aplastic anemia that shares many features with 15% of MDS cases characterized by hypocellularity [46, 47]. Numerous abnormalities in immune function appear to contribute to impaired hematopoiesis in MDS including elevated plasma levels of several cytokines such as tumor necrosis factor-alpha (TNF-α) [48, 49] and interferon-gamma (IFN-γ) [50], which are well-known contributors to aplastic anemia pathogenesis [35, 51]. Many investigators have now confirmed that cytopenias are corrected by T cell depleting immunotherapy in both aplastic anemia and MDS [52-54]. Autologous T cells appear to directly suppress bone marrow progenitor cell differentiation [55]. Sloand confirmed the identity of one bone marrow-associated antigen, Wilms-tumor 1 (WT1), which is overexpressed due to trisomy 8 cytogenetic abnormality in MDS and aplastic anemia [56, 57]. Direct cytotoxicity of autologous trisomy 8 hematopoietic progenitors was observed *in vitro* by clonaly expanded $CD8^+$ cells with select TCR-Vβ repertoires [56, 58, 59]. It was hypothesized that the lymphocytic response was triggered by the presence of the abnormal stem cells which contributed to this T cell expansion and cytotoxic response [60]. Additional antigens that have been linked to MDS include c-MYC, CD1, and surviving [61-63]. Trisomy 8 occurs in 5–10% of MDS cases in the United States, but more frequently in those that have evolved from aplastic anemia. As such, other antigens are likely to be present and responsible for the aberrant TCR-Vβ repertoires.

5. *STAT3* MUTATIONS IN LGL LEUKEMIA AND MDS

In LGLL, clonal expansion has been linked to somatic driver mutations in the transcription factor *STAT3*. In 2001, a study showed that *STAT3* is constitutively activated in peripheral blood mononuclear cells from patients with T cell LGLL, [64] and the molecular basis of this clinically heterogenous, but morphologically distinct entity, remained enigmatic until an international group of investigators identified somatic mutations in *STAT3* [65, 66]. Originally identified as an acute phase response factor central to the transcriptional activation of downstream molecular pathways that mediate signaling by the IL-6-family of cytokines [67-70], *STAT3* is one member of a family of STAT-family proteins that act as signaling intermediates for many cytokine receptors. Cytokine receptor subunits bind to their respective ligands and induce receptor dimerization leading to activation of members of the Janus kinase family (Jak1, Jak2, Jak3, and Tyk2 signaling molecules. These, in turn, cause STAT protein dimerization, nuclear translocation, DNA binding, and transcriptional activation of target genes. Somatic mutations were identified by both Koskela [65] and Jerez [66] in patients with LGLL. These mutations reside within the Src homology 2 (SH2) phosphotyrosine-binding domains near the dimerization interface. Of 49 *STAT3* mutations identified by Jerez and colleagues [66], 80% were either Y640F or D661Y. These mutations result in amino acid substitutions in the major protein-protein interaction domain in which an interface is formed with the carboxy-terminal phospho-tyrosine 705 (Y705). Constitutive *STAT3* DNA binding [64] and increased expression of *STAT3*-responsive genes [65, 66] suggest that *STAT3* mutations in LGLL contribute to leukemic LGL pathogenesis.

The first linkage between *STAT3* signaling and T cell leukemia pathogenesis was based on studies of HTLV-1-mediated adult T cell leukemia (ATL) where constitutive phosphorylation of JAK proteins was shown to mediate tumor growth by HTLV-1 [71, 72]. Targeted deletion of *STAT3* using the Cre-*loxP* recombination system demonstrated the importance of this transcription factor in T cell cytokine signaling [73]. The Cre-Lox system is a site-specific recombinase technology used to delete, insert, and translocate specific DNA sequences. This system consists of a Cre recombinase that, when expressed, recognizes LoxP sequences that are derived from bacteriophage P1. The Cre-Lox system is popular in mouse genetics to deplete genes in specific cell types and was used to specifically delete *STAT3* in thymocytes by expressing the Cre recombinase under the promoter control of the Lck gene that is selectively expressed early during T cell differentiation in the thymus. Lck-Cre/*STAT3*$^{\text{flox}/-}$ mice maintained normal function in response to another STAT-family protein, *STAT5* activated by the cytokines IL-2 and IL-7, but a markedly reduced proliferative response to *STAT3*-specific IL-6 stimulation. *STAT3*-deficient T cells were resistant to IL-6 induced anti-apoptotic responses, which is consistent with the proposed role of this molecule in LGLL. In the case of LGLL, *STAT3* activation in patients with or without the mutation is associated with an anti-apoptotic phenotype [64-66].

6. FREQUENCY OF *STAT3* AND *STAT5* MUTATIONS IN LGL LEUKEMIA AND MDS

Acquired somatic mutations in signal transducer and activator of transcription 3 gene (*STAT3*) [66], or its related family member *STAT5* [65, 74], contribute to the clonal expansion of LGL cells in a large fraction of patients with LGLL. Of 367 MDS and 140 aplastic anemia cases, *STAT3* mutant clones were found in 7% and 2.5%, respectively [75]. Similar somatic *STAT3* mutations have not been identified in the neoplastic myeloid populations suggesting that this may be acquired directly in the T cell or NK cells in this disease. IL-21 is a critical determinant of T cell-derived cytokines, regulation of NK and T cell function, and is a strong activator of *STAT3* [76, 77]. IL-21 stimulates a receptor complex that is shared with IL-2, IL-4, IL-7, IL-9, and IL-15[78]. While IL-15 primarily signals through *STAT5*, both IL-15 and IL-21 activates *STAT3* [77, 79]. Persistence of normal $CD8^+$ T cell memory populations is dependent of signaling through IL-21 and *STAT3* [76, 80]. Control of the memory T cell response is obliterated in IL-21 deficient mice [76, 77]. Interestingly, patients with autosomal-dominant hyper-IgE syndrome (AD-HIES) carry a dominant-negative *STAT3* mutation which contributes to enhanced susceptibility to a variety of bacterial and fungal infections and poor recall memory responses to varicella zoster virus (VZV) and Epstein-Barr virus (EBV) caused by a deficiency in memory T cells [81]. Collectively, this information suggests that *STAT3* is a central player in formation and persistence of memory T cells in both mouse and humans and that it may be the presence of a continued signaling response that leads to the T cell clonal expansion in both LGLL and MDS [82]. While this provides a potential mechanism for co-existing disease, roughly 50-70% of all MDS cases display clonal T cell expansion but lack the *STAT3* mutation [10, 11, 35, 75]. Gain-of-function mutations in the *STAT5* gene were also demonstrated, but this too was in a small proportion of LGLL patients and MDS and other autoimmune disorders suggesting that these events may be linked to subclinical and clinical expansion of T cell clones in some cases [74, 83, 84]. Additional mechanisms leading to LGLL or T cell and NK cell expansion in MDS are likely to be explained through common mechanisms of pathogenesis.

7. IL-15 AND IL-7 IN MDS AND LGL LEUKEMIA

In MDS, an inflammatory bone marrow microenvironment is pivotal for initiation and progression. Namely, IL-1, TNF-α, iNOS, IL-18, IL-6, IL-10, and TGF-β, have been detected at increased concentrations and participate in the induction of dysplastic bone marrow features [85-92]. IL-15 is a critical inflammatory cytokine that is elevated in both LGLL and MDS [93]. This cytokine is structurally similar to IL-2 and other cytokine family members that interact and activate *STAT3* and *STAT5* downstream of the IL2/IL-15 receptor beta chain (CD122) and the common gamma chain (γ_c, CD132) [94-96]. Mice constitutively overexpressing IL-15 develop a syndrome that is very similar to LGLL suggesting that there is a causative linkage [97, 98]. Given that myeloid differentiation and function are modulated in both MDS and LGLL, IL-15 has been studied in relationship to the initiation of both diseases [3, 93, 99]. Within the IL-2R$\beta\gamma_c$-common family, IL-7 appears to primarily promote the naïve state of T cells rather than impact their memory differentiation [100]. Increased IL-15 concentrations in the plasma of MDS patients was examined and compared to healthy donors (n = 20 in both groups). Reduced naïve CD4$^+$ and CD8$^+$ T cells [16.11 ± 6.56 vs. 24.11 ± 7.18 for CD4$^+$ T cells ($p < 0.001$) and 13.15 ± 5.67 vs. 23.51 ± 6.25 for CD8$^+$ T cells ($p < 0.001$)] were observed, while an increase in memory T cells significantly correlated with IL-15 plasma levels [93]. Treatment of peripheral blood cells with IL-15 decreased naïve CD4 and CD8 cells and strongly increases memory T cells [101]. Alternatively, treatment with IL-7 increased naïve CD4$^+$ ($p < 0.05$) and CD8$^+$ ($p < 0.001$) T cells suggesting that exposure to high levels of IL-15 may be involved in the T cell phenotype conversion observed in MDS and in LGLL. We and others have accurately verified discordance in naïve and memory sub-populations and identification of the pathways driving these phenotypes [102].

7.1. Common IL-15-Directed Phenotype May Underlie Similar Pathological Features of LGL Leukemia and MDS

The regulation of IL-15 is very complex, but is secreted by myeloid cells following viral infection [103]. Prolonged *in vitro* exposure to IL-15 results in c-MYC upregulation which induces the activation of many genes including Aurora Kinase A (*AURKA*) and B (*AURKB*) [104]. The pathway activated in response to persistently elevated levels of IL-15 is tightly linked to the overexpression of DNA (cytosine-5)-methyltransferase 3B (Dnmt3b)-mediated DNA hypermethylation. Interestingly, alteration in DNA methylation is a hallmark of MDS. Methylation of CpG dinucleotides is mediated by DNA methyltransferase including *DNMT1*, *DNMT3A*, and *DNMT3B*. DNMT3 mutations, and associated hypermethylation, occur early in the course of MDS [23, 28]. Adoptive transfer of IL-15-cultured mouse LGL cells leads to malignant transformation *in vivo* suggesting that the common pathway of DNA hypermethylation caused by the DNMT-family underlies the phenotype. Aberrant DNA hypermethylation is targetable therapeutically by two nucleoside analog DNA methylation inhibitors, 5-aza-2'deoxycytidine (decitabine) and 5-azacytidine (azacitidine). Clinical data shows response rates in approximately half of MDS cases, but it not restricted to patients with epigenetic effector mutations such as *DNMT3A, TET2, ASXL1* or *EZH2*, which are all common in MDS and are likely linked to the transforming process [23]. Evaluation of LGLL clone size or association with demethylating agent response may be informative in understanding the disease mechanisms. As a critical cytokine for the genesis and homeostasis of normal LGL cells, IL-15 may be able to initiate the clonal expansion of clonal LGL cells in MDS [105]. Interestingly, the global hypermethylation that occurs in DNMT3B transgenic mice leads to an increase in the incidence of LGLL clones [104].

7.2. IL-15 as a Therapeutic Target

Treatment of LGLL primarily consists of immunosuppressive agents such as low-dose methotrexate, cyclophosphamide or cyclosporine which has been associated with an approximate 50% response rate in retrospective studies. A prospective trial conducted by the Eastern Cooperative Oncology Group (ECOG) cooperative group was the first prospective clinical trial in LGLL. In this study, response to methotrexate was demonstrated to be 39% while treatment with an anti-CD52 antibody (alemtuzumab) showed a response rate of 50% (four out of eight patients) that were refractory to other immunosuppressive drugs. As mentioned above, the IL-15 receptor or IL-15 cytokine may be valid therapeutic targets in both MDS and LGLL. Monocytes and dendritic cells express the IL-15-specific subunit (IL15Rα) and secrete IL-15 locally [103, 106, 107]. IL15Rα presents IL-15 to the other two receptor subunits, IL-2/IL-15Rβ (specific to IL-2 and IL-15) and γ-c common subunits expressed on NK and cytotoxic T cells. The presentation of IL-15 from one receptor subunit on one cell type to the two other receptor subunits is known as *trans* presentation of IL-15. Interestingly, it has recently been identified that in some patients with T-LGLL, IL-15Rα is expressed in the T-LGL cells, leading to all three subunits being expressed in *cis*. Dysregulated IL-15 has been reported in patients with autoimmune diseases (e.g., rheumatoid arthritis, multiple sclerosis and Celiac's disease), as well as HTLV-1 infection. Based on this data, a phase I trial of the IL-2/IL-15Rβ antibody (Hu-Mikβ1) was conducted [99, 108]. Nine T cell LGLL patients were enrolled and given a single dose of the antibody intravenously at three dosage ranges, 0.5, 1.0 and 1.5 mg/kg administered over a 90 min period with a 42-day observation period for toxicity and response. While there were no acute toxicities reported, one patient developed an immune response due to drug administration. Although there were transient increases in neutrophil counts in three patients and an increase in platelet counts in one patient, further investigations with this agent were not conducted due to the complexity in IL-15 regulation.

8. THERAPEUTIC IMPLICATION OF LGL LEUKEMIA AND IMMUNE PATHOLOGY IN MDS

Based on the co-existence of LGLL cells in MDS and aplastic anemia, several clinical trials were launched as early as 1998 to test anti-thymocyte globulin (ATG) to induce immune suppression [52]. The goals of MDS therapy are to prolong survival, delay or prevent AML progression, and to improve quality of life (QOL). With the success of ATG in aplastic anemia, there have been several studies of not only ATG but other ATG-combination therapies in MDS [35, 52, 53, 56, 57, 109-114]. In the studies using ATG, a mixture of purified polyclonal IgG from the sera of rabbits (rATG, Thymoglobulin, Genzyme, Cambridge, MA) or horses (eATG) immunized with human thymocytes (Lymphoglobulin, and Atgam) or the Jurkat cell line (ATG Fresenius, Fresenius SE, Bad Homburg, Germany), clinical benefit has been observed. ATG has diverse effects on the immune system including; (1) T cell depletion (2) modulation of key cell surface molecules that mediate leukocyte/epithelium interactions; (3) induction of apoptosis in B-cell lineages (4) interference with dendritic cell functional properties; (5) induction of regulatory T cells and natural killer T cells, (6) direct effect on hematopoietic progenitor cell colony formation from primitive hematopoietic cells and (7) possibly, elimination of the Fas-Fas-L interactions [58, 114]. In addition to ATG treatment, clinical trials of CsA have also been conducted in MDS either alone or in combination [110]. CsA has a potent immunosuppressive agent that blocks IL-2 production. While there has been an increase in overall survival (OS) and progression free survival (PFS) observed after r-ATG therapy [115], a randomized phase III [116] trial in MDS combining ATG and CsA failed to show an increase in two-year transformation-free survival or overall survival compared to best supportive care (BSC) although this study allowed for cross-over to ATG/CsA upon disease progression on the BSC arm. There has also been a campaign to identify biomarkers with positive association to response to ATG among MDS patients independent of age or other covariates [115]. The presence of LGLL clonal variants have failed to discriminate responders from non-responders prior to treatment although there was a clear elimination of the population after treatment in responding patients [52, 115]. Recognition that the dysplastic phenotype, which characterizes MDS, may arise from diverse biological processes, including an immune mechanism associated with T cell clonal expansion, strengthens the need for conducting prospective clinical trials based on biomarker-assigned therapy and identification of the molecular mechanisms responsible for co-existing LGLL and MDS.

8.1. ATG Based Regimens to Modify the Immune System in MDS

The goals of MDS therapy are to prolong survival, delay or prevent AML progression, and to improve QOL. Although allogeneic hematopoietic stem cell transplantation (HSCT) is the only curative treatment in MDS, eligibility is limited by several factors including the identification of HLA-matched donor and the procedure-related co-morbidities, which is particularly important in this older patient population[117]. ATG is a mixture of purified polyclonal IgG from the sera of rabbits (rATG, Thymoglobulin, Genzyme, Cambridge, MA) or horses (eATG) immunized with human thymocytes (Lymphoglobulin, and Atgam) or the Jurkat cell line (ATG Fresenius, Fresenius SE, Bad Homburg, Germany) that induces significant therapeutic improvement in aplastic anemia [118, 119]. ATG depletes T cells in blood and peripheral lymphoid tissues by a mechanism dependent on complement-mediated lysis [119]. This pharmacological modality also modulates key cell surface molecules that stimulate leukocyte/epithelium interactions involved in T cell activation [120]. Finally, ATG eliminate other cellular populations that may be important in the induction of an immune response including 1) B-cells [121], 2) dendritic cells [122], and natural killer T cells (NKT) [123]. Direct effects on hematopoietic progenitor cells and expansion of regulatory T cells may aide in the suppression of the effector T cells [124]. Depending on the product, differential effects have been demonstrated with the eATG significantly more active in aplastic anemia. Although the mechanisms for the differential effect are unknown, the immune microenvironment and homeostasis are most likely important contributing factors.

In MDS, the first ATG clinical trial was conducted at the National Institute of Health (NIH) in 1997 [125] and the mature data (median follow-up: 30 months) with a larger sample size was reported in 2002 [126]. In this single-arm prospective study, 61 transfusion-dependent patients with MDS (with <20% blasts) were treated with one cycle of eATG at 40 mg/kg/d for four days [63]. Response criteria included independence from transfusion for a minimum of six weeks with a sustained increase in hemoglobin, or stable hemoglobin within eight months as measured from the time the patient last received a transfusion until reinstitution of RBC transfusions. Within eight months of treatment, 21 of 61 MDS patients (34%) no longer required red blood cell transfusions. Independence from transfusion was maintained in 17 of the 21 responders (81%) for a median of 36 months (range 3–72 months). Ten of 21 patients (47.5%) with severe thrombocytopenia had a sustained increase in platelet counts, and 6 of 11 patients (55%) with severe neutropenia had sustained increase in neutrophil counts.

Yazji [127], Killick [128-132], and Steensma [113] conducted similar studies with varied success. Steensma terminated the trial early due to a lack of clinical efficacy and reported infusion-related toxicity. Compared to the previous trials, this cohort exhibited unfavorable characteristics as all patients exhibited a hemaglobin under 9 g/dL, older age (range 62–74 years), and had higher risk disease classification using the IPSS system. Based on IPSS, 63% were intermediate-1 and 36% were intermediate-2 and only 2 had a normal karyotype. This highlights an important factor related to MDS pathogenesis. While clonal T cell expansion appears to be prevalent in all subtypes, the therapeutic implications may diverge in accordance with leukemia progression. Stadler compared the efficacy of eATG (lymphoglobulin, 15 mg/kg/d for five days, n = 20) to rATG (thymoglobulin, 3.75 mg/kg/d for five days, n = 15) [112]. Unlike aplastic anemia where eATG has superior efficacy [133], no significant difference was observed between the two ATG products with regard to responses or adverse effects.

8.2. CsA Usage in MDS

In addition to ATG, cyclosporine (CsA) has also been used through rational study designs motivated by responses in aplastic anemia patients [134]. Broliden reported the efficacy of ATG plus CsA [135] to be greater than ATG alone in MDS. Twenty patients (17 RA, 3 RAEB) received treatment with rATG (ATG-Fresenius) plus CsA and while the overall response rate was 30% (6/20); 3 of the 6 responders had a complete response. The responses lasted 2–58 months, and 2 patients remained in a complete remission for 42 and 58 months, respectively.

Several clinical trials of CsA, most focused on hypoplastic MDS, have been conducted in MDS [50, 136-139], but Janasova [136] performed the first clinical trial in 17 MDS patients and reported a durable response rate of 82%. This surprisingly high response rate may have been observed due to patient selection since 16 out of the 17 subjects had refractory anemia. Catalano treated nine MDS patients with refractory anemia and found a similar response rate [137]. Compared to studies conducted in the United States, large multicenter Japanese trials have reported consistent responses above 50% [139, 140]. The dose of CsA used in these trials has generally been 6 mg/kg/d. Hematologic improvement is superior in patients with a favorable karyotype, low IPSS score, and HLA-DRB1*1501 genotype [141, 142]. Inconsistent differences in CsA response have been reported when stratified by age, bone marrow cellularity, bone marrow blast percentage, dose and CsA blood concentration. The disease course and median age of MDS patients differs by geographical region suggesting that this difference in therapeutic response may align with altered mechanistic contributions [114].

9. BIOMARKER-BASED PATIENT SELECTION

In the Japanese trial, CsA response was significantly correlated CD4/CD8 ratio and presence of TCR-V/β and –γ gene rearrangements [140]. Although correlative studies were carried out in only a few patients (n = 4), these results corroborate the findings by Zou using samples from patients at the NHLBI [102]. Ishikawa demonstrated a significant association with CsA response and clonal expansion of bone marrow cells carrying *PIG-A* genetic mutations[143]. In these clones, the surface expression of all glycosylphosphatidylinositol (GPI)-anchored proteins is quenched and the clinical presentation overlaps with paroxysmal nocturnal hemoglobinuria (PNH) [143]. In this study, 20 MDS patients were treated with CsA (4 mg/kg/d) and among 19 patients evaluated, 10 showed hematologic improvement. Toxicity associated with CsA usage was manageable and median follow up was 30 months. Here, the presence of PNH clones, a shorter duration of disease and minimal evidence of dysplasia were significantly associated with improved platelet responses. From this study, several important clinical standards were established; 1) immunosuppressive therapy may be more prevalent in Japan and possibly other countries in Asia, and 2) PNH may overlap with aberrant T cell phenotypes in aplastic anemia, LGLL and MDS. Saunthararajah then focused on biomarker discovery in ATG and CsA-treated patients [111]. HLA-DR15 and PNH were selected as potential biomarkers for validation because HLA-DR15 is overrepresented in patients with aplastic anemia and PNH [141, 142, 144, 145]. Sloand confirmed findings by Saunthararajah in a study of 129 MDS patients receiving equine antithymocyte globulin (eATG, Atgam, Pfizer, New York, NY) with or without CsA (Novartis, Basel, Switzerland) at the National Heart Lung Blood Institute (NHLBI) [146]. Of 129 patients on either eATG or CsA, 39 (30%) achieved a hematologic response. The median follow-up was three years (range 0.03–11.3 years). The strongest linkage to response was observed in younger patients (under 61 years of age) and in those that have a shorter duration of transfusion dependence, and HLA-DR15 genotype. Despite the strong correlation between the biomarker prediction and response, standardized usage of this biomarker-based patient selection has not been widely implemented. Recently, Haider reported sixty-six MDS patients treated with immunosuppressive therapy (ATG and CsA) at a single institution. The median age was 61 years, and the majority had low risk disease. The median time to initiate therapy with ATG or CsA was 1 year. Erythroid improvement was evaluated in 30 patients and 60% responded. Neutrophil improvement was evaluated in 15 patients, and 39% responded while platelet improvement was observed in 18 patients (57%). The presence of a poor-risk karyotype was associated with significantly lower response rate of 25% compared to 41% and 44% for intermediate and good karyotypes, respectively. CsA provided a clear advantage in the regimen with 51% response rate compared to a 27% response observed with ATG alone. Thus, immunosuppressive regimens clearly have a response rate in the range of or superior to other treatments in lower-risk MDS. Despite these promising results, the treatment still remains underutilized in MDS.

To examine more precise characteristics of the T cells and ATG response, Zou analyzed the age-adjusted CD4/CD8 ratio in 54 MDS patients compared to 37 healthy controls which revealed that inadequate CD4$^+$ count rather than expansion of CD8$^+$ T cells was associated with a lower ratio [102]. This T cell phenotype was present in both lower and higher risk MDS patients as defined by the IPSS. Inversion of the CD4/CD8 ratio was strongly associated with response to ATG therapy (P < 0.001). The loss of CD4-cells was inversely correlated to the proliferative T cell index before treatment. Accelerated CD4$^+$ T cell turnover is also evident in LGLL and may be important in disease pathogenesis. In many autoimmune diseases, there is a correlation between the loss of CD4$^+$ T cells and the expansion of autoreactive CD8$^+$ T cells [12, 13, 16]. This abnormality supersedes the simple loss of CD4$^+$ regulatory T cells (Tregs) from the peripheral or tissue compartment. Reduction in CD4$^+$ T cells may initiate a cytokine-dependent pathway known as "homeostatic proliferation" in which the interleukin (IL)-2Rγ common cytokines such as IL-2, IL-7, IL-15 and/or IL-21 non-specifically expand antigen-specific and self-reactive T cells leading to an increased risk for evasion of peripheral tolerance mechanisms leading to autoimmunity [102, 147]. Results by Zou are the first to demonstrate involvement of CD4$^+$ T cells and response to ATG. Since the loss of CD4$^+$ T cells is strongly associated with impaired T cell homeostasis and accumulation of self-reactive CD8$^+$ T cells it contributes to autoimmunity in many models of human diseases. This mechanism may explain immune pathogenesis from a global perspective [102]. The highest homeostatic proliferative index is attributed to T cells with the highest affinity to self-antigens, explaining not only trisomy 8 -associated autoimmunity, but also autoimmune pathogenesis in other settings. A discovery of TCR antigen reactivity in patients with aggressive homeostatic proliferation, without trisomy 8 has not been studied. Kordasti showed that the numbers of CD3$^+$ CD4$^+$ IL-17 producing T cells (Th17) were markedly increased in MDS. FoxP3$^+$ regulatory T cells (Tregs) were associated with higher IPSS risk stratification [148, 149]. Delineation of unique Treg subsets revealed that an increase in the absolute number of CD4($^+$)FoxP3($^+$)CD25($^+$)CD127(^{low}) CD45RA($^-$)CD27($^-$) Tregs (effector memory Tregs; Treg^{EM}) was associated with anemia ($p = 0.046$), reduced hemoglobin ($p = 0.038$), and blast counts $\geq$5% ($p = 0.006$). Treg^{EM} constitutes only 2% of Tregs in healthy donors [150]. With a median follow-up of 3.1 years (range-2.7 to 4.9) from sample acquisition, increased numbers of Treg^{EM} cells proved to have independent prognostic importance for survival. Multivariate analyses showed that Treg^{EM} cells impacted survival independently from myeloblast characteristics. Based on these findings, clonal expansion of effector CD8$^+$ T cells and the accumulation of CD4$^+$ T cells with the Treg^{EM} phenotype may indicate microenvironmental changes conducive to transformation in MDS and reflects the overlapping disease with LGLL.

CONCLUSION

MDS is associated with immune deregulation and inflammation. Coincidently with the occurrence of this disease, there is overlapping amplification of T-LGL clones. The frequency of this phenomenon has been documented in at least 50% of MDS patients, but its impact on survival is still unknown. Clonal disease may be initiated through somatic driver mutations, autoimmune reactivity, or other selective pressures induced by aging or the microenvironment. The frequent overlap suggest that there could be causative relationships between these two diseases resulting in therapeutic implications. Additional studies are needed to understand the impact of T-LGL clones in MDS.

REFERENCES

[1] Loughran TP, Jr., Kadin ME, Starkebaum G, et al. Leukemia of large granular lymphocytes: association with clonal chromosomal abnormalities and autoimmune neutropenia, thrombocytopenia, and hemolytic anemia. *Ann Intern Med.* 1985;102(2):169-175.

[2] Lamy T, Loughran TP, Jr. Pathogenesis of Autoimmune Diseases in Large Granular Lymphocyte Leukemia. *Hematology.* 1998;3(1):17-29.

[3] Lamy T, Loughran TP. Large Granular Lymphocyte Leukemia. *Cancer Control.* 1998;5(1):25-33.

[4] Lamy T, Loughran TP, Jr. Current concepts: large granular lymphocyte leukemia. *Blood Rev.* 1999;13(4):230-240.

[5] Lamy T, Loughran TP, Jr. How I treat LGL leukemia. *Blood.* 2011;117(10):2764-2774.

[6] Loughran TP, Jr. Clonal diseases of large granular lymphocytes. *Blood.* 1993;82(1):1-14.

[7] Lieber MR. Mechanisms of human lymphoid chromosomal translocations. *Nat Rev Cancer.* 2016;16(6):387-398.

[8] Chen X, Bai F, Sokol L, et al. A critical role for DAP10 and DAP12 in CD8$^+$ T cell-mediated tissue damage in large granular lymphocyte leukemia. *Blood.* 2009;113(14):3226-3234.

[9] Epling-Burnette PK, Painter JS, Rollison DE, et al. Prevalence and clinical association of clonal T-cell expansions in Myelodysplastic Syndrome. *Leukemia.* 2007;21(4):659-667.

[10] Maciejewski JP, O'Keefe C, Gondek L, Tiu R. Immune-mediated bone marrow failure syndromes of progenitor and stem cells: molecular analysis of cytotoxic T cell clones. *Folia Histochem Cytobiol.* 2007;45(1):5-14.

[11] Plasilova M, Risitano A, Maciejewski JP. Application of the molecular analysis of the T-cell receptor repertoire in the study of immune-mediated hematologic diseases. *Hematology*. 2003;8(3):173-181.

[12] Goronzy JJ, Bartz-Bazzanella P, Hu W, Jendro MC, Walser-Kuntz DR, Weyand CM. Dominant clonotypes in the repertoire of peripheral CD4$^+$ T cells in rheumatoid arthritis. *J Clin Invest*. 1994;94(5):2068-2076.

[13] Goronzy JJ, Zettl A, Weyand CM. T cell receptor repertoire in rheumatoid arthritis. *Int Rev Immunol*. 1998;17(5-6):339-363.

[14] Weyand CM, Goronzy JJ. Pathogenesis of rheumatoid arthritis. *Med Clin North Am*. 1997;81(1):29-55.

[15] Weyand CM, Klimiuk PA, Goronzy JJ. Heterogeneity of rheumatoid arthritis: from phenotypes to genotypes. *Springer Semin Immunopathol*. 1998;20(1-2):5-22.

[16] Rittner HL, Zettl A, Jendro MC, Bartz-Bazzanella P, Goronzy JJ, Weyand CM. Multiple mechanisms support oligoclonal T cell expansion in rheumatoid synovitis. *Mol Med*. 1997;3(7):452-465.

[17] Gurney M, Patnaik MM, Hanson CA, et al. The 2016 revised World Health Organization definition of 'myelodysplastic syndrome with isolated del(5q)'; prognostic implications of single versus double cytogenetic abnormalities. *Br J Haematol*. 2017.

[18] Estey E. Acute myeloid leukemia and myelodysplastic syndromes in older patients. *J Clin Oncol*. 2007;25(14):1908-1915.

[19] Kosmider O, Gelsi-Boyer V, Cheok M, et al. TET2 mutation is an independent favorable prognostic factor in myelodysplastic syndromes (MDSs). *Blood*. 2009;114(15):3285-3291.

[20] Chesnais V, Kosmider O, Damm F, et al. Spliceosome mutations in myelodysplastic syndromes and chronic myelomonocytic leukemia. *Oncotarget*. 2012;3(11):1284-1293.

[21] Bejar R. Splicing Factor Mutations in Cancer. *Adv Exp Med Biol*. 2016;907:215-228.

[22] Chen TC, Hou HA, Chou WC, et al. Dynamics of ASXL1 mutation and other associated genetic alterations during disease progression in patients with primary myelodysplastic syndrome. *Blood Cancer J*. 2014;4:e177.

[23] Graubert T, Walter MJ. Genetics of myelodysplastic syndromes: new insights. *Hematology Am Soc Hematol Educ Program*. 2011;2011:543-549.

[24] Graubert TA, Mardis ER. Genomics of acute myeloid leukemia. *Cancer J*. 2011;17(6):487-491.

[25] Graubert TA, Shen D, Ding L, et al. Recurrent mutations in the U2AF1 splicing factor in myelodysplastic syndromes. *Nat Genet*. 2011;44(1):53-57.

[26] Link DC, Schuettpelz LG, Shen D, et al. Identification of a novel TP53 cancer susceptibility mutation through whole-genome sequencing of a patient with therapy-related AML. *JAMA*. 2011;305(15):1568-1576.

[27] Patel JP, Gonen M, Figueroa ME, et al. Prognostic relevance of integrated genetic profiling in acute myeloid leukemia. *N Engl J Med*. 2012;366(12):1079-1089.

[28] Walter MJ, Ding L, Shen D, et al. Recurrent DNMT3A mutations in patients with myelodysplastic syndromes. *Leukemia*. 2011;25(7):1153-1158.

[29] Cogle CR. Incidence and Burden of the Myelodysplastic Syndromes. *Curr Hematol Malig Rep*. 2015;10(3):272-281.

[30] Rollison DE, Howlader N, Smith MT, et al. Epidemiology of myelodysplastic syndromes and chronic myeloproliferative disorders in the United States, 2001-2004, using data from the NAACCR and SEER programs. *Blood*. 2008;112(1):45-52.

[31] Ma X, Does M, Raza A, Mayne ST. Myelodysplastic syndromes: incidence and survival in the United States. *Cancer*. 2007;109(8):1536-1542.

[32] Bassan R, Rambaldi A, Allavena P, Abbate M, Marini B, Barbui T. Association of large granular lymphocyte/natural killer cell proliferative disease and second hematologic malignancy. *Am J Hematol*. 1988;29(2):85-93.

[33] Karadimitris A, Li K, Notaro R, et al. Association of clonal T-cell large granular lymphocyte disease and paroxysmal nocturnal haemoglobinuria (PNH): further evidence for a pathogenetic link between T cells, aplastic anaemia and PNH. *Br J Haematol*. 2001;115(4):1010-1014.

[34] Matsutani T, Yoshioka T, Tsuruta Y, et al. Determination of T-cell receptors of clonal CD8-positive T-cells in myelodysplastic syndrome with erythroid hypoplasia. *Leuk Res*. 2003;27(4):305-312.

[35] Saunthararajah Y, Molldrem JL, Rivera M, et al. Coincident myelodysplastic syndrome and T-cell large granular lymphocytic disease: clinical and pathophysiological features. *Br J Haematol*. 2001;112(1):195-200.

[36] Zhang X, Sokol L, Bennett JM, Moscinski LC, List A, Zhang L. T-cell large granular lymphocyte proliferation in myelodysplastic syndromes: Clinicopathological features and prognostic significance. *Leuk Res*. 2016;43:18-23.

[37] Bennett JM, Catovsky D, Daniel MT, et al. Proposals for the classification of the acute leukaemias. French-American-British (FAB) co-operative group. *Br J Haematol*. 1976;33(4):451-458.

[38] Bennett JM, Catovsky D, Daniel MT, et al. Proposals for the classification of the myelodysplastic syndromes. *Br J Haematol*. 1982;51(2):189-199.

[39] Harris NL, Jaffe ES, Diebold J, et al. World Health Organization classification of neoplastic diseases of the hematopoietic and lymphoid tissues: report of the Clinical Advisory Committee meeting-Airlie House, Virginia, November 1997. *J Clin Oncol*. 1999;17(12):3835-3849.

[40] Vardiman JW, Harris NL, Brunning RD. The World Health Organization (WHO) classification of the myeloid neoplasms. *Blood.* 2002;100(7):2292-2302.

[41] Vardiman JW, Thiele J, Arber DA, et al. The 2008 revision of the World Health Organization (WHO) classification of myeloid neoplasms and acute leukemia: rationale and important changes. *Blood.* 2009;114(5):937-951.

[42] Greenberg P, Cox C, LeBeau MM, et al. International scoring system for evaluating prognosis in myelodysplastic syndromes. *Blood.* 1997;89(6):2079-2088.

[43] Greenberg PL, Stone RM, Al-Kali A, et al. Myelodysplastic Syndromes, Version 2.2017, NCCN Clinical Practice Guidelines in Oncology. *J Natl Compr Canc Netw.* 2017;15(1):60-87.

[44] Greenberg PL, Stone RM, Bejar R, et al. Myelodysplastic syndromes, version 2.2015. *J Natl Compr Canc Netw.* 2015;13(3):261-272.

[45] Kantarjian H, O'Brien S, Ravandi F, et al. Proposal for a new risk model in myelodysplastic syndrome that accounts for events not considered in the original International Prognostic Scoring System. *Cancer.* 2008;113(6):1351-1361.

[46] Schemenau J, Baldus S, Anlauf M, et al. Cellularity, characteristics of hematopoietic parameters and prognosis in myelodysplastic syndromes. *Eur J Haematol.* 2015;95(3):181-189.

[47] Young NS, Maciejewski J. The pathophysiology of acquired aplastic anemia. *N Engl J Med.* 1997;336(19):1365-1372.

[48] Kitagawa M, Saito I, Kuwata T, et al. Overexpression of tumor necrosis factor (TNF)-alpha and interferon (IFN)-gamma by bone marrow cells from patients with myelodysplastic syndromes. *Leukemia.* 1997;11(12):2049-2054.

[49] Molnar L, Berki T, Hussain A, Nemeth P, Losonczy H. [The role of TNF-alpha in myelodysplastic syndrome: immunoserologic and immunohistochemical studies]. *Orv Hetil.* 2000;141(33):1807-1811.

[50] Selleri C, Maciejewski JP, Catalano L, et al. Effects of cyclosporine on hematopoietic and immune functions in patients with hypoplastic myelodysplasia: in vitro and in vivo studies. *Cancer.* 2002;95(9):1911-1922.

[51] Gaman A, Gaman G, Bold A. Acquired aplastic anemia: correlation between etiology, pathophysiology, bone marrow histology and prognosis factors. *Rom J Morphol Embryol.* 2009;50(4):669-674.

[52] Molldrem JJ, Jiang YZ, Stetler-Stevenson M, Mavroudis D, Hensel N, Barrett AJ. Haematological response of patients with myelodysplastic syndrome to antithymocyte globulin is associated with a loss of lymphocyte-mediated inhibition of CFU-GM and alterations in T-cell receptor Vbeta profiles. *Br J Haematol.* 1998;102(5):1314-1322.

[53] Kochenderfer JN, Kobayashi S, Wieder ED, Su C, Molldrem JJ. Loss of T-lymphocyte clonal dominance in patients with myelodysplastic syndrome responsive to immunosuppression. *Blood.* 2002;100(10):3639-3645.

[54] Kook H, Zeng W, Guibin C, Kirby M, Young NS, Maciejewski JP. Increased cytotoxic T cells with effector phenotype in aplastic anemia and myelodysplasia. *Exp Hematol*. 2001;29(11):1270-1277.

[55] Baumann I, Scheid C, Koref MS, Swindell R, Stern P, Testa NG. Autologous lymphocytes inhibit hemopoiesis in long-term culture in patients with myelodysplastic syndrome. *Exp Hematol*. 2002;30(12):1405-1411.

[56] Sloand EM, Mainwaring L, Fuhrer M, et al. Preferential suppression of trisomy 8 compared with normal hematopoietic cell growth by autologous lymphocytes in patients with trisomy 8 myelodysplastic syndrome. *Blood*. 2005;106(3):841-851.

[57] Sloand EM, Kim S, Fuhrer M, et al. Fas-mediated apoptosis is important in regulating cell replication and death in trisomy 8 hematopoietic cells but not in cells with other cytogenetic abnormalities. *Blood*. 2002;100(13):4427-4432.

[58] Sloand EM, Melenhorst JJ, Tucker ZC, et al. T-cell immune responses to Wilms tumor 1 protein in myelodysplasia responsive to immunosuppressive therapy. *Blood*. 2011;117(9):2691-2699.

[59] Sloand EM, Pfannes L, Chen G, et al. CD34 cells from patients with trisomy 8 myelodysplastic syndrome (MDS) express early apoptotic markers but avoid programmed cell death by up-regulation of antiapoptotic proteins. *Blood*. 2007;109(6):2399-2405.

[60] Chen G, Zeng W, Miyazato A, et al. Distinctive gene expression profiles of CD34 cells from patients with myelodysplastic syndrome characterized by specific chromosomal abnormalities. *Blood*. 2004;104(13):4210-4218.

[61] Sloand EM, Rezvani K. The role of the immune system in myelodysplasia: implications for therapy. *Semin Hematol*. 2008;45(1):39-48.

[62] Olnes MJ, Sloand EM. Targeting immune dysregulation in myelodysplastic syndromes. *JAMA*. 2011;305(8):814-819.

[63] Sloand EM, Barrett AJ. Immunosuppression for myelodysplastic syndrome: how bench to bedside to bench research led to success. *Hematol Oncol Clin North Am*. 2010;24(2):331-341.

[64] Epling-Burnette PK, Liu JH, Catlett-Falcone R, et al. Inhibition of STAT3 signaling leads to apoptosis of leukemic large granular lymphocytes and decreased Mcl-1 expression. *J Clin Invest*. 2001;107(3):351-362.

[65] Koskela HL, Eldfors S, Ellonen P, et al. Somatic STAT3 mutations in large granular lymphocytic leukemia. *N Engl J Med*. 2012;366(20):1905-1913.

[66] Jerez A, Clemente MJ, Makishima H, et al. STAT3 mutations unify the pathogenesis of chronic lymphoproliferative disorders of NK cells and T cell large granular lymphocyte leukemia. *Blood*. 2012.

[67] Kishimoto T. Signal transduction through homo- or heterodimers of gp130. *Stem Cells*. 1994;12 Suppl 1:37-44; discussion 44-35.

[68] Endo TA, Masuhara M, Yokouchi M, et al. A new protein containing an SH2 domain that inhibits JAK kinases. *Nature.* 1997;387(6636):921-924.

[69] Raz R, Durbin JE, Levy DE. Acute phase response factor and additional members of the interferon-stimulated gene factor 3 family integrate diverse signals from cytokines, interferons, and growth factors. *J Biol Chem.* 1994;269(39):24391-24395.

[70] Starr R, Willson TA, Viney EM, et al. A family of cytokine-inducible inhibitors of signalling. *Nature.* 1997;387(6636):917-921.

[71] Xu X, Kang SH, Heidenreich O, Okerholm M, O'Shea JJ, Nerenberg MI. Constitutive activation of different Jak tyrosine kinases in human T cell leukemia virus type 1 (HTLV-1) tax protein or virus-transformed cells. *J Clin Invest.* 1995;96(3):1548-1555.

[72] Yu CL, Meyer DJ, Campbell GS, et al. Enhanced DNA-binding activity of a Stat3-related protein in cells transformed by the Src oncoprotein. *Science.* 1995;269(5220):81-83.

[73] Takeda K, Kaisho T, Yoshida N, Takeda J, Kishimoto T, Akira S. Stat3 activation is responsible for IL-6-dependent T cell proliferation through preventing apoptosis: generation and characterization of T cell-specific Stat3-deficient mice. *J Immunol.* 1998;161(9):4652-4660.

[74] Rajala HL, Eldfors S, Kuusanmaki H, et al. Discovery of somatic STAT5b mutations in large granular lymphocytic leukemia. *Blood.* 2013;121(22):4541-4550.

[75] Jerez A, Clemente MJ, Makishima H, et al. STAT3 mutations indicate the presence of subclinical T-cell clones in a subset of aplastic anemia and myelodysplastic syndrome patients. *Blood.* 2013;122(14):2453-2459.

[76] Cui W, Liu Y, Weinstein JS, Craft J, Kaech SM. An interleukin-21-interleukin-10-STAT3 pathway is critical for functional maturation of memory CD8[+] T cells. *Immunity.* 2011;35(5):792-805.

[77] Habib T, Nelson A, Kaushansky K. IL-21: a novel IL-2-family lymphokine that modulates B, T, and natural killer cell responses. *J Allergy Clin Immunol.* 2003;112(6):1033-1045.

[78] Ozaki K, Kikly K, Michalovich D, Young PR, Leonard WJ. Cloning of a type I cytokine receptor most related to the IL-2 receptor beta chain. *Proc Natl Acad Sci U S A.* 2000;97(21):11439-11444.

[79] Nielsen M, Svejgaard A, Skov S, Odum N. Interleukin-2 induces tyrosine phosphorylation and nuclear translocation of stat3 in human T lymphocytes. *Eur J Immunol.* 1994;24(12):3082-3086.

[80] Olson JA, Jameson SC. Keeping STATs on memory CD8[+] T cells. *Immunity.* 2011;35(5):663-665.

[81] Siegel AM, Heimall J, Freeman AF, et al. A critical role for STAT3 transcription factor signaling in the development and maintenance of human T cell memory. *Immunity.* 2011;35(5):806-818.

[82] Agarwal A. MDS: roadblock to differentiation. *Blood.* 2012;120(10):1968-1969.

[83] Andersson EI, Rajala HL, Eldfors S, et al. Novel somatic mutations in large granular lymphocytic leukemia affecting the STAT-pathway and T-cell activation. *Blood Cancer J.* 2013;3:e168.

[84] Rajala HL, Porkka K, Maciejewski JP, Loughran TP, Jr., Mustjoki S. Uncovering the pathogenesis of large granular lymphocytic leukemia-novel STAT3 and STAT5b mutations. *Ann Med.* 2014;46(3):114-122.

[85] Chen X, Eksioglu EA, Zhou J, et al. Induction of myelodysplasia by myeloid-derived suppressor cells. *J Clin Invest.* 2013;123(11):4595-4611.

[86] Zoumbos N, Symeonidis A, Kourakli A, et al. Increased levels of soluble interleukin-2 receptors and tumor necrosis factor in serum of patients with myelodysplastic syndromes. *Blood.* 1991;77(2):413-414.

[87] Verhoef GE, De Schouwer P, Ceuppens JL, Van Damme J, Goossens W, Boogaerts MA. Measurement of serum cytokine levels in patients with myelodysplastic syndromes. *Leukemia.* 1992;6(12):1268-1272.

[88] Seipelt G, Ganser A, Duranceyk H, Maurer A, Ottmann OG, Hoelzer D. Induction of TNF-alpha in patients with myelodysplastic syndromes undergoing treatment with interleukin-3. *Br J Haematol.* 1993;84(4):749-751.

[89] Benesch M, Platzbecker U, Ward J, Deeg HJ, Leisenring W. Expression of FLIP(Long) and FLIP(Short) in bone marrow mononuclear and CD34$^+$ cells in patients with myelodysplastic syndrome: correlation with apoptosis. *Leukemia.* 2003;17(12):2460-2466.

[90] Plasilova M, Zivny J, Jelinek J, et al. TRAIL (Apo2L) suppresses growth of primary human leukemia and myelodysplasia progenitors. *Leukemia.* 2002;16(1):67-73.

[91] Koike M, Ishiyama T, Tomoyasu S, Tsuruoka N. Spontaneous cytokine overproduction by peripheral blood mononuclear cells from patients with myelodysplastic syndromes and aplastic anemia. *Leuk Res.* 1995;19(9):639-644.

[92] Koschmieder S, Hofmann WK, Kunert J, et al. TGF beta-induced SMAD2 phosphorylation predicts inhibition of thymidine incorporation in CD34$^+$ cells from healthy donors, but not from patients with AML after MDS. *Leukemia.* 2001;15(6):942-949.

[93] Dong W, Ding T, Wu L, Ren X, Epling-Burnette PK, Yang L. Effect of IL-7 and IL-15 on T cell phenotype in myelodysplastic syndromes. *Oncotarget.* 2016;7(19):27479-27488.

[94] Wu Z, Xue HH, Bernard J, et al. The IL-15 receptor {alpha} chain cytoplasmic domain is critical for normal IL-15R alpha function but is not required for trans-presentation. *Blood.* 2008;112(12):4411-4419.

[95] Noguchi M, Yi H, Rosenblatt HM, et al. Interleukin-2 receptor gamma chain mutation results in X-linked severe combined immunodeficiency in humans. *Cell.* 1993;73(1):147-157.

[96] Ring AM, Lin JX, Feng D, et al. Mechanistic and structural insight into the functional dichotomy between IL-2 and IL-15. *Nat Immunol.* 2012;13(12):1187-1195.

[97] Fehniger TA, Suzuki K, Ponnappan A, et al. Fatal leukemia in interleukin 15 transgenic mice follows early expansions in natural killer and memory phenotype CD8+ T cells. *J Exp Med.* 2001;193(2):219-231.

[98] Fehniger TA, Suzuki K, VanDeusen JB, Cooper MA, Freud AG, Caligiuri MA. Fatal leukemia in interleukin-15 transgenic mice. *Blood Cells Mol Dis.* 2001;27(1):223-230.

[99] Steinway SN, Loughran TP. Targeting IL-15 in large granular lymphocyte leukemia. *Expert Rev Clin Immunol.* 2013;9(5):405-408.

[100] Nguyen ML, Jones SA, Prier JE, Russ BE. Transcriptional Enhancers in the Regulation of T Cell Differentiation. *Front Immunol.* 2015;6:462.

[101] O'Sullivan D, van der Windt GJ, Huang SC, et al. Memory CD8(+) T cells use cell-intrinsic lipolysis to support the metabolic programming necessary for development. *Immunity.* 2014;41(1):75-88.

[102] Zou JX, Rollison DE, Boulware D, et al. Altered naive and memory CD4+ T-cell homeostasis and immunosenescence characterize younger patients with myelodysplastic syndrome. *Leukemia.* 2009;23(7):1288-1296.

[103] Zhang Y, Tian S, Liu Z, et al. Dendritic cell-derived interleukin-15 is crucial for therapeutic cancer vaccine potency. *Oncoimmunology.* 2014;3(10):e959321.

[104] Mishra A, Liu S, Sams GH, et al. Aberrant overexpression of IL-15 initiates large granular lymphocyte leukemia through chromosomal instability and DNA hypermethylation. *Cancer Cell.* 2012;22(5):645-655.

[105] Fehniger TA, Caligiuri MA. Ontogeny and expansion of human natural killer cells: clinical implications. *Int Rev Immunol.* 2001;20(3-4):503-534.

[106] Rochman Y, Spolski R, Leonard WJ. New insights into the regulation of T cells by gamma(c) family cytokines. *Nat Rev Immunol.* 2009;9(7):480-490.

[107] Russell SM, Tayebi N, Nakajima H, et al. Mutation of Jak3 in a patient with SCID: essential role of Jak3 in lymphoid development. *Science.* 1995;270(5237):797-800.

[108] Steinway SN, LeBlanc F, Loughran TP, Jr. The pathogenesis and treatment of large granular lymphocyte leukemia. *Blood Rev.* 2014;28(3):87-94.

[109] Aivado M, Rong A, Stadler M, et al. Favourable response to antithymocyte or antilymphocyte globulin in low-risk myelodysplastic syndrome patients with a

'non-clonal' pattern of X-chromosome inactivation in bone marrow cells. *Eur J Haematol.* 2002;68(4):210-216.

[110] Haider M, Al Ali N, Padron E, et al. Immunosuppressive Therapy: Exploring an Underutilized Treatment Option for Myelodysplastic Syndrome. *Clin Lymphoma Myeloma Leuk.* 2016;16 Suppl:S44-48.

[111] Saunthararajah Y, Nakamura R, Nam JM, et al. HLA-DR15 (DR2) is overrepresented in myelodysplastic syndrome and aplastic anemia and predicts a response to immunosuppression in myelodysplastic syndrome. *Blood.* 2002;100(5):1570-1574.

[112] Stadler M, Germing U, Kliche KO, et al. A prospective, randomised, phase II study of horse antithymocyte globulin vs rabbit antithymocyte globulin as immune-modulating therapy in patients with low-risk myelodysplastic syndromes. *Leukemia.* 2004;18(3):460-465.

[113] Steensma DP, Dispenzieri A, Moore SB, Schroeder G, Tefferi A. Antithymocyte globulin has limited efficacy and substantial toxicity in unselected anemic patients with myelodysplastic syndrome. *Blood.* 2003;101(6):2156-2158.

[114] Sugimori C, List AF, Epling-Burnette PK. Immune dysregulation in myelodysplastic syndrome. *Hematol Rep.* 2010;2(1):e1.

[115] Komrokji RS, Mailloux AW, Chen DT, et al. A phase II multicenter rabbit anti-thymocyte globulin trial in patients with myelodysplastic syndromes identifying a novel model for response prediction. *Haematologica.* 2014;99(7):1176-1183.

[116] Passweg JR, Giagounidis AA, Simcock M, et al. Immunosuppressive therapy for patients with myelodysplastic syndrome: a prospective randomized multicenter phase III trial comparing antithymocyte globulin plus cyclosporine with best supportive care--SAKK 33/99. *J Clin Oncol.* 2011;29(3):303-309.

[117] Luger S, Sacks N. Bone marrow transplantation for myelodysplastic syndrome--who? when? and which? *Bone Marrow Transplant.* 2002;30(4):199-206.

[118] Mohty M. Mechanisms of action of antithymocyte globulin: T-cell depletion and beyond. *Leukemia.* 2007;21(7):1387-1394.

[119] Bonnefoy-Berard N, Vincent C, Revillard JP. Antibodies against functional leukocyte surface molecules in polyclonal antilymphocyte and antithymocyte globulins. *Transplantation.* 1991;51(3):669-673.

[120] Michallet MC, Preville X, Flacher M, Fournel S, Genestier L, Revillard JP. Functional antibodies to leukocyte adhesion molecules in antithymocyte globulins. *Transplantation.* 2003;75(5):657-662.

[121] Zand MS, Vo T, Huggins J, et al. Polyclonal rabbit antithymocyte globulin triggers B-cell and plasma cell apoptosis by multiple pathways. *Transplantation.* 2005;79(11):1507-1515.

[122] Haidinger M, Geyeregger R, Poglitsch M, et al. Antithymocyte globulin impairs T-cell/antigen-presenting cell interaction: disruption of immunological synapse and conjugate formation. *Transplantation*. 2007;84(1):117-121.

[123] Lan F, Zeng D, Higuchi M, Huie P, Higgins JP, Strober S. Predominance of NK1.1+TCR alpha beta+ or DX5+TCR alpha beta+ T cells in mice conditioned with fractionated lymphoid irradiation protects against graft-versus-host disease: "natural suppressor" cells. *J Immunol*. 2001;167(4):2087-2096.

[124] Lopez M, Clarkson MR, Albin M, Sayegh MH, Najafian N. A novel mechanism of action for anti-thymocyte globulin: induction of CD4+CD25+Foxp3+ regulatory T cells. *J Am Soc Nephrol*. 2006;17(10):2844-2853.

[125] Molldrem JJ, Caples M, Mavroudis D, Plante M, Young NS, Barrett AJ. Antithymocyte globulin for patients with myelodysplastic syndrome. *Br J Haematol*. 1997;99(3):699-705.

[126] Molldrem JJ, Leifer E, Bahceci E, et al. Antithymocyte globulin for treatment of the bone marrow failure associated with myelodysplastic syndromes. *Ann Intern Med*. 2002;137(3):156-163.

[127] Yazji S, Giles FJ, Tsimberidou AM, et al. Antithymocyte globulin (ATG)-based therapy in patients with myelodysplastic syndromes. *Leukemia*. 2003;17(11):2101-2106.

[128] Killick SB, Cavenagh JD, Davies JK, Marsh JC. Low dose antithymocyte globulin for the treatment of older patients with aplastic anaemia. *Leuk Res*. 2006;30(12):1517-1520.

[129] Killick SB, Marsh JC, Gordon-Smith EC, Sorlin L, Gibson FM. Effects of antithymocyte globulin on bone marrow CD34+ cells in aplastic anaemia and myelodysplasia. *Br J Haematol*. 2000;108(3):582-591.

[130] Killick SB, Mufti G, Cavenagh JD, et al. A pilot study of antithymocyte globulin (ATG) in the treatment of patients with 'low-risk' myelodysplasia. *Br J Haematol*. 2003;120(4):679-684.

[131] Lim ZY, Killick S, Germing U, et al. Low IPSS score and bone marrow hypocellularity in MDS patients predict hematological responses to antithymocyte globulin. *Leukemia*. 2007;21(7):1436-1441.

[132] Marsh JC, Bacigalupo A, Schrezenmeier H, et al. Prospective study of rabbit antithymocyte globulin and cyclosporine for aplastic anemia from the EBMT Severe Aplastic Anaemia Working Party. *Blood*. 2012;119(23):5391-5396.

[133] Shin SH, Yoon JH, Yahng SA, et al. The efficacy of rabbit antithymocyte globulin with cyclosporine in comparison to horse antithymocyte globulin as a first-line treatment in adult patients with severe aplastic anemia: a single-center retrospective study. *Ann Hematol*. 2013;92(6):817-824.

[134] Frickhofen N, Heimpel H, Kaltwasser JP, Schrezenmeier H, German Aplastic Anemia Study G. Antithymocyte globulin with or without cyclosporin A: 11-year

follow-up of a randomized trial comparing treatments of aplastic anemia. *Blood.* 2003;101(4):1236-1242.

[135] Broliden PA, Dahl IM, Hast R, et al. Antithymocyte globulin and cyclosporine A as combination therapy for low-risk non-sideroblastic myelodysplastic syndromes. *Haematologica.* 2006;91(5):667-670.

[136] Jonasova A, Neuwirtova R, Cermak J, et al. Cyclosporin A therapy in hypoplastic MDS patients and certain refractory anaemias without hypoplastic bone marrow. *Br J Haematol.* 1998;100(2):304-309.

[137] Catalano L, Selleri C, Califano C, et al. Prolonged response to cyclosporin-A in hypoplastic refractory anemia and correlation with in vitro studies. *Haematologica.* 2000;85(2):133-138.

[138] Atoyebi W, Bywater L, Rawlings L, Brunskill S, Littlewood TJ. Treatment of myelodysplasia with oral cyclosporin. *Clin Lab Haematol.* 2002;24(4):211-214.

[139] Chen SC, Jiang B, Da WM, Gong M, Guan M. [Curative effects of cyclosporin A therapy upon myelodysplastic syndrome]. *Zhonghua Yi Xue Za Zhi.* 2006;86(38):2711-2715.

[140] Shimamoto T, Iguchi T, Ando K, et al. Successful treatment with cyclosporin A for myelodysplastic syndrome with erythroid hypoplasia associated with T-cell receptor gene rearrangements. *Br J Haematol.* 2001;114(2):358-361.

[141] Nakao S, Takamatsu H, Chuhjo T, et al. Identification of a specific HLA class II haplotype strongly associated with susceptibility to cyclosporine-dependent aplastic anemia. *Blood.* 1994;84(12):4257-4261.

[142] Kapustin SI, Popova TI, Lyschov AA, Togo AV, Abdulkadyrov KM, Blinov MN. HLA-DR2 Frequency Increase in Severe Aplastic Anemia Patients is Mainly Attributed to the Prevalence of DR15 Subtype. *Pathol Oncol Res.* 1997;3(2):106-108.

[143] Ishikawa T, Tohyama K, Nakao S, et al. A prospective study of cyclosporine A treatment of patients with low-risk myelodysplastic syndrome: presence of CD55(-)CD59(-) blood cells predicts platelet response. *Int J Hematol.* 2007;86(2):150-157.

[144] Kook H, Risitano AM, Zeng W, et al. Changes in T-cell receptor VB repertoire in aplastic anemia: effects of different immunosuppressive regimens. *Blood.* 2002;99(10):3668-3675.

[145] Maciejewski JP, Follmann D, Nakamura R, et al. Increased frequency of HLA-DR2 in patients with paroxysmal nocturnal hemoglobinuria and the PNH/aplastic anemia syndrome. *Blood.* 2001;98(13):3513-3519.

[146] Sloand EM, Wu CO, Greenberg P, Young N, Barrett J. Factors affecting response and survival in patients with myelodysplasia treated with immunosuppressive therapy. *J Clin Oncol.* 2008;26(15):2505-2511.

[147] Parrish-Novak J, Foster DC, Holly RD, Clegg CH. Interleukin-21 and the IL-21 receptor: novel effectors of NK and T cell responses. *J Leukoc Biol.* 2002;72(5):856-863.

[148] Kordasti SY, Afzali B, Lim Z, et al. IL-17-producing CD4$^{(+)}$ T cells, pro-inflammatory cytokines and apoptosis are increased in low risk myelodysplastic syndrome. *Br J Haematol.* 2009;145(1):64-72.

[149] Kordasti SY, Ingram W, Hayden J, et al. CD4$^+$CD25high Foxp3$^+$ regulatory T cells in myelodysplastic syndrome (MDS). *Blood.* 2007;110(3):847-850.

[150] Mailloux AW, Sugimori C, Komrokji RS, et al. Expansion of effector memory regulatory T cells represents a novel prognostic factor in lower risk myelodysplastic syndrome. *J Immunol.* 2012;189(6):3198-3208.

In: Benign and Malignant Disorders …
Editors: Ling Zhang and Lubomir Sokol

ISBN: 978-1-53612-999-1
© 2018 Nova Science Publishers, Inc.

Chapter 5

BENIGN T-LGL AND NK CELL PROLIFERATIONS EVOLVED AFTER HEMATOPOIETIC CELL TRANSPLANTATION, AND ANTI-NEOPLASTIC AGENTS

Taiga Nishihori, MD
Department of Blood and Marrow Transplant and Cellular Immunotherapy,
H. Lee Moffitt Cancer Center and Research Institute, Tampa, FL, US

ABSTRACT

Expansion of large granular lymphocytes(LGL), T- or NK-type, defined as >15% of total peripheral blood mononuclear cells, is not uncommonly associated with post autologous or allogeneic hematopoietic cell transplantation (auto- or allo-HCT), post chemotherapy including cytoreduction and tyrosine kinase inhibitors, and post immunotherapy for various benign or malignant disorders. Increased LGL count after allo-HCT is considered a normal immune response to alloantigen exposure, viral infection or reactivation, or the immune reconstitution following lymphodepletion. An increase of LGL count post auto-HCT is likely due to T-cell stimulation. Reactive LGL proliferations secondary to dasatinib therapy in Philadelphia chromosome positive chronic myelogenous leukemia (CML) and acute lymphoblastic leukemia is mostly NK cell lineage but the exact mechanisms underlying the proliferation of clonal LGLs have not been fully understood. Expanded LGL population due to aging might be attributed to putative extrinsic or intrinsic antigen stimulation. The mechanisms of T- or NK-cell expansion following immunotherapy or immunomodulation could be complex and might depend on their response to activated or inhibited signaling pathways. Nevertheless, the expansion of LGLs is regarded as a benign process in the aforementioned setting, unlike T-LGL leukemia (LGLL), and no therapeutic intervention is necessary.

1. INTRODUCTION

Large granular lymphocytes (LGL) typically refer to the lymphoid proliferation of either T-cell or natural killer (NK)-cell lineages [1]. In healthy individuals, LGLs are a minor population of peripheral blood mononuclear cells. T-cell LGLs (CD3+CD8+) are mature post-thymic, antigen-experienced cytotoxic T-cells, and NK-cell LGLs are those surface CD3-CD56+ cells that belong to the innate immune system [2]. LGLs likely represent approximately 10% to 15% of the total peripheral blood mononuclear cells in healthy individuals [1]. Most LGL-associated lymphoproliferative conditions may be known as T-cell leukemia (LGLL), however, several benign LGL-associated conditions have also been described after chemotherapy, immunotherapy, and transplantation. Aging related LGL increase has also been documented although the exact mechanisms are not clear. In this chapter, benign LGL expansions following medical interventions and conditions are described and reviewed. LGLL occurring after transplantation as a part of the post-transplant lymphoproliferative disorder (PTLD) is not covered [3-7]. Detailed immunophenotyping of LGLLs is described elsewhere in this book. Benign expansion of LGLs typically refers to the identification of CD3+CD8+CD57+ T-cell LGL or CD2+CD3-CD16+CD56+ NK cell population with negative T-cell receptor (TCR) gene rearrangement studies.

2. LGL EXPANSIONS AFTER HEMATOPOIETIC CELL TRANSPLANTATION

2.1. Following Allogeneic Hematopoietic Cell Transplantation

Expansion of LGL population following hematopoietic cell transplantation (HCT) has been reported in numerous studies; however, a development of definitive malignant clonal LGL disorder has not been described. Gorochov et al. described nine HCT recipients where CD8+CD57+ cells expanded to >15% of their total peripheral blood lymphocytes [8]. This study showed a restricted use of Vβ segments where Vβ16 and Vβ17 were overexpressed in the CD8+CD57+ cells in six out of 9 patients and there was an oligoclonal pattern observed on the αβ TCR gene rearrangement studies [8]. In another study, Dolstra et al. reported that the early repopulation of CD8+CD57+ T-cells expressing the αβ TCR in the peripheral blood was associated with lower risk of leukemia relapse in recipients of lymphocyte-depleted bone marrow allografts [9]. However, those patients also had a higher incidence of cytomegalovirus (CMV) infection [9]. This report did not include TCR gene rearrangement studies [9].

Mohty et al. reviewed six cases of LGL expansion in 201 consecutive patients (approximately 3%) undergoing allogeneic HCT in France [10]. Those with absolute lymphocyte count > 2 x 10^9/L with LGL features (expressing CD57) were retained in their study [10]. Expansion of LGL was seen between 3 and 15 months following allogeneic HCT [10]. LGL expansions were more commonly found in patients receiving reduced intensity conditioning with recurrent viral infections, especially CMV, and also in those who achieved complete response (CR) after allogeneic HCT (in five of six patients) [10]. Of these patients, two developed severe neutropenia and one experienced autoimmune hemolytic anemia requiring treatment. It was not clear whether these LGL expansions were polyclonal or oligoclonal [10].

In a single center study from Switzerland, Nann-Rutti et al. evaluated LGL expansions in 215 allogeneic HCT recipients. Those with persistent lymphocytosis (> 3.0 x 10^9/L for more than 3 months) and abnormal CD4/CD8 ratios (defined as CD4/CD8 ratio < 1 or CD4/CD8 > 1.5) underwent extensive immunophenotyping of the peripheral blood [11]. T-LGL expansion was defined as the presence of an abnormal T-cell population with CD3+CD8+ or CD3+CD4+ with expression of at least 1 of the NK markers (CD16, CD57, or CD56), and with the presence of LGLs on the peripheral blood films [11]. Fourteen patients (7%) developed LGL expansions 13 of them expressed CD8, and 5 demonstrated clonal TCR-γ rearrangement [11]. The lymphocytes appeared at a median of 16 months (range, 3-58 months) after allogeneic HCT and interestingly lasted for a median of 31 months (range, 2-179 months) [11]. CMV reactivation ($P = 0.001$) and acute graft-versus-host disease (GVHD) were associated with LGL expansion ($P = 0.02$) [11]. In the multivariate analysis, only CMV reactivation showed a significant association with T-LGL expansion (relative risk 5.063, $P = 0.006$) [11].

Kim et al. from Princess Margaret Hospital in Canada evaluated 418 patients for large granular lymphocytosis after allogeneic HCT [12]. They defined LGL lymphocytosis as the presence of at least two of the following criteria: (a) sustained lymphocytosis > 3.0 x 10^9/L at least observed on three consecutive occasions over 2-3 months, (b) > 30% LGLs in peripheral blood, (c) confirmation of monoclonality by TCR gene analysis using polymerase chain reaction (PCR). Seventy-seven patients (18.4%) developed LGL lymphocytosis with a median of 312 days (range, 26-1840 days) [12]. The incidence of LGL lymphocytosis increased over time with a cumulative incidence of 23.6% at 3 years. This study demonstrated that patients with LGL lymphocytosis had better overall survival (OS) (86.2% vs. 53.8%, $P < 0.001$), lower non-relapse mortality (NRM) (3.2 vs. 27.3%, $P < 0.001$) and lower relapse rate (9.6 vs. 29.4%, $P < 0.001$) [12]. There were three clinical factors associated with LGL lymphocytosis: (a) CMV seropositive recipients regardless of donor CMV serological status, (b) CMV reactivation and (c) chronic GVHD [12]. This study showed favorable outcomes in recipients with LGL lymphocytosis after allogeneic HCT [12].

In a recent study, Munoz-Ballester et al. from Spain evaluated peripheral expansion of cytotoxic T lymphocytes (CTL) derived from the graft in 154 recipients of allogeneic HCT where lymphocyte subpopulation was available for analysis and unmanipulated graft was infused [13]. When a persistent CTL expansion was observed together with a higher CD8+/CD4+ ratio (> 1.5), then it was termed *"relative cytotoxic T-lymphocyte expansion, CTLe"* and when a number of CD8+ cells was > 2 x 10^9/L, then it was called *"absolute cytotoxic T-lymphocytes expansion, CTLe"* [13]. A persistence (> 6 months) of CD8+/CD4+ ratio > 1.5 was noted in 75 out of 154 patients (48%: *relative CTLe*) and 14 patients (9%) had *absolute CTLe* with CD57 expressed invariably in *CTLe* cases [13]. Persistence of *relative CTLe* was more frequently seen with thymoglobulin prophylaxis, acute GVHD and reduced intensity conditioning. *Absolute CTLe* was associated with chronic GVHD [13]. All 14 cases of *absolute CLTe* patients had clonal TCR rearrangement [13]. Somatic mutations in the SH2 dimerization and activation domain of signal transducer and activator of transcription 3 (*STAT3*) were identified in 30% to 40% of LGL leukemias of both NK- and T-cell lineages [14, 15]. *STAT3* exon 21 mutations were assessed with negative result supporting the benign nature of the post allo-HCT lymphocytosis [13].

Thymic-independent peripheral expansion of CD8+ T cells derived from the donor stem cell graft during the initial recovery phase after allogeneic HCT has been well documented. The study by Munoz-Ballester concluded that the presence of CD8+ T-cells with increased CD8+/CD4+ ratio was more frequent than previously thought. Due to the differences in the definition of LGL expansions in reported studies, the true incidence of LGL expansion after allogeneic HCT is not known, though these studies reported approximately 10% to 20% occurrence. Additionally, these observations suggested that LGL appearing after allogeneic HCT might have chronic and indolent presentation with persistence. The driving force behind generation of LGLs in allograft recipients remains somewhat unclear. However, it was postulated that the alloantigen exposure and viral reactivation, in addition to the immune reconstitution following lymphodepletion conditioning regimen especially in long-term, might play a role in the LGL expansion derived from graft [10-12]. The presence of LGL expansions might be associated with better allogeneic HCT outcomes implicating potential of the graft-versus-tumor effects [12]. Although earlier studies reported a few cases of autoimmune conditions associated with LGL expansion, subsequent studies did not seem to replicate this observation. Generally speaking, the persistence of LGL expansion after allogeneic HCT is a benign condition and does not herald the future development of LGLL. Monitoring of LGL after allogeneic HCT is not performed routinely and further study to elucidate its role in immune reconstitution would be necessary.

2.2. Following Autologous Hematopoietic Cell Transplantation

Expansion of LGLs after autologous HCT has also been described [16]. Wolniak et al. evaluated 20 multiple myeloma patients undergoing autologous HCT and showed that the LGLs were increased in HCT recipients between days 45 and 90 with an average of 590/μL (range, 164-3,225/μL) as compared to 195/μL (range, 50-340/μL) for myeloma patients without autologous HCT [17]. In the bone marrow aspirate, flow cytometric relative quantification of the CD8+ cells showed that the percentage of CD8+ cells was increased and within the CD8+ population, the proportion of CD57+ cells was also significantly increased compared to control (39% vs. 18%) [17]. Immunophenotyping of the LGLs showed predominant subtype of CD5+/CD8+/CD57partial+/CD56dim+/CD16-/TIA-1+ LGLs with negative granzyme B [17]. It appears that these expanded LGLs persisted at least for 4 years in some cases with no demonstrable morphologic increase in peripheral blood [17]. It suggests that LGLs may initially expand into the peripheral blood compartment but they would subsequently remain in the bone marrow niche. In the TCR gene rearrangement analysis, 65% of patients had clonal TCR in the marrow aspirate [17]. There were no clear correlations with LGL expansion and clinical outcomes such as neutropenia and infections in the post autologous HCT setting.

Maggi et al. made a unique observation where torquetenovirus (TTV) viremia after autologous HCT correlated with CD8+CD57+ viremia [18]. TTV is a non-enveloped virus with a small single-stranded circular DNA genome, which belongs to the *Anellovirus* genus [18]. Chronic TTV viremia is extremely common and about 90% of all population have the condition [18]. The authors evaluated 19 consecutive multiple myeloma patients undergoing tandem autologous HCT with high-dose melphalan. Serum TTV viral load using PCR was assessed along with circulating CD8+CD57+ T lymphocytes [18]. TTV viremia at day +70 was approximately 2 log higher than at baseline and at day +40, and this was sustained at day +100 [18]. CD8+CD57+ T lymphocyte percentage was over 20% at day +40 and this further increased to 25% at day +100 which correlated with TTV viremia [18]. The significance of this correlation is unknown but it is suggested that it might help to assess the functional immune status after autologous HCT.

The mechanisms of LGL expansion following autologous HCT remain unclear as there is no alloantigen exposure in the autologous setting. It is possible that the LGL expansion may result from the T-cell immune reconstitution and expansion following HCT [19]. The phenotype of CD8+ LGLs could be similar to pre-existing cytotoxic T cells and lymphodepletion by autologous HCT may facilitate the clonal expansion of this cell population. The clinical implication of LGL expansion following autologous HCT requires additional studies. It is crucial to determine whether LGL expansions after HCT are neoplastic or reactive as it would change the therapeutic decisions. LGLL requires treatment in majority of patients but benign LGL expansion after HCT without evidence of PTLD or leukemia could be observed without specific interventions.

3. LGL EXPANSIONS AFTER TYROSINE KINASE INHIBITORS OR OTHER ANTI-NEOPLASTIC AGENTS

3.1. Following Tyrosine Kinase Inhibitor (TKI) Therapy

Some chemotherapy agents have been associated with the development of LGL expansion after administration. Dasatinib, a dual tyrosine kinase inhibitor (TKI), is known to modulate T-cell activation and proliferation. Dasatinib therapy associated LGL lymphocytosis have been well described [20-26]. Kim et al. reported a series of eight patients (chronic myeloid leukemia (CML) = 7 and Philadelphia chromosome (Ph) positive acute lymphoblastic leukemia (ALL) = 1) receiving dasatinib who developed LGL lymphocytosis. They defined LGL lymphocytosis as (a) lymphocytes > 3×10^9/L for at least 3 months and (b) predominance of LGLs in the peripheral blood smear samples [27]. The median onset was 4 months after the initiation of dasatinib therapy (range, 1.5-15 months) and the median duration was 9 months (range, 6-24 months) [27]. None of these patients had symptoms suggestive of LGLL, and immunophenotype suggested NK-cell lineage in seven and NK/T-cell type in one [27]. LGL expansion persisted in four patients who had optimal molecular responses compared to those who did not develop LGL [27]. In the NK cell cytotoxicity testing with ^{51}Cr release assays using two types of target cells (K562 cells, a BCR/ABL1 positive blastic phase cell line) and T2 cells (an acute lymphoblastic cell line expressing HLA-A2) with negatively selected NK cells expressing the CD16+/CD56+/CD3- phenotype as effector cells, NK cells exhibited moderate to high cytotoxic effects, especially against T2 cell lines, compared to NK cells from healthy donors [27].

This observation was replicated by many different groups. Mustjoki et al. identified 22 patients with Ph+ leukemia receiving dasatinib who developed marked lymphoproliferation with a median of 3 months from the start of dasatinib therapy [28]. Fifteen patients had a cytotoxic T-cell and seven had NK-cell immunophenotype [28]. All T-cell expansions were clonal based on TCR-γ/δ gene rearrangement analysis [28].

Of note, colitis and pleuritis were common (18 out of 22 patients) which were preceded by LGL lymphocytosis [28]. Further workup also uncovered that identical cytotoxic T cells were identified in pleural effusion and colonic biopsy [28]. Similar to the prior study, development of LGL lymphocytosis was associated with long-lasting remission [28]. These findings were intriguing and suggested the development of aberrant immune reactivity in the context of dasatinib exposure but they were associated with distinct adverse events.

This finding was expanded by evaluating the presence of LGL at diagnosis of CML and during therapy with dasatinib in 34 CML patients [29]. Surprisingly, 15 out of 18 patients (83%) had a sizeable clonal, BCR-ABL1 negative lymphocyte population with TCR rearrangements [29]. The same clone persisted in most of imatinib treated patients; however, the clone markedly expanded with dasatinib therapy resulted in absolute lymphocytosis [29]. Most LGL expansion was seen with TCR δ rearrangements and TCR δ clones were confined to γδ+ T-cell or NK-cell compartments while TCR γ clones were confined to CD4+/CD8+ αβ+ fractions [29].

Ito et al. reported nine patients with Ph+ALL who relapsed after allogeneic HCT and received dasatinib for their treatment [30]. Six out of nine patients developed marked increase in LGLs but all six patients discontinued dasatinib due to adverse events [30]. Four patients were able to resume dasatinib and three remained alive in molecular remission with persistent LGL lymphocytosis [30]. Immunophenotype of LGL population (n = 3) was CD3-CD16+CD56+ NK cell type [30]. This study illustrates the potential impact of dasatinib on allogeneic HCT recipients where both conditions may contribute to the increased frequency of LGL lymphocytosis.

LGL expansion rarely happens with other TKIs, and broader spectrum inhibitory effect of dasatinib on the kinome may contribute to the development of LGL rather specifically after dasatinib exposure. It was hypothesized that TKI therapy may restore the function and proliferative capacity of NK cells while CML cells could produce reactive oxygen species with inhibitory effects on NK cells [31], leading to profoundly inhibited function and decreased number of NK cells [32, 33]. Dasatinib might also directly activate or modulate the proliferation and function of LGLs as several SRC kinases (such as Fyn, Lck, Btk, Tec, EphB4, Hck, Zak, and Src) are involved in the regulation of NK cells. Additionally, imatinib, another TKI, can also induce NK cell activation and it has been shown to correlative with enhanced response against gastrointestinal stromal tumors [34]. Observations that CD4+CD25+FOXP3+ regulatory T-cells are reduced in patients with LGL lymphocytosis receiving dasatinib could also suggest potential mechanisms explaining the favorable responses with dasatinib in these patients [28, 35].

In vivo and *in vitro* studies demonstrated that dasatinib has the potential to modulate the immune response by T- or NK cells [36, 37]. A subsequent LGL expansion is predominantly found in CMV seropositive patients who were treated with dasatinib [38]. However, detectable CMV reactivation was only noted in a small population of such patients [23]. It was postulated that CMV herein might play an essential role in T- or NK-cell proliferation process. A recent study from Ishiyama et al. proved the hypothesis by using principal component analysis in dasatinib induced LGL cases [39]. The study suggested that a subset of NK cells, which was CMV associated, was attributed to dasatinib-induced LGL expansion through subclinical CMV reactivation [39].

As LGL lymphocytosis was seen in some patients with adverse events while receiving dasatinib (including pleural effusion and colitis), close attention and careful evaluation of these patients are required while they receive dasatinib. Besides aforementioned CMV reactivation, precise mechanisms underlying the proliferation of clonal LGLs in patients receiving dasatinib have not been fully elucidated and further clinical and laboratory research is needed to uncover molecular mechanisms including the association with viral infections and genetic predisposition.

3.2. Following Other Anti-Neoplastic and Biologic Agents

There are other anti-neoplastic therapies and biologic agents associated with LGL expansion. Rituximab, a genetically engineered, chimeric, monoclonal antibody directed against the CD20 B-cell antigen, has been reported to cause late-onset neutropenia when used either alone or in combination with other chemotherapeutic agents [40, 41]. Some suggested the possibility of suppression of neutrophils by LGLs as a mechanism for late-onset neutropenia [42]. Papadaki et al. described two cases of late-onset neutropenia following rituximab therapy in patients who had evidence of LGLs in the peripheral blood and bone marrow [42]. These LGLs were CD3+CD8+CD57+ and CD28-. The direct causation of LGL and late-onset neutropenia following rituximab cannot be proven, but it is possible that LGL expansion in the context of hemostatic proliferation may follow rituximab administration.

In a single case report, Theodoridou described a patient with rheumatoid arthritis who was treated with adalimumab, a tumor necrosis factor alpha (TNFα) inhibitor, and developed a prolonged neutropenia in the setting of reversible LGL expansion [43]. The LGLs noted were predominantly CD3+CD8+CD7+CD56- cells and were polyclonal based on specific TCR αβ+ monoclonal antibodies [43]. This report suggests the potential role of the expanded T-LGL population in the pathogenesis of anti-TNF-induced neutropenia. Covach et al. reported additional 2 patients with autoimmune disorders (rheumatoid arthritis and HLA-B27 associated spondyloarthropathy) who received adalimumab and developed CD4+ LGL lymphocytosis [44]. In one of the cases, gene rearrangement analysis of TCR γ by PCR showed a monoclonal amplicon within a polyclonal background [44]. These T-LGLs were composed of CD4+ T cells that coexpressed dim CD8 but lacked CD56 expression [44]. It is speculated that TNF-α inhibition may be shifting the T-cell selection pressure in patients with underlying autoimmune disorders to favor development of a CD4+ T-LGL population.

Use of methotrexate is an independent risk factor of development of lymphoproliferative disorders in patients with rheumatoid arthritis [45]. Ureshino et al.

reported a case of rheumatoid arthritis and the development of transient LGL lymphocytosis induced by methotrexate withdrawal following the spontaneous regression of methotrexate-related lymphoproliferative disorder (i.e., diffuse large B cell lymphoma in this case) [46]. The predominant LGLs were CD8+ and a southern blot analysis of both bone marrow and peripheral blood cells revealed the presence of monoclonal TCR-β gene rearrangement [46]. They speculated that withdrawal of methotrexate raised the plasma levels of interleukin-6 (IL-6), and increased IL-6 activated *STAT3*, thus leading to LGL lymphocytosis through the inhibition of apoptosis [47]. It is also thought that the occurrence of T-LGL lymphocytosis is a favorable prognostic factor in patients with methotrexate-related lymphoproliferative disorder.

Additionally, various other hematologic malignancies have been associated with occurrence of LGL lymphocytosis after different anti-neoplastic treatments. A refractory multiple myeloma patient who received lenalidomide and low-dose dexamethasone was reported to be associated with increased LGLs [48]. In this patient, LGLs were present up to 8% in the peripheral blood prior to treatment and LGLs increased to 40% following lenalidomide treatment [48]. In this case, LGLs had NK-cell phenotype with CD16 and CD56 expression, and TCR β gene rearrangement was not detected by PCR [48]. Although lenalidomide has been known to possess the immunomodulatory property, the exact mechanisms facilitating the LGL lymphocytosis in this context remains to be elucidated. Reda et al. reported a case of acute promyelocytic leukemia (APL) with neutropenia following treatment with multiple chemotherapeutic agents including all-trans retinoic acid and mitoxantrone [49]. The patient subsequently developed CD8+ T-LGL lymphocytosis and complete remission was maintained for 21 months after completing chemotherapy [49]. In retrospect, there was approximately 10% T-LGL infiltrate in the bone marrow at the time of APL diagnosis but it was missed initially [49]. It was postulated that anti-APL chemotherapy may have conferred a growth advantage and possibly led to LGL clone expansion.

4. LGL EXPANSION WITH AGE

Non-malignant clonal CD8-αβ-T-cell expansions are relatively common phenomenon in elder population. In some studies, expansion of CD8+ T-cells with restricted clonality was observed in one third of total population over the age of 65 years [50]. Increased clonal restriction of CD8+ T-cells in turn correlates with reduced proportions of naïve CD8+ T-cells as well as reversed CD4/CD8 ratio in these population [51]. For γδ-T-cells, increased proportions have undergone previous activation [52] and a total number of γδ-T-cells was lower with increasing age [53]. The development of T-cell expansion may result from immune senescence and could be associated with life time exposure to infections though no clear common antigen specificity has been observed. Aging have likely some impact on intrinsic CD8+ T-cell molecular alternations coupled with extrinsic factors such as infections. This observation has implications in understanding the development of LGL expansion after certain medical interventions including HCT and chemotherapy where additional extrinsic or antigen stimulation may be introduced to the immune system.

REFERENCES

[1] Loughran TP. Clonal diseases of large granular lymphocytes. *Blood.* 1993;82(1):1-14.
[2] Alekshun TJ, Sokol L. Diseases of large granular lymphocytes. *Cancer Control.* 2007;14(2):141-150.
[3] Swerdlow SH. T-cell and NK-cell posttransplantation lymphoproliferative disorders. *Am J Clin Pathol.* 2007;127(6):887-895.
[4] Hanson MN, Morrison VA, Peterson BA, et al. Posttransplant T-cell lymphoproliferative disorders--an aggressive, late complication of solid-organ transplantation. *Blood.* 1996;88(9):3626-3633.
[5] Natkunam Y, Warnke RA, Zehnder JL, Cornbleet PJ. Aggressive natural killer-like T-cell malignancy with leukemic presentation following solid organ transplantation. *Am J Clin Pathol.* 1999;111(5):663-671.
[6] Tiede C, Maecker-Kolhoff B, Klein C, Kreipe H, Hussein K. Risk factors and prognosis in T-cell posttransplantation lymphoproliferative diseases: reevaluation of 163 cases. *Transplantation.* 2013;95(3):479-488.
[7] Kwong YL, Lam CC, Chan TM. Post-transplantation lymphoproliferative disease of natural killer cell lineage: a clinicopathological and molecular analysis. *Br J Haematol.* 2000;110(1):197-202.
[8] Gorochov G, Debré P, Leblond V, Sadat-Sowti B, Sigaux F, Autran B. Oligoclonal expansion of CD8+ CD57+ T cells with restricted T-cell receptor beta chain variability after bone marrow transplantation. *Blood.* 1994;83(2):587-595.
[9] Dolstra H, Preijers F, Van de Wiel-van Kemenade E, Schattenberg A, Galama J, de Witte T. Expansion of CD8+CD57+ T cells after allogeneic BMT is related with a low incidence of relapse and with cytomegalovirus infection. *Br J Haematol.* 1995;90(2):300-307.
[10] Mohty M, Faucher C, Vey N, et al. Features of large granular lymphocytes (LGL) expansion following allogeneic stem cell transplantation: a long-term analysis. *Leukemia.* 2002;16(10):2129-2133.
[11] Nann-Rütti S, Tzankov A, Cantoni N, et al. Large granular lymphocyte expansion after allogeneic hematopoietic stem cell transplant is associated with a

cytomegalovirus reactivation and shows an indolent outcome. *Biol Blood Marrow Transplant*. 2012;18(11):1765-1770.

[12] Kim D, Al-Dawsari G, Chang H, et al. Large granular lymphocytosis and its impact on long-term clinical outcomes following allo-SCT. *Bone Marrow Transplant*. 2013;48(8):1104-1111.

[13] Muñoz-Ballester J, Chen-Liang TH, Hurtado AM, et al. Persistent cytotoxic T lymphocyte expansions after allogeneic haematopoietic stem cell transplantation: kinetics, clinical impact and absence of STAT3 mutations. *Br J Haematol*. 2016;172(6):937-946.

[14] Jerez A, Clemente MJ, Makishima H, et al. STAT3 mutations unify the pathogenesis of chronic lymphoproliferative disorders of NK cells and T-cell large granular lymphocyte leukemia. *Blood*. 2012;120(15):3048-3057.

[15] Koskela HL, Eldfors S, Ellonen P, et al. Somatic STAT3 mutations in large granular lymphocytic leukemia. *N Engl J Med*. 2012;366(20):1905-1913.

[16] Sajeva MR, Greco MM, Cascavilla N, et al. Effective autologous peripheral blood stem cell transplantation in plasma cell leukemia followed by T-large granular lymphocyte expansion: a case report. *Bone Marrow Transplant*. 1996;18(1):225-227.

[17] Wolniak KL, Goolsby CL, Chen YH, et al. Expansion of a clonal CD8+CD57+ large granular lymphocyte population after autologous stem cell transplant in multiple myeloma. *Am J Clin Pathol*. 2013;139(2):231-241.

[18] Maggi F, Fabrizio M, Ricci V, et al. Changes In CD8+57+ T lymphocyte expansions after autologous hematopoietic stem cell transplantation correlate with changes in torquetenovirus viremia. *Transplantation*. 2008;85(12):1867-1868.

[19] Porter DL, June CH. T-cell reconstitution and expansion after hematopoietic stem cell transplantation: 'T' it up! *Bone Marrow Transplant*. 2005;35(10):935-942.

[20] Qiu ZY, Xu W, Li JY. Large granular lymphocytosis during dasatinib therapy. *Cancer Biol Ther*. 2014;15(3):247-255.

[21] Paydas S. Dasatinib, large granular lymphocytosis, and pleural effusion: useful or adverse effect? *Crit Rev Oncol Hematol*. 2014;89(2):242-247.

[22] Nagata Y, Ohashi K, Fukuda S, Kamata N, Akiyama H, Sakamaki H. Clinical features of dasatinib-induced large granular lymphocytosis and pleural effusion. *Int J Hematol*. 2010;91(5):799-807.

[23] Tanaka H, Nakashima S, Usuda M. Rapid and sustained increase of large granular lymphocytes and rare cytomegalovirus reactivation during dasatinib treatment in chronic myelogenous leukemia patients. *Int J Hematol*. 2012;96(3):308-319.

[24] Valent JN, Schiffer CA. Prevalence of large granular lymphocytosis in patients with chronic myelogenous leukemia (CML) treated with dasatinib. *Leuk Res*. 2011;35(1):e1-3.

[25] Lee SJ, Jung CW, Kim DY, et al. Retrospective multicenter study on the development of peripheral lymphocytosis following second-line dasatinib therapy for chronic myeloid leukemia. *Am J Hematol*. 2011;86(4):346-350.

[26] Powers JJ, Dubovsky JA, Epling-Burnette PK, et al. A molecular and functional analysis of large granular lymphocyte expansions in patients with chronic myelogenous leukemia treated with tyrosine kinase inhibitors. *Leuk Lymphoma*. 2011;52(4):668-679.

[27] Kim DH, Kamel-Reid S, Chang H, et al. Natural killer or natural killer/T cell lineage large granular lymphocytosis associated with dasatinib therapy for Philadelphia chromosome positive leukemia. *Haematologica*. 2009;94(1):135-139.

[28] Mustjoki S, Ekblom M, Arstila TP, et al. Clonal expansion of T/NK-cells during tyrosine kinase inhibitor dasatinib therapy. *Leukemia*. 2009;23(8):1398-1405.

[29] Kreutzman A, Juvonen V, Kairisto V, et al. Mono/oligoclonal T and NK cells are common in chronic myeloid leukemia patients at diagnosis and expand during dasatinib therapy. *Blood*. 2010;116(5):772-782.

[30] Ito Y, Miyamoto T, Kamimura T, et al. Characteristics of patients with development of large granular lymphocyte expansion among dasatinib-treated patients with relapsed Philadelphia chromosome-positive acute lymphoblastic leukemia after allogeneic stem cell transplantation. *Clin Lymphoma Myeloma Leuk*. 2015;15(3):e47-54.

[31] Mellqvist UH, Hansson M, Brune M, Dahlgren C, Hermodsson S, Hellstrand K. Natural killer cell dysfunction and apoptosis induced by chronic myelogenous leukemia cells: role of reactive oxygen species and regulation by histamine. *Blood*. 2000;96(5):1961-1968.

[32] Chang WC, Hsiao MH, Pattengale PK. Natural killer cell immunodeficiency in patients with chronic myelogenous leukemia. IV. Interleukin-1 deficiency, gamma-interferon deficiency and the restorative effects of short-term culture in the presence of interleukin-2 on natural killer cytotoxicity, natural killer-target binding and production of natural killer cytotoxic factor. *Nat Immun Cell Growth Regul*. 1991;10(2):57-70.

[33] Pierson BA, Miller JS. CD56+bright and CD56+dim natural killer cells in patients with chronic myelogenous leukemia progressively decrease in number, respond less to stimuli that recruit clonogenic natural killer cells, and exhibit decreased proliferation on a per cell basis. *Blood*. 1996;88(6):2279-2287.

[34] Borg C, Terme M, Taïeb J, et al. Novel mode of action of c-kit tyrosine kinase inhibitors leading to NK cell-dependent antitumor effects. *J Clin Invest*. 2004;114(3):379-388.

[35] Rohon P, Porkka K, Mustjoki S. Immunoprofiling of patients with chronic myeloid leukemia at diagnosis and during tyrosine kinase inhibitor therapy. *Eur J Haematol*. 2010;85(5):387-398.

[36] Fraser CK, Blake SJ, Diener KR, et al. Dasatinib inhibits recombinant viral antigen-specific murine CD4+ and CD8+ T-cell responses and NK-cell cytolytic activity in vitro and in vivo. *Exp Hematol.* 2009;37(2):256-265.

[37] Uchiyama T, Sato N, Narita M, et al. Direct effect of dasatinib on proliferation and cytotoxicity of natural killer cells in in vitro study. *Hematol Oncol.* 2013;31(3):156-163.

[38] Kreutzman A, Ladell K, Koechel C, et al. Expansion of highly differentiated CD8+ T-cells or NK-cells in patients treated with dasatinib is associated with cytomegalovirus reactivation. *Leukemia.* 2011;25(10):1587-1597.

[39] Ishiyama K, Kitawaki T, Sugimoto N, et al. Principal component analysis uncovers cytomegalovirus-associated NK cell activation in Ph(+) leukemia patients treated with dasatinib. *Leukemia.* 2017;31(1):203-212.

[40] Voog E, Morschhauser F, Solal-Céligny P. Neutropenia in patients treated with rituximab. *N Engl J Med.* 2003;348(26):2691-2694; discussion 2691-2694.

[41] Lai GG, Lim ST, Tao M, Chan A, Li H, Quek R. Late-onset neutropenia following RCHOP chemotherapy in diffuse large B-cell lymphoma. *Am J Hematol.* 2009;84(7):414-417.

[42] Papadaki T, Stamatopoulos K, Stavroyianni N, Paterakis G, Phisphis M, Stefanoudaki-Sofianatou K. Evidence for T-large granular lymphocyte-mediated neutropenia in Rituximab-treated lymphoma patients: report of two cases. *Leuk Res.* 2002;26(6):597-600.

[43] Theodoridou A, Kartsios C, Yiannaki E, Markala D, Settas L. Reversible T-large granular lymphocyte expansion and neutropenia associated with adalimumab therapy. *Rheumatol Int.* 2006;27(2):201-202.

[44] Covach A, Leith CP, Rajguru SA, Yang DT. A unique CD4+ large granular lymphocytosis occurring in patients treated with tumor necrosis factor α inhibitors: report of 2 cases. *Hum Pathol.* 2015;46(8):1237-1241.

[45] Wolfe F, Michaud K. Lymphoma in rheumatoid arthritis: the effect of methotrexate and anti-tumor necrosis factor therapy in 18,572 patients. *Arthritis Rheum.* 2004;50(6):1740-1751.

[46] Ureshino H, Kadota C, Kurogi K, Miyahara M, Kimura S. Spontaneous Regression of Methotrexate-related Lymphoproliferative Disorder with T-cell Large Granular Lymphocytosis. *Intern Med.* 2015;54(17):2235-2239.

[47] Schade AE, Wlodarski MW, Maciejewski JP. Pathophysiology defined by altered signal transduction pathways: the role of JAK-STAT and PI3K signaling in leukemic large granular lymphocytes. *Cell Cycle.* 2006;5(22):2571-2574.

[48] Hashiguchi M, Okamura T, Nomura K, et al. A case of refractory multiple myeloma with proliferation of large granular lymphocytes by lenalidomide treatment and its association with clinical efficacy. *Mol Clin Oncol.* 2016;4(4):574-578.

[49] Reda G, Fattizzo B, Cassin R, et al. Multifactorial neutropenia in a patient with acute promyelocytic leukemia and associated large granular lymphocyte expansion: A case report. *Oncol Lett*. 2017;13(3):1307-1310.

[50] Ricalton NS, Roberton C, Norris JM, Rewers M, Hamman RF, Kotzin BL. Prevalence of CD8+ T-cell expansions in relation to age in healthy individuals. *J Gerontol A Biol Sci Med Sci*. 1998;53(3):B196-203.

[51] Effros RB, Dagarag M, Spaulding C, Man J. The role of CD8+ T-cell replicative senescence in human aging. *Immunol Rev*. 2005;205:147-157.

[52] Re F, Poccia F, Donnini A, Bartozzi B, Bernardini G, Provinciali M. Skewed representation of functionally distinct populations of Vgamma9Vdelta2 T lymphocytes in aging. *Exp Gerontol*. 2005;40(1-2):59-66.

[53] Argentati K, Re F, Donnini A, et al. Numerical and functional alterations of circulating gammadelta T lymphocytes in aged people and centenarians. *J Leukoc Biol*. 2002;72(1):65-71.

In: Benign and Malignant Disorders …
Editors: Ling Zhang and Lubomir Sokol

ISBN: 978-1-53612-999-1
© 2018 Nova Science Publishers, Inc.

Chapter 6

ROUTINE DIAGNOSTIC APPROACHES OF T-CELL LARGE GRANULAR LYMPHOCYTIC LEUKEMIA

Ling Zhang, MD
Department of Hematopathology and Laboratory Medicine,
H. Lee Moffitt Cancer Center and Research Institute, Tampa, FL, US

ABSTRACT

T-cell large granular lymphocytic leukemia (T-LGLL) is chronic lymphoproliferative disorder derived from effector memory cytotoxic T cells. Clinically, T-LGLL manifests cytopenia, splenomegaly, and persistent expansion of circulating large granular lymphocytes ($>0.5\times10^9$/L to 2×10^9/L) without any explainable etiology, and is often associated with autoimmune disorders. It was hypothesized that prolonged stimulation with putative antigen is the initiating trigger resulting in altered apoptosis of LGLs via constitutive activation of several survival signalling pathways such as JAK/STAT, MAPK, RAS-RAF, phosphatidylinositol 3-kinase (PI3K)-AKT and NF-κB. Additionally, increased cytokine release (e.g., IL15), and acquired somatic mutations in *signal transducer and activator of transcription-3 and -5B (STAT3* and *STAT5B*) or tumor necrosis factor alpha induced protein 3 (*TNFA-IP3*) are potent drivers of leukemogenesis. Cytomorphologic assessment is insufficient for distinction between T-LGLL, reactive LGL proliferation and other T/NK cell neoplasms in that all these diseases can share similar morphology. Immunophenotyping is considered the most useful and feasible method to differentiate T-LGLL from chronic lymphoproliferative disorder of NK cells (CLPD-NK), aggressive NK cell leukemia (ANKL) and extranodal NK/T cell lymphoma (ENKL). T-LGLL shows typically surface CD3(+), dim CD5(+), dim CD7(+), CD8(+), CD57(+), and T-cell receptors, TCR αβ (+) or γδ (+) while CLPD-NK is usually negative for surface CD3, CD5, CD57, and TCR but expresses cytoplasmic CD3ε, CD16+ and CD56-/+. ANKL and ENKL exhibit cytoplasmic CD3ε(+), bright CD56(+), and CD57(-). TCR gene rearrangement occurs frequently in T-LGLL whereas it is always in germline configuration in NK cell lineage derived disorders. Epstein-Barr virus (EBV) plays a critical role in development of aggressive NK cell neoplasm, but is usually absent in LGLL or CLPD-NK. There are no specific recurrent cytogenetic abnormalities identified in the aforementioned T-/NK cell disorders. Frequent gene mutations of *STAT3*, *STAT5B*, and *TNF-AIP3* have been identified in approximately 50% of T-LGLL and CLPD-NK and can be useful in differential diagnosis of LGLL from reactive LGL expansions. Accurate diagnosis of T-LGLL is based on clinicopathological characteristics that are included in current diagnostic algorithm (NCCN guidelines T-LGLL). It is important to have the knowledge of the disease course, pathogenesis, immunophenotyping, molecular signatures and other available diagnostic methods.

1. INTRODUCTION

Mature T/NK-cell lymphomas comprise a heterogeneous group of peripheral T cell lymphomas and leukemias with distinct pathobiology and prognosis [1]. The T/NK cell neoplasms account for approximately 6% of all lymphoid malignancies with an estimated incidence rate of 2.09 cases per 100,000 persons according to data collected between 1997 and 2006 and posted in the United States Surveillance, Epidemiology and End Results (SEER) [2]. T-cell large granular lymphocytic leukemia (T-LGLL) is an extremely rare entity, with an incidence rate of only 0.2 cases per 1,000,000 individuals per 2000-2011 SEER registration [3], while the incidence of aggressive NK cell leukemia (ANKL), extranodal NK cell lymphoma (ENKL) or chronic lymphoproliferative disorder of NK (CLPD-NK) was not documented in the SEER data pool. Among all T-cell lymphoproliferative disorders, LGLL represents approximately 3% of patients diagnosed in the United States [4].

T-LGLL is a low grade lymphoproliferative disorder characterized by increased circulating T-cell large granular lymphocytes ($>0.5\times10^9$/L), often associated with cytopenia, systemic symptoms, bone marrow infiltrate and splenomegaly [4-7]. The exact etiopathogenesis of T-LGLL is not well understood. It is hypothesized that chronic stimulation with putative autoantigen or viral antigen results in resistance to FAS/FASL mediated apoptosis of LGLs. As a consequence of chronic exposure to exogenous antigens and release of inflammatory cytokines such as IL15, the survival pathways including JAK/STAT, MAPK, MEK1, RAS-RAF-1, PI3K (phosphatidylinositol 3-kinase)-Akt, NFkB (nuclear factor-kB), and sphingolipid are constitutively activated leading to malignant phenotype of T-LGLL [8].

T-LGLL can affect subjects of any age, but the majority of patients fall between 45-75 years old (median 65 years) [6]. No gender predilection is noted. The clinical course of T-LGLL is indolent with median overall survival (OS) of >10 years [9]. Clinically T-LGLL is frequently associated with autoimmune disorders [rheumatoid arthritis, Sjogren's syndrome, systemic lupus erythematosus (SLE)], pulmonary artery hypertension, status post treatment response to anti-neoplastic or monoclonal antibody therapy, and hematopoietic stem cell transplantation [5, 8, 10-13]. There is also increased frequency of monoclonal gammopathy (MGUS) (3-9%), B-cell lymphoproliferative disorders (such as chronic lymphocytic leukemia, 2-5%, follicular lymphoma and hairy cell leukemia) in patients with LGLL [5, 10, 14-17]. Given its indolent clinical nature, up to 1/3 of patients diagnosed with T-LGLL do not require specific treatment during a course of their disease. Ten-year OS was 70% and only approximately 10% of patients died of the disease, mostly secondary to severe neutropenia leading to severe infection [8, 10, 18].

A comprehensive evaluation including accurate documentation of a patient's current and past medical history, imaging study, laboratory data, histopathology, and cytogenetic and molecular profiles is necessary. The chapter will focus on diagnostic approach of T-LGLL and its differential diagnosis from other indolent or aggressive NK-cell lymphomas/leukemias: CLPD-NK, an provisional entity in World Health Organization of Classification of Haematopoietic and Lymphoid Tissue, as well as two aggressive forms of NK cell disorder including ANKL and ENKL. Other nodal T-cell lymphomas with features that can cause diagnostic dilemma are also included in differential diagnoses herein.

2. Clinical Features

T-LGLL is defined as a clonal proliferation of T-cell large granular lymphocytes greater than 2×10^9/L lasting more than 6 months after exclusion of reactive T-cell large granular lymphocytic proliferation. Given that T-LGL count $<1\times10^9$/L can be seen in up to one third of patients with LGLL, the original absolute T-LGL count is not anymore considered mandatory for definitive diagnosis of LGLL. A new cut-off LGL count of 0.5×10^9/L is arbitrarily selected the upper normal range of LGLs observed in normal subjects [9, 19, 20], while the LGL count beyond 0.5×10^9/L is adopted for diagnosis of LGLL for those who present with laboratory abnormalities or systemic symptoms characteristic for LGLL. LGLs often constitute >50% of the circulating lymphocytes in majority of such cases [21].

The patients with indolent T-LGLL or NK cell proliferation have similar clinical presentation [10]. Increased number of circulating T-LGLs could just be an incidental laboratory finding during work-up of asymptomatic lymphocytosis or investigation of cytopenias. Mature lymphocytosis composed of T-LGLs is the most common laboratory finding. A variable degree of neutropenia is frequently seen while anemia may or may not be present [21, 22]. When associated with hemolytic anemia or pure red blood cell aplasia, a subset of patients (approximately 20%) often shows moderate to severe anemia [23]. Approximately 60-70% of patients with T-LGLL could be asymptomatic [20]. However, a subset of them shows recurrent bacterial infection involving skin, subcutaneous tissue, or urinary tract. Rarely bacteremia or perirectal abscesses can happen. Constitutional symptoms such as fevers, chills, and night sweats can be found in

20-30% of cases [20]. Approximately 20-30% of T-LGLL patients have palpable splenomegaly [24] and 10% of the patients have hepatomegaly [20, 25]. Very rarely lymphadenopathy is observed. It was reported that approximately 40% of patients with Felty's syndrome have diagnosis of T-LGLL [26].

3. ROUTINE LABORATORY FINDINGS

Large granular lymphocytes in healthy subjects account for a small subset of lymphocytes in peripheral blood (0.22-0.25×10^9/L), which play important roles in immunosurveillance by releasing cytotoxic granules to kill virally infected cells or transformed tumor cells [4]. LGLs are derived from two major lineages: surface CD3+ LGLs (activated cytotoxic T-cells) and surface CD3- NK cells, together comprising 10-15% of total white blood cells [20].

Initial evaluation of complete blood count with differential (CBC/Diff) and a review of peripheral blood smear are the most two important diagnostic methods. Neutropenia is the most common cytopenia that accompanies expanded clonal T-LGL cells in peripheral blood. It is not uncommon to see severe neutropenia with an absolute neutrophil count less than 0.5×10^9/L [5]. Since patients with T-LGLL can also have other autoimmune disorders, laboratory studies should include rheumatoid factor, autoantibodies (antinuclear antibody, antineutrophil antibody, and antiplatelet antibody), circulating immune complexes, β-2 macroglobulin, direct Coombs test, and soluble Fas-ligand, which are often positive or elevated in T-LGLL [7, 16, 26, 27]. Protein electrophoresis is performed for evaluation of hyper- or hypo-gammaglobinemia or monoclonal gammopathy. Elevated rheumatoid factor and antinuclear antibodies were detected in 60% and 40% of patients with LGLL, respectively [20, 28].

HLA typing may be considered to identify autoimmunity in T-LGLL. A high frequency of the HLA-DR4 haplotype is found in patients with LGLL (90%) and rheumatoid arthritis (86%) [29]. Overexpression of HLA-DR4 may be linked to an immune mediated neutrophil destruction although the exact mechanism is unclear. Patients with T-LGLL have a higher level of cytokine, chemokine and death receptor ligand, Fas ligand (FasL) that is measurable in the patients's sera [28, 30].

It is critical to exclude transient polyclonal T-LGL proliferation secondary to viral infection before rendering a diagnosis of T-LGLL. Laboratory virology tests commonly include the DNA titers of Epstein-Barr virus and cytomegalovirus (CMV), serology evaluation of anti-hepatitis A/B/C antibodies, and enzyme-linked immunosorbent assay (ELISA) or Western blotting for human immunodeficiency virus (HIV), etc. Parvovirus B-19 needs to be tested when bone marrow shows an erythroid aplasia. Assessment of episomal EBV genome is critical to exclude ANKL or leukemic phase of ENKL. As far as human T-cell leukemia virus 1(HTLV-1) is concerned there was not definitive confirmation that this virus plays an important role in etiopathogenesis of LGLL. However, in selected patients from regions with high prevalence of HTLV-1 infection this test can be useful [22].

A panel including ferritin level, triglyceride, anti-CD25, NK cell function tests, and liver function profile can be ordered when more aggressive NK cell neoplasms or hepatosplenic T-cell lymphoma and accompanying hemophagocytic lymphohistiocytosis (HLH) are suspected clinically [31].

4. CYTOMORPHOLOGY

Of note, normal circulating LGLs are 15-18μm in size, round to orally indented nuclei and contain reddish cytoplasmic cytotoxic granules and pale cytoplasm (Figure 1A and 1B). LGLs in T-LGLL could resemble their normal counterparts without significant morphologic differences between each other. Peripheral blood smear of patients with T-LGLL reveals that the T-LGLL cells are medium in size with round to oval nuclei, condense chromatin, smooth nuclear contour, inconspicuous nucleoli, and a moderate amount of clear cytoplasm containing reddish cytotoxic granules. However, morphologic variants are also identified [20], which can share CD3+/CD8+/CD57+ immunophenotype but distinct LGL morphology [7, 32]. In some occasions cytotoxic granules in T-cell LGLL are decreased or even absent. Aggressive variant of T-LGLL demonstrates more overt cytologic atypia, including nuclear irregularity, visible to prominent nucleoli, reduced cytoplasmic to nuclear ratio, and less condense chromatin (Figure 2A and B).

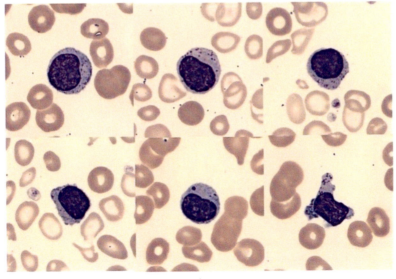

A

Figure 1A and B. (Continued).

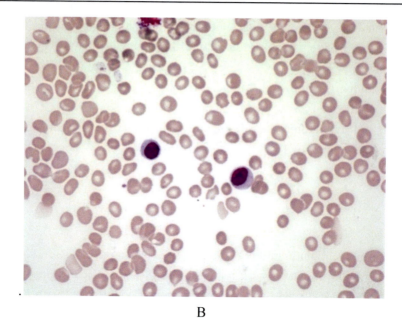

B

Figure 1A and B. Normal large granular lymphocytes contain variable level of cytoplasmic red to purple cytotoxic granules and display slight variation of size and shape from normal adults (image collection via Cellavision) (1A) or Wright stained peripheral blood smear (1B, 600x).

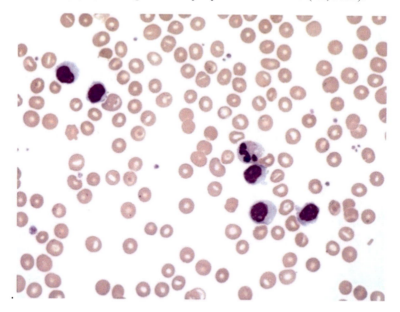

Figure 2A. The peripheral blood smear (Wright stain, 600x) shows increased circulating large granular lymphocytes (LGLs) with oval to minimally irregular nuclear contour and condensed chromatin. Cytoplasmic reddish cytotoxic granules are barely identified. Neutrophils are decreased in number. Occasional mature esoinophil is present. Platelets appear adequate in number. Red blood cells display minimal to mild anisiopoikilocytosis.

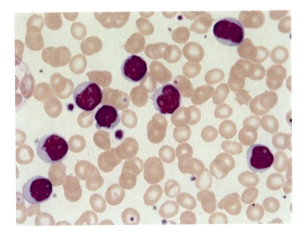

Figure 2B. The peripheral blood smear shows predominantly mature lymphocytosis consisting of LGLs in a patient with aggressive T-LGLL. These cells are nearly identical in size, slightly larger than red blood cells, and containing barely visible cytoplasmic cytotoxic granules. Some LGLs display relatively high nuclear to cytoplasmic (N: C) ratio, irregular contours, prominent nucleoli or blastoid morphology (Wright stain, 1000x).

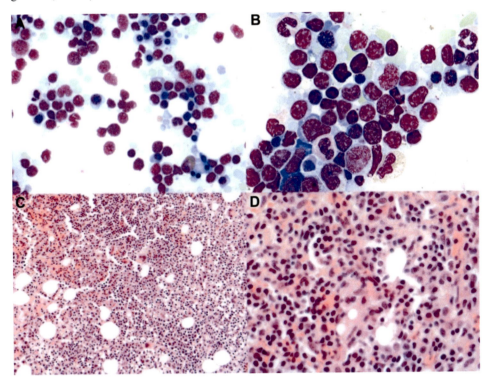

Figure 3. A and B. The bone marrow aspirate smears from a patient with T-LGLL show overt mature lymphocytosis associated with myeloid hypoplasia and relative erythroid preponderance (Wright Giemsa, 600× and 1000×, respectively). Smudged nuclei and few normal appearing small lymphocytes are present in the background. The atypical lymphoid cells are slightly larger than normal lymphocytes in size with normal or less cytoplasm. They show condensed chromatin, round to slightly irregular nuclei and occasional identifiable cytoplasmic cytotoxic granules. No dysplasia is present in the background hematopoietic cells. C and D. Low and high power view of bone marrow infiltrated by small lymphoid cells in interstitial and/or perisinasoidal patterns (H&E, 200× and 600×, respectively).

Even though bone marrow biopsy is not routinely necessary to make diagnosis of T-LGLL, it can be indicated especially in patients with lower LGL count than 0.5×10^9/L in peripheral blood and/or clinical suspicion of a concomitant distinct bone marrow disorder, e.g., myelodysplastic syndrome, pure red cell aplasia, lymphoma, or plasma cell dyscrasia. Examination of T-LGL on Wright-Giemsa stained bone marrow aspirate smears shows findings similar to those noted in peripheral blood smear. However, given background of other hematopoietic elements and cell debris, morphologic distinction between indolent T-LGLL and normal appearing reactive lymphocytes is more difficult, particularly when there is only a low level involvement by T-LGLL. In bone marrow, a large subset of LGLs in T-LGLL shows only minimal to mild cytologic atypia although cytologic variants are present, similar to peripheral blood findings. Cytologic granules may not be easily visualized in the core biopsy. In view of core biopsy, the bone marrow involvement of T-LGLL is insidious and often missed without performing additional immunohistochemical staining. Regardless indolent or aggressive variants of T-LGLL, infiltrating pattern is predominantly interstitial or perisinasoidal. Reactive lymphoid aggregate, monoclonal B-cell lymphocytosis or polyclonal or monoclonal plasmacytosis has been reported [14, 15]. Patchy increase of reticulin fibrosis is also observed in a subset of patients [33]. In most cases of T-LGLL, bone marrow involvement is approximately 10-15% of total cellularity. Bone marrow hypercellularity associated with decreased myeloid precursors or maturation arrest is identified in 55% of patients with T-LGLL [16]. Sometimes confluent lymphoid infiltrate is present in indolent T-LGLL (Figure 3A-D). Of note, the level of bone marrow involvement may be disproportional to the peripheral circulating T-LGL count or the degree of peripheral cytopenia.

There is an overlap between T-LGLL and aplastic anemia, pure red blood cell aplasia, paroxysmal nocturnal hemoglobinuria (PNH), and hypoplastic myelodysplastic syndrome (MDS). These diseases can manifest with small LGL clones or develop overt LGLL. A search for morphologic and laboratory features for other co-existent hematopoietic disorders is obligated. Moreover, T-LGLL can also be associated with reduction of single or multiple lineage hematopoietic precursors, resulting in lineage specific hypoplasia [34, 35].

Nodal involvement by T-LGLL or CLPD-NK, though rare, has been reported, usually indicating more aggressive clinical behaviour or transformation [36]. Transformed LGL show a morphologic change ranging from normal LGLs to blastoid cells with dispersed chromatin, mixed normal LGL and blast looking cells, or large atypical lymphoid cells resembling peripheral T-cell lymphoma (PTCL) [36-38]. Nonetheless, aggressive variant of LGLL could manifest normal LGL morphology in lymph node, which is difficult to separate it from reactive counterpart and requires a correlation with clinical history and flow cytometry findings. When transformed, the neoplastic LGLs can show original phenotype or atypical phenotype different from the original one. Frequently, increased number of circulating LGLs is present at the time when LGLL involves lymph node.

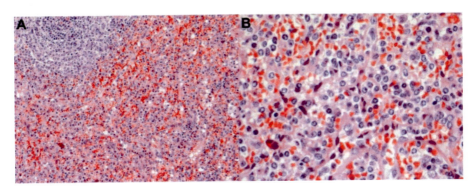

Figure 4. A. low power view of splenic parenchyma (Wright Giemsa, 200×) shows intact white pulp and adjacent expanded red pulp filled with mature-appearing small lymphoid cells, in a perisinusoidal distribution. B. High power view reveals these small lymphoid cells with round to oval nuclei and scant eosinophilic to clear cytoplasm intermingled with sinus histiocytes, scattered mature plasma cells, endothelial cells (some with prominent nuclei) and intrasinusoidal red blood cells.

Splenic involvement of T-LGLL is very common. The neoplastic T-cells are mainly found in red pulps resulting in expansion of red pulps while white pulps are identifiable or focally decreased depending on the level of involvementt (Figure 4A and B). LGLL cells in spleen are also in perisinasoidal arrangement. By touch imprint, T-LGLs are medium in size and mature in appearance. Of importance, a variable degree of cytologic atypia can be seen with conventional or aggressive variant of T-LGLL. Furthermore, a concurrent diagnosis of T-LGLL with low grade B-cell lymphoma and gamma heavy chain diseases have been reported [39].

5. IMMUNOPHENOTYPING

5.1. Flow Cytometry Analysis

Flow cytometry is essential to identify the phenotypic features of T-LGLL. The majority of LGL cells in T-LGLL show an activated T-cell phenotype with characteristic expression of surface CD3(+), CD8(+), CD4(-), CD16(+), CD27(-), CD45RO(-), CD57(+), and CD94(+). The LGLL cells are often dim CD5(+), dim CD7(+), CD2(+), CD45RA(+), CD62L+(subset), and HLA-DR(+) [7, 32, 40] (Figure 5). The most prevalent NK-associated marker is CD57 (90%), followed by CD16 (80%) and CD94/NKG2A (50%) [21]. Cases with expression of CD16 and CD57 account for more than ¾ of the cases while CD56 is infrequently detected in LGLL (reportedly 20%) [9, 20, 21]. Decreased or lost expression of other pan-T-cell markers such as CD2 or CD3 has also been reported [41, 42]. Decreased expression of surface CD2 is present in approximately 20% of the patients. Occasionally, diminished or loss of CD3 expression is also observed [41, 42]. Other markers, which are not commonly adopted in routine laboratory but expressed in LGLL, include CD25, CD69, and CD122 [20, 43]. Approximately 50% of LGLL expresses KIR families of NK-associated MHC-class I receptor and shows single isoform of KIR expression which indicates clonality when using antibodies against CD158a, CD158b, CD158e, CD158i, and CD158k [6, 41, 42]. Of these antibodies, CD158b is dominant. Few cases (approximately 10%) exhibit 2 KIR patterns [21]. Gamma-delta (γδ) variant of T-LGLL is present in a minority of patients (<5%) [44, 45], which exhibits similar phenotype to TCR αβ T-LGLL including surface CD3, dim CD5, dim CD7, and also demonstrates other unique features including CD4-, CD8-/+, and TCR γδ (Figure 6). Given lacking CD4 and CD8 expression in the subtype of T-LGLL, a differential diagnosis should include hepatosplenic γδ T-cell lymphoma [46-48]. CD4(+), dual CD4(+)/CD8(+), and dual CD4(-)/CD8(-) LGLL have been reported [6, 49, 50]. In contrast to the classical CD8(+) T-LGLL, the CD4(+) variant shows uniform, moderate or bright CD56 [50]. Other phenotypic variation has been observed in aggressive variants of T-LGLL such as acquired CD56 expression [21], which should be cautiously differentiated from other CD56 positive lymphomas [51]. Of note, there are overlapping immunophenotype features between reactive LGLs and T-LGLL. For example, weak expression of CD5 and CD7 can be also seen with reactive LGLs [52]. Flow cytometry with a panel of monoclonal antibodies against variable β-chain repertoire is considered as another option for assessment of clonality in addition to T-cell αβ and γδ gene rearrangement. Even though, this test is infrequently used in routine clinical practice. An antibody against variable region for families of the beta chain (V beta) has been adopted for diagnosis of T-LGLL since approximately 70% of LGLL cases display V beta restriction [53, 54, 55]. Qiu's group indicated that flow cytometry V beta assay showed identical sensitivity and specificity to PCR with Gene Scanning but was more sensitive than PCR with heteroduplex study [53].

5.2. Immunohistochemical Staining

LGLs contain cytotoxic granules such as perforin, granzyme and TIA1, which can be highlighted by immunohistochemical staining. Perforin, a pore-forming protein belongs to a family of serine proteases, directly inducing cell lysis through increased osmolality after cell membrane pore formation and permit enzyme delivery to the targeted cells [56]. Granzymes M or granzyme B shows protease activity that will cause cell death by activating apoptotic caspase [57, 58]. TIA1 is recognized as a member of a RNA-binding protein family and have a function of nucleolysis against cytotoxic lymphocyte target cells, also casting an important role in eliminating LGL targeted cells [59, 60]. Performing immunohistochemical staining for cytotoxic markers is feasible in tissue block or bone marrow in addition to the common T/NK-cell markers CD3, CD8 and CD57. The LGLL cells show cytoplasmic granules associated proteins, TIA1(+), perforin (+) and granzyme B(+) (Figure 7) [7, 43, 61]. The expression pattern is also useful to discriminate from inactive (immature) cytotoxic granules from hepatosplenic T-cell lymphoma, which show usually TIA1(+), and perforin(-), and granzyme B(-) [62-64]. Of note, CD57 positive LGL cells are also detectable in the normal, reactive, as well as pathologic bone marrow with cytopenia [65].

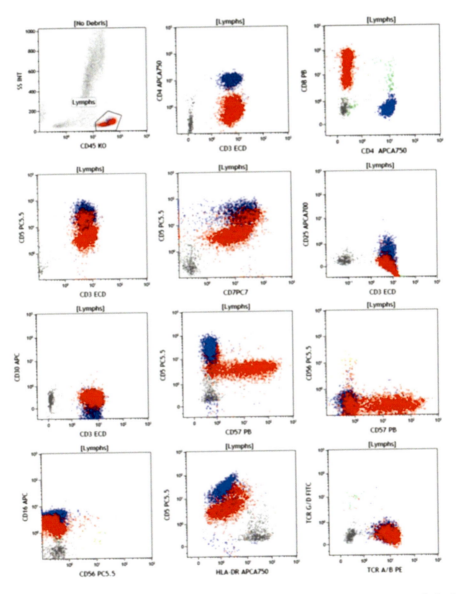

Figure 5. Flow cytometry study identifies a distinct population of mature T-cells composed of mixed CD4 (blue), CD8 (red) and dual CD4/CD8 (green) cells. The CD8 positive cytotoxic T-cells co-express surface CD3, CD5 (dim), CD7, CD16 (dim), CD57, HLA-DR, and TCRαβ and are negative for CD25, CD30, CD56 and TCR-γδ, characteristic for αβ LGLL. These T-LGLL cells are also positive for CD2, negative for CD1a and TdT (data not shown).

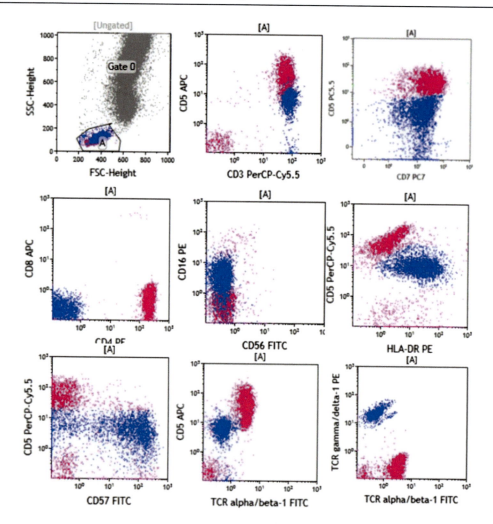

Figure 6. Flow cytometry study identifies a distinct population of mature T-cells phenotypically shows surface CD3(+), CD5 dim(+), CD16(+), CD57(+), HLA-DR(+), and TCR γδ (+) and CD4(-), CD8(-), CD56(-) and TCRαβ(-), characteristic for γδ variant of T-LGLL. These T-LGLL cells are also positive for CD2 and negative for CD25 and CD30 (data not shown).

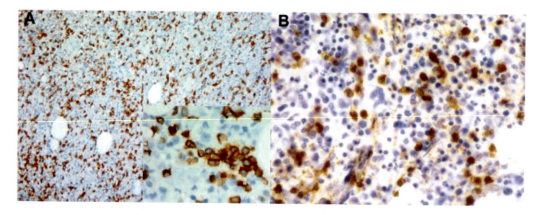

Figure 7. (Continued).

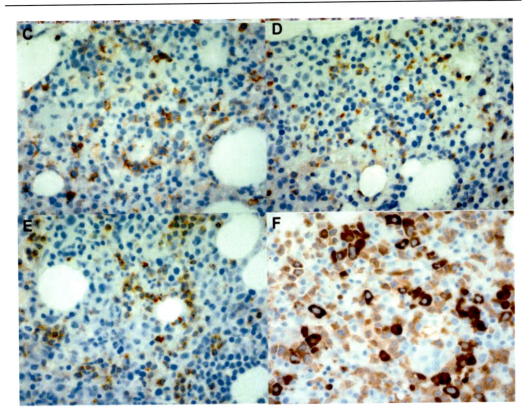

Figure 7. A panel of immunohistochemical stains was performed in a patient with bone marrow involvement by T-LGLL. The staining suggested that CD3 positive T-cells were increased in the bone marrow, approximately 15-20% of marrow space (Immunoperoxidase, 200×). Inset shows the CD3 positive T-cells are interstitial and perisinasoidal infiltrating pattern, focally forming small clusters. The T-LGLL cells were positive for CD8 (B, 200×) and CD57 (C, 200×). Intracellular cytotoxic granules (TIA, perforin and granzyme B) were identified (D-E, 200×).

6. MOLECULAR STUDY

6.1. T-Cell Gene Rearrangements and Clonality of T-LGLL

Polymerase chain reaction (PCR) is the most common diagnostic tool for assessment of T-cell receptor (TCR) gene rearrangements. The presence of clonal TCR gene rearrangement is also a feature of T-LGLL and may be useful to separate this disease from reactive LGL proliferations with increased circulating T-LGLs. However, interpretation of this test should be done with a caution since some T-LGLL patients do not exhibit TCR gene rearrangements [21]. Besides PCR, other methods have also been utilized in assessment of T-cell clonality. As aforementioned, flow cytometry is alternative way to identify T-cell clonality via measuring TCR beta V region restriction pattern [66, 67]. Traditionally, Southern blot or isolated complementary DNA clones was employed [20, 68]. Even though, how to correctly interpret the clonality remains controversial. The absence of so called "clonality" is observed in a subset of T-LGLL [20], leading an unsolved puzzle regarding whether clonality is equal to malignancy in this setting. A novel method of high-throughput sequencing of TCR gene might improve sensitivity of clonality testing in patients with T-LGLL [69].

6.2. Mutation Study

Following a wide use of next generation sequencing technology in lymphoma, more and more gene mutations have been detected in T/NK cell lymphomas/leukemias. Mutations identified in NK/T cell disease include *DDX3X, JAK3, STAT3, STAT5B, BCOR, MLL2, ASXL3, ARID1A, EP300* gene mutations or alterations [70]. It is of notion that activation of the JAK/STAT pathway, and over-expression of NK-κB and aurora kinase A play critical roles in oncogenesis of NK/T-cell lymphomas [2, 71], which is partially attributed to mutations such as *JAK3, STAT3* or *STAT5B* mutations [72-74]. Recently several studies have shown that *STAT3* mutation is frequently seen in T-LGLL (25-78%, on average 50%) [75-79]. *STAT5B* gene is also mutated in a minor subset (approximately 5%), mutual exclusively with *STAT3* mutations [76, 79]. Specific *STAT3* mutation (e.g., Y640E) may predict a therapeutic response to methotrexate as a frontline therapy and N642 mutations appear to be linked to a unfavorable clinical nature in CD3+/CD56+ aggressive LGLL [75, 80]. *STAT5B* mutation was associated with aggressive CD3+/CD56+ T-LGLL [76, 81]. *TNFA-IP3* mutation is detected in approximately 8% of T-LGLL, which acts as an NF-kB signaling inhibitor [8]. However, these aforementioned mutations are not specific to T-LGLL, but may support a diagnosis of neoplastic LGL proliferation/leukemia over reactive LGL expansion if integrated with clinical and laboratory features.

6.3. Cytogenetic Study

Conventional karyotyping or FISH study is not useful in differential diagnosis of T/NK cell lymphoma/leukemia since no specific cytogenetic aberrations are identified in T-LGLL, CLPD-NK, ENKL, and ANKL. The majority of T-LGLL patients exhibit normal karyotype but a minority of cases (<10%) might carry sporadic cytogenetic abnormalities involving 7p14-p15 (TCR-γ gene loci), 14q11 (TCR-α/TCR-δ gene loci) [82], or other loci with unknown significances including +3, inv(4)(p14q12), del(5q), del(6)(q21), +8, inv(12p), inv(14q), +14, -X, or complex aberrations [23, 40, 83, 84].

7. Differential Diagnoses

7.1. Benign LGL Proliferation

Benign LGL proliferations are frequently seen in post viral infections (e.g., CMV, EBV, and hepatitis), post solid organ or hematopoietic stem cell transplantation, post immunotherapy, or concurrent with skin lesions, lymphomas, and solid tumors [7, 85-89]. The LGL proliferation is often polyclonal and transient (<6 months). The LGL count usually does not exceed $3\text{-}4 \times 10^9$/L [20].

Of note, an increase of monoclonal CD3/CD8+ T-cells can be identified in some elderly individuals who are otherwise healthy, which, however, do not exhibit similar phenotypic findings to those observed in T-LGLL. The clinical significance of such a benign proliferation of T-cells is uncertain. In addition, clonal or non-clonal T-LGLs are also seen in patients infected with a virus. The increase of T-LGLs is usually transient [90].

In normal individual, circulating T-LGLs, γδ subtype, can be detected in approximately 5% of T-LGLs, which are phenotypically similar to T-LGLL γδ variant. In addition, some normal γδ T-LGLs could show dim CD5 as well as V-delta 2 [91]. Due to aberrant expression of KIRs it was recommended to perform KIR test in order to differentiate normal from neoplastic LGL proliferation/leukemia [21].

7.2. Chronic Lymphoproliferation of NK Cells

Chronic lymphoproliferative disorder of NK cells (CLPD-NK) that is listed as a provisional entity in WHO classification is even rarer than T-LGLL. The latter comprise 85-90% of cases with expansion of circulating LGLs [9]. Similar to T-LGLL, CLPD-NK has indolent clinical course with the median overall survival of 94% at 5 years [92].

CLPD-NK also shows increased number of circulating NK-cells (>0.5×10^9/L) that is sustained for more than 6 months without any explainable etiology [6, 93]. NK cell proliferations secondary to virus infection should be excluded [13]. Given its rarity, only case report or small case series were published. A larger retrospective multi-institutional cohort study of 70 patients with CLPD-NK confirmed the similarities with T-LGLL regarding association with autoimmunity and hematopoietic neoplasms [92]. CLPD-NK is immunophenotypically positive for CD16, CD8 (75%), and CD94, and dim to negative for CD56, which resembles T-LGLL while the unique phenotypic features can be used to differentiate from T-LGLL: The cells are negative for surface CD3 expression, absence of expression of the KIR CD158a, CD158b, and CD158e and TCR αβ or γδ [21]. CLPD-NK also does not show any recurrent karyotypic abnormalities. Clonal origin of NK cells in informative female patients with CLPD-NK was confirmed with use of X-chromosome polymorphism inactivation assay [94-96]. Unlike ANKL or ENKL, the majority of which display a clonal episomal form, EBV genome is never identified in CLPD-NK [93].

7.3. Extranoal NK/T Cell Lymphoma

Extranoal NK/T cell lymphoma is an aggressive type of NK cell neoplasm with a majority of patients exhibiting NK-cell phenotype and frequently associated with clonal episomal EBV. Unlike T-LGLL, ENKL shows a geographic predilection. The incidence is 10-20 times higher in Asian and South American than in North American and European [70, 97]. Clinically it should not be difficult to distinguish T-LGLL from ENKL in light of the latter's tissue base infiltrate but rarely involving spleen, liver, and peripheral blood. ENKL is typically found in nasal cavity, pharynx or upper aerodigestive tract and often presents with nasal congestion, bleeding, obstructive symptoms and signs [98]. Extranasal dissemination of this disease is most commonly located in skin, gastrointestinal tracts, testis and soft tissue [99-101]. Imaging study using fluorodeoxyglucose (FDG) positron emission tomography/computed tomography (PET/CT) helps to identify an occult nasal or non-nasal involvement [70, 102]. Bone marrow involvement is less frequent (16%) than in LGLL. Differential diagnosis of ENKL in case of bone marrow involvement should be made by aid of cytology (large in size, irregular nuclei, prominent nuclei and basophilic cytoplasm) and unique immunophenotypes (CD2+, surface CD3-, CD56+, CD4-, CD5-, CD8-, CD16- and CD57-) [103]. Of note, ENKL can originate from T cell lineage in a minority of patients which are phenotypically positive for surface CD3, TCR-αβ or TCR γδ. However, they, different from LGLL, display bright CD56 [103-105].

In contrast to T-LGLL with indolent clinical course and >10 year OS in majority of patients, ENKL shows more aggressive clinical behavior and shorter OS especially in advanced stage disease. Vasquez et al. recently reported results of the 153 patients with aggressive NK/T cell lymphoma that showed the median OS of 49 months and five year OS was 48.9% for non-Asian group [106], with not significantly different from the previous studies, with the OS ranging from 19.6 months to 50 months [107-109].

When atypical LGLs present in peripheral blood, peripheral blood EBV DNA viral titer by PCR and/or in situ hybridization using EBV encoded RNA probe (EBER) would be helpful in differential diagnosis of EBV associated ENNK and ANKL. Due to apoptosis of malignant cells, a small EBV DNA fragments (usually <500 base-pairs) are detectable in the peripheral blood of these patients [110-112]. To avoid interference with EBV infected memory B-cells, plasma, instead of whole blood sample, is considered the more suitable material for quantification of circulating EBV DNA [110]. Monitoring plasma EBV DNA titers s is also used for therapeutic response assessment of NK/T lymphoma/leukemia to chemotherapy as well as for a detection of a minimal residual disease [111, 113]. Comparative genomic hybridization (CGH) study done in ENKL shows various cytogenetic abnormalities, such as a gain of 2q, and loss of other chromosomal materials including 1p36, 4q12, 5q34-35, 6q16-q27, 7q21-22, 11q22-23,and 15q11-14 [114], of which deletion of 6q is the most common one. However, these changes are not specific and of unknown prognostic significance [115].

7.4. Aggressive NK Cell Leukemia

Aggressive NK cell leukemia (ANKL) is extremely rare malignancy with estimated incidence of <0.1% of all lymphoma/leukemia [116]. Geographic preference includes Far East, South and Central America. The leukemia shows a strong association with EBV [117]. Patients with ANKL presents with an abnormal proliferation of NK cells found in peripheral blood and bone marrow, the circulating atypical lymphoid cells vary from 5% to 80% [118]. A median survival is about 2 months [116, 119, 120]. The majority of patients are younger in ages with median age of 39 years [117], and men and women are equally affected [6]. It is not uncommon for ANKL cells to have bizarre cytology such as enlarged cell size, markedly irregular or lobated nuclei, frequent mitosis, karyolysis, karyorrhexis, pyknosis, and increased apoptosis. In particular, ANKL is often accompanied with hemophagocytosis with increased histiocytes/macrophages engulfing hematopoietic elements, which is absolutely not a feature for either indolent T-LGLL or CLPD-NK. In addition, the presence of fever of unknown origin, progressive cytopenia (e.g., anemia, thrombocytopenia) and accompanying liver dysfunction, rapid hepatosplenomegaly, disseminated intravascular coagulation (DIC), hemophagocytic lymphohistiocytosis (HLH) and multiorgan failure found in ANKL are not seen with T-LGLL. A manifestation of aggressive variant of T-LGLL resembles of ANKL. However, transformed LGLL should have a known history of prior indolent T-LGLL.

Li et al. recently reported that flow cytometry is the most sensitive way for an early diagnosis of ANKL (97.4%) in comparison to immunohistochemical study (90%), morphologic assessment (89.5%), and cytogenetics (56.5%) [121]. In general, NK cells in ANKL express surface CD45, CD2, CD7, cytoplasmic CD3, bright CD56 and lack expression of surface CD3, CD4, CD5, CD57, TCR$\alpha\beta$ and TCR$\gamma\delta$. CD8 can be variably positive in a subset of NK cell disorders. In Li's study, they also reported intact CD94 expression in ANKL; the majority of cells express strikingly bright CD56, dim CD16, and absence of CD57 (91.9%) with an entire loss of NK cell receptors (CD158a/h, CD158b and CD158e) (72.7%) and a partial loss of CD161 (33%). Decreased CD7, CD8 and perforin expressions were noted in 27.9%, 78.4% and 50% of patients, respectively [121]. Recent study by del Mel et al. demonstrated that CLPD-NK shared a phenotype similar to reactive NK cells with CD56+, CD16 dim+, CD57 dim+ and CD94 dim+ whereas the NK cell leukemia/lymphoma (ENKL or ANKL) demonstrated bright

CD56+, dim CD16+, CD94+, and absence of CD57, which completely distinct from T-LGLL phenotype. ANKL and ENKL are phenotypically positive for CD2, CD7 and HLA-DR [122], which, can be also observed in LGLL. TCR gene germline configurations help to confirm the neoplastic cells to be of NK cell origin. However, the presence of TCR gene rearrangements should not be used as a sole marker to exclude NK cell origin of any neoplasms as the TCR β or γ gene rearrangement could be from the by standing T-cells as a consequence of reactive process in tumor microenvironment [6]. Tables 1 and 2 have summarized the similar or distinguishable clinical and immunophenotypic features among ANKL, ENKL, T-LGLL and CLPD-NK.

Table 1. Key clinical features identified in T-LGLL, CLPD-NK, ANKL, and ENKL

	T-LGLL	CLPD-NK	ANKL	ENKL
Cytopenia	Present	Present	Pancytopenia	May be present
Circulating LGLs	yes	yes	yes	Rarely when disseminated disease
Bone marrow infiltration	Yes, interstitial and focally aggregate	Yes, interstitial and focally aggregate	Yes, interstitial and focally aggregate, often associate with hemophagocytosis	May occur, interstitial and focally aggregate, could associate with hemophagocytosis
Splenomegaly	Yes (often)	Yes (infrequently)	Yes (often)	No or rarely
PCR for TCR gene rearrangement	TCRαβ and/or TCR γδ gene rearranged	TCR gene germline configuration	TCR gene germline configuration	TCRαβ and/or TCR γδ gene germline configuration (NK cells) or rearranged (T-cells)

Table 2. Phenotypic differences among T-LGLL, CLPD-NK, ANKL and ENKL [121-123]

	T-LGLL	CLPD-NK	ANKL	ENKL
CD2	+	+	+	+
Surface CD3	+	-	-	sub+
Cytoplasmic CD3	-	+	+	+
CD4	Minority +	-	-	-/+
CD8	+	+/-	-/+	-/+
CD5	Dim+	-	-	-/+
CD7	Dim+	+	+/-	+/-
CD16	+/-	+	Dim +	Dim +
CD25	-	-	+	+
CD26	+/-	+/-	+	+
CD30	-	-	-	+/
CD56	-/ +	dim+/-	Bright +	Bright +
CD57	+	-/+	-	-
CD94	-	+	+/-	-/+
CD161	-	+	-	-/+
KIR	+	-/+	-/+	+/-
HLA-DR	dim+	+/-	+	+

7.5. Peripheral T-Cell Lymphoma, NOS

Peripheral T-cell lymphoma, not otherwise specified (PTCL-NOS) is a lymphoma originating most commonly in lymph nodes. Disseminate PTCL, NOS to peripheral blood and bone marrow occurs in a majority of cases (approximately 70%) during a course of the disease [124]. CD4 positive PTCL, NOS, is the most common subtype while cytotoxic PTCL, NOS, have also been reported in 15-30% of cases [125, 126]. Immunohistochemical stains performed on these cases show the neoplastic cells containing cytotoxic granules as described in LGLL but phenotypically they can be CD4+, CD8+ or double CD4- and CD8- T-cells [126, 127]. The presence of CD4+ LGLs with diminished CD7 expression could result in a diagnostic dilemma [125, 126]. However, in contrast to CD4 positive LGLL, PTCL, NOS, does not co-express CD57 [125] and usually shows more pleomorphic morphology with moderate nuclear irregularity [128, 129]. Generalized lymphadenopathy is characteristic for PTCL, NOS, but not for LGLL [6]. Concurrent T-LGLL or clonal T-LGL proliferation with any subtype of peripheral T cell lymphoma or hematological malignancy is not uncommon [13, 130]. A case with donor-derived T-cell LGLL in a patient with PTCL was also reported [131]. Thus, benign or neoplastic proliferations of LGLs must be distinguished from PTCL, NOS. Figure 8 summarizes a diagnostic algorithm of circulating LGLs in selected types of T- and NK cell lymphoproliferative disorder.

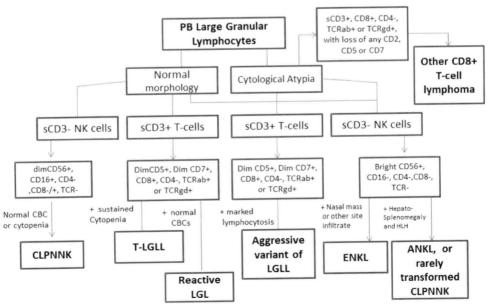

Figure 8. Schematic diagnostic approaches of circulating large granular lymphocytes in peripheral blood.

7.6. Hepatosplenic T-Cell Lymphoma

Similar to T-LGLL, hepatosplenic T-cell lymphoma (HSTL) could occur in immunocompromised subjects, and manifest cytopenias and hepatosplenomegaly [132]. The bone marrow and extramedullary tissue infiltrating pattern of HSTL shows almost no differences from T-LGLL, which often exhibits interstitial and sinusoidal arrangement of T-cells and infrequent lymphoid aggregates in bone marrow and liver, and both cord and sinus involvement of spleen [132]. A majority of HSTL express T-cell receptor γδ phenotype (CD4-/CD8-) with a minority of HSTL having αβ receptor expression [132]. In addition, HSTL cells express surface CD3(+), CD5(-), CD7(-), CD4(-), CD8(-/+), TCR γδ(+), CD56(+), subset CD16(+), and CD57(-) and contain inactive cytotoxic granules in their cytoplasm [63, 64]. Different from LGLL, regardless of γδ or αβ types, HSTL shows a more aggressive clinical picture, and is often associated with hemophagocytosis [132]. A multi-center study demonstrated that HSTCL patients more frequently manifested massive hepatosplenomegaly, significantly increased atypical T-cells that are devoid of azurophilic cytoplasmic inclusion and showed predominantly sinusoid infiltrate [46]. HSTCL cells appear more atypical with easily identifiable nuclear irregularity than conventional T-LGLL. Thus, touch imprint of splenic tissue is very useful to assess cytological details than histological section. When splenectomy is no longer the only way for diagnosis of both diseases or in post splenectomy patients, a correct diagnosis can also be made using liver biopsy, bone marrow biopsy, or peripheral blood specimen in conjunction with the corresponding immunophenotypic and genetic profiles [62]. Due to its feasibility and frequent involvement by T-LGLL and HSTL, a bone marrow biopsy often yields positive results. Aggressive clinical course and the presence of isochrosome 7q or other chromosome 7 anomalies support a diagnosis of HSTL rather than T-LGLL [48, 123, 133]. An interpretation of a low level of peripheral blood involvement by γδ HSTL must be careful since there is a notable population of normal counterpart of γδ T-cells as well as reactive γδ T-LGLs in circulation [134, 135]. Table 3 includes the features useful to differentiate hepatosplenic T-cell lymphoma from T-LGLL.

7.7. Mycosis Fungoides/Sezary Syndrome

There is a diagnostic pitfall in assessment of circulating Sezary cells in patients with Sezary syndrome/mycosis fungoides (SS/MF) by using limited flow cytometry panel without a peripheral blood smear review. Concurrent LGL proliferation or LGLL with syndromes/MF has been rarely reported [136]. Zhang et al. [130] reported a case with increased CD4(+)/CD7 dim (+)/CD57+ LGLs with an absolute count of the LGLs up to 5.5×10^9/L in a patient with early stage MF. The accurate assessment of the finding prevented the patient from can prompt a systemic treatment for SS/MF.

Table 3. Differential diagnosis of T-LGLL and HSTL

	T-LGLL	HSTL [62, 64]
Cell Nature	Active cytotoxic T-cells	Nonactive cytotoxic memory T-cells
TCR	majority: TCR αβ minority: TCR γδ	majority: TCR γδ minority: TCR αβ
Age	50-60 years old	20% in younger age
Gender	Male and female equally affected	Male predominant
Clinical symptoms and signs	Weakness, fever secondary to infection	Weight loss, fever of unknown origin
Associated diseases	Autoimmune disorder, e.g., Rheumatoid arthritis	Immunocompromised status, e.g., long time on immunosuppressant(s), post transplantation, IBD
Complication	Infection, bone marrow failure, enlarged spleen	hemophagocytic syndrome, bone marrow failure, hypersplenism
Circulating neoplastic T-cells	Always present	1-3%
Absolute lymphocytosis >2.0 x 10 ^{9}/L	A subset	infrequent
Cytology	Small to medium, round to oval nuclei, inconspicuous nucleoli, and cytoplasmic reddish granules	Medium in size, round to slight irregular nuclei, inconspicuous nucleoli, cytotoxic granules, sometimes with blastoid chromatin, pleomorphic or engulfed erythrocytes
LDH	Normal	High
Lymphadenopathy	Rare	Rare
BM, Liver and Spleen infiltration	Linear arrays in the sinusoids	Expansion or packed atypical cells in the sinusoids
Immunophenotype	Surface CD3(+), dim CD5(+), dim CD7(+), CD8(+), HLA-DR(+), CD57(+), CD16(+) and TCRαβ (+); minority: CD4(-)/CD8(-)/TCRγδ(+)	Surface CD3(+), CD5(-), CD7(-), CD4(-), CD8(-/+), TCR γδ(+), CD56(+), subset CD16(+), and CD57(-); minority: TCRαβ(+)
Cytotoxic granules	TIA1(+), Perforin(+), Granzyme B(+)	TIA1(+), perforin(-), and granzyme B(-)
Cytogenetic alterations	None or nonspecific cytogenetic findings	Isochromosome 7q, ring chromosome 7 or del (7q)
Gene mutation	*STAT3*, infrequent *STAB5B*	*STAB5B*
Treatment	MTX, cyclosporine, GCSF, transfusion, splenectomy if symptomatic	CHOP and HyperCVAD followed by autologous or allogeneic stem cell transplantation.
Clinical course	Indolent	Aggressive, with rapid progression
Overall 5-year survival	Nearly 99%	7%

MTX: methotrexate; GCSF: granulocyte-colony stimulating factor; CHOP: (cyclophosphamide, doxorubicin, vincristine and prednisone); HyperCVAD (fractionated cyclophosphamide, vincristine, doxorubicin, dexamethasone, alternating with high-dose methotrexate and cytarabine).

7.8. Blastic Plasmacytoid Dendritic Cell Neoplasm

Given coexpression of CD4/CD56 in some LGLL cases, it is noteworthy to point out the importance to tell it apart from circulating blastic plasmacytoid dendritic cell neoplasm (BPDCN) cells [137]. BPDCN is hematopoietic neoplasm listed under the category of myeloid neoplasm and regarded as a clonal proliferation of early precursors or immature forms of plasmacytoid dendritic cells [138]. The disease often involves predominantly skin followed by bone marrow and peripheral blood and less often lymph node. In contrast to BPDCN skin involvement has not been reported in patient with LGLL. Thus, a search for characteristic dark purple/bruise-like skin lesion and a referral for punch skin biopsy are essential for diagnosis of BPDCN. Similar to the findings observed in skin biopsy, the circulating BPDCN cells are phenotypically positive for dendritic markers such as CD123, TCL1, and BDCA2/CD303, in addition to the coexpression of CD4 and CD56 [139]. TdT expression is identified in 1/3 of cases with BPDCN, which is also indicative of malignancy similar to CD56 in this setting.

CONCLUSION

A correct diagnostic approach of T-cell LGLL should follow a clinical suspicion of the disease based on persistent cytopenia, peripheral blood lymphocytosis or recurrent mucocutaneous infections with unexplainable etiology. Reactive LGL conditions should be excluded in cases with paraneoplastic syndrome, post transplantation, immunotherapy or viral infection. A careful investigation of concomitant autoimmunity, hematopoietic or solid tumors, bone marrow failure syndromes etc. should be attempted to narrow diagnosis. Integrating clinical information with cytomorphology, immunophenotyping, and molecular profiles is required for a correct diagnosis and differential diagnosis. It should be alerted for the hematopathologists to differentiate LGLL from all morphologic and phenotypic mimickers of benign or malignant processes. It is imperative to immediately recognize aggressive T/NK cell leukemia/lymphoma, e.g., ANKL and ENKL and HSTL, which warrants an immediate intensive therapeutic intervention.

REFERENCES

[1] Swerdlow SH, Elias. C, Harris NL, et al. *WHO Classification of Tumours of Haematopoietic and Lymphoid Tissues.* 4th ed: WHO publications Center; 2008.

[2] Wang SS, Vose JM. Epidemiology and Prognosis of T-cell lymphoma. In: Foss F, ed. *T-cells Lymphomas, Contemporary Hematology*: Springer Science + Business Media 2013:25-39.

[3] Shah MV, Hook CC, Call TG, Go RS. A population-based study of large granular lymphocyte leukemia. *Blood Cancer J.* 2016;6(8):e455.

[4] Zhang R, Shah MV, Loughran TP, Jr. The root of many evils: indolent large granular lymphocyte leukaemia and associated disorders. *Hematol Oncol.* 2010;28(3):105-117.

[5] Lamy T, Loughran TP, Jr. How I treat LGL leukemia. *Blood.* 2011;117(10):2764-2774.

[6] Chan WC, Foucar K, Morice WG, Catovsky D. T-cell large granular lymphocytic leukemia. In: Swerdlow SH, Elias. C, Harris NL, et al., eds. *WHO Classification of Tumours of Haematopoietic and Lymphoid Tissues*. 4th ed: WHO publications Center; 2008:272-273.

[7] Loughran TP, Jr. Clonal diseases of large granular lymphocytes. *Blood.* 1993;82(1):1-14.

[8] Lamy T, Moignet A, Loughran TP, Jr. LGL leukemia: from pathogenesis to treatment. *Blood.* 2017;129(9):1082-1094.

[9] Matutes E. Large granular lymphocytic leukemia. Current diagnostic and therapeutic approaches and novel treatment options. *Expert Rev Hematol.* 2017;10(3):251-258.

[10] Bareau B, Rey J, Hamidou M, et al. Analysis of a French cohort of patients with large granular lymphocyte leukemia: a report on 229 cases. *Haematologica.* 2010;95(9):1534-1541.

[11] Epling-Burnette PK, Sokol L, Chen X, et al. Clinical improvement by farnesyltransferase inhibition in NK large granular lymphocyte leukemia associated with imbalanced NK receptor signaling. *Blood.* 2008;112(12):4694-4698.

[12] Rossoff LJ, Genovese J, Coleman M, Dantzker DR. Primary pulmonary hypertension in a patient with CD8/T-cell large granulocyte leukemia: amelioration by cladribine therapy. *Chest.* 1997;112(2):551-553.

[13] Viny AD, Maciejewski JP. High rate of both hematopoietic and solid tumors associated with large granular lymphocyte leukemia. *Leuk Lymphoma.* 2015;56(2):503-504.

[14] Matos DM, de Oliveira AC, Tome Mde N, Scrideli CA. Monoclonal B-cell lymphocytosis (MBL, CD4+/CD8 weak T-cell large granular lymphocytic leukemia (T-LGL leukemia) and monoclonal gammopathy of unknown significance (MGUS): molecular and flow cytometry characterization of three concomitant hematological disorders. *Med Oncol.* 2012;29(5):3557-3560.

[15] Viny AD, Lichtin A, Pohlman B, Loughran T, Maciejewski J. Chronic B-cell dyscrasias are an important clinical feature of T-LGL leukemia. *Leuk Lymphoma.* 2008;49(5):932-938.

[16] Dhodapkar MV, Li CY, Lust JA, Tefferi A, Phyliky RL. Clinical spectrum of clonal proliferations of T-large granular lymphocytes: a T-cell clonopathy of undetermined significance? *Blood.* 1994;84(5):1620-1627.

[17] Papadaki T, Stamatopoulos K, Kosmas C, et al. Clonal T-large granular lymphocyte proliferations associated with clonal B cell lymphoproliferative disorders: report of eight cases. *Leukemia.* 2002;16(10):2167-2169.

[18] Pandolfi F, Loughran TP, Jr., Starkebaum G, et al. Clinical course and prognosis of the lymphoproliferative disease of granular lymphocytes. A multicenter study. *Cancer.* 1990;65(2):341-348.

[19] Semenzato G, Zambello R, Starkebaum G, Oshimi K, Loughran TP, Jr. The lymphoproliferative disease of granular lymphocytes: updated criteria for diagnosis. *Blood.* 1997;89(1):256-260.

[20] Lamy T, Loughran TP, Jr. Clinical features of large granular lymphocyte leukemia. *Semin Hematol.* 2003;40(3):185-195.

[21] Morice WG. T-cell and NK-cell large granular lymphocyte proliferations. In: Jaffe ES, Arber DAC, D. A, Harris NL, Quintanilla-Martinez L, eds. *Hematopathology*: Elsevier; 2017:599-608.

[22] Loughran TP, Jr., Hadlock KG, Perzova R, et al. Epitope mapping of HTLV envelope seroreactivity in LGL leukaemia. *Br J Haematol.* 1998;101(2):318-324.

[23] Loughran TP, Jr., Kadin ME, Starkebaum G, et al. Leukemia of large granular lymphocytes: association with clonal chromosomal abnormalities and autoimmune neutropenia, thrombocytopenia, and hemolytic anemia. *Ann Intern Med.* 1985;102(2):169-175.

[24] Neben MA, Morice WG, Tefferi A. Clinical features in T-cell vs. natural killer-cell variants of large granular lymphocyte leukemia. *Eur J Haematol.* 2003;71(4):263-265.

[25] Agnarsson BA, Loughran TP, Jr., Starkebaum G, Kadin ME. The pathology of large granular lymphocyte leukemia. *Hum Pathol.* 1989;20(7):643-651.

[26] O'Malley DP. T-cell large granular leukemia and related proliferations. *Am J Clin Pathol.* 2007;127(6):850-859.

[27] Bassan R, Pronesti M, Buzzetti M, et al. Autoimmunity and B-cell dysfunction in chronic proliferative disorders of large granular lymphocytes/natural killer cells. *Cancer.* 1989;63(1):90-95.

[28] Loughran TP, Jr., Starkebaum G. Large granular lymphocyte leukemia. Report of 38 cases and review of the literature. *Medicine (Baltimore).* 1987;66(5):397-405.

[29] Battiwalla M, Melenhorst J, Saunthararajah Y, et al. HLA-DR4 predicts haematological response to cyclosporine in T-large granular lymphocyte lymphoproliferative disorders. *Br J Haematol.* 2003;123(3):449-453.

[30] Lamy T, Liu JH, Landowski TH, Dalton WS, Loughran TP, Jr. Dysregulation of CD95/CD95 ligand-apoptotic pathway in CD3(+) large granular lymphocyte leukemia. *Blood.* 1998;92(12):4771-4777.

[31] Zhang L, Zhou J, Sokol L. Hereditary and acquired hemophagocytic lymphohistiocytosis. *Cancer Control.* 2014;21(4):301-312.

[32] Lamy T, Loughran TP, Jr. Current concepts: large granular lymphocyte leukemia. *Blood Rev.* 1999;13(4):230-240.

[33] Mailloux AW, Zhang L, Moscinski L, et al. Fibrosis and subsequent cytopenias are associated with basic fibroblast growth factor-deficient pluripotent mesenchymal stromal cells in large granular lymphocyte leukemia. *J Immunol.* 2013;191(7):3578-3593.

[34] Zhang X, Sokol L, Bennett JM, Moscinski LC, List A, Zhang L. T-cell large granular lymphocyte proliferation in myelodysplastic syndromes: Clinicopathological features and prognostic significance. *Leuk Res.* 2016;43:18-23.

[35] Hansen RM, Lerner N, Abrams RA, Patrick CW, Malik MI, Keller R. T-cell chronic lymphocytic leukemia with pure red cell aplasia: laboratory demonstration of persistent leukemia in spite of apparent complete clinical remission. *Am J Hematol.* 1986;22(1):79-86.

[36] Matutes E, Wotherspoon AC, Parker NE, Osuji N, Isaacson PG, Catovsky D. Transformation of T-cell large granular lymphocyte leukaemia into a high-grade large T-cell lymphoma. *Br J Haematol.* 2001;115(4):801-806.

[37] Tagawa S, Mizuki M, Onoi U, et al. Transformation of large granular lymphocytic leukemia during the course of a reactivated human herpesvirus-6 infection. *Leukemia.* 1992;6(5):465-469.

[38] Brito-Babapulle V, Matutes E, Foroni L, Pomfret M, Catovsky D. A t(8;14)(q24;q32) in a T-lymphoma/leukemia of CD8+ large granular lymphocytes. *Leukemia.* 1987;1(12):789-794.

[39] Zhang L, Sotomayor EM, Papenhausen PR, et al. Unusual concurrence of T-cell large granular lymphocytic leukemia with Franklin disease (gamma heavy chain disease) manifested with massive splenomegaly. *Leuk Lymphoma.* 2013;54(1):205-208.

[40] Dallapiccola B, Alimena G, Chessa L, et al. Chromosome studies in patients with T-CLL chronic lymphocytic leukemia and expansions of granular lymphocytes. *Int J Cancer.* 1984;34(2):171-176.

[41] Morice WG, Kurtin PJ, Leibson PJ, Tefferi A, Hanson CA. Demonstration of aberrant T-cell and natural killer-cell antigen expression in all cases of granular lymphocytic leukaemia. *Br J Haematol.* 2003;120(6):1026-1036.

[42] Lundell R, Hartung L, Hill S, Perkins SL, Bahler DW. T-cell large granular lymphocyte leukemias have multiple phenotypic abnormalities involving pan-T-cell antigens and receptors for MHC molecules. *Am J Clin Pathol.* 2005;124(6):937-946.

[43] Lauria F, Foa R, Migone N, et al. Heterogeneity of large granular lymphocyte proliferations: morphological, immunological and molecular analysis in seven patients. *Br J Haematol.* 1987;66(2):187-191.

[44] Yabe M, Medeiros LJ, Wang SA, et al. Clinicopathologic, Immunophenotypic, Cytogenetic, and Molecular Features of gammadelta T-Cell Large Granular Lymphocytic Leukemia: An Analysis of 14 Patients Suggests Biologic Differences With alphabeta T-Cell Large Granular Lymphocytic Leukemia [corrected]. *Am J Clin Pathol.* 2015;144(4):607-619.

[45] Sandberg Y, Almeida J, Gonzalez M, et al. TCRgammadelta+ large granular lymphocyte leukemias reflect the spectrum of normal antigen-selected TCRgammadelta+ T-cells. *Leukemia.* 2006;20(3):505-513.

[46] Yabe M, Medeiros LJ, Wang SA, et al. Distinguishing Between Hepatosplenic T-cell Lymphoma and gammadelta T-cell Large Granular Lymphocytic Leukemia: A Clinicopathologic, Immunophenotypic, and Molecular Analysis. *Am J Surg Pathol.* 2017;41(1):82-93.

[47] Morice WG, Macon WR, Dogan A, Hanson CA, Kurtin PJ. NK-cell-associated receptor expression in hepatosplenic T-cell lymphoma, insights into pathogenesis. *Leukemia.* 2006;20(5):883-886.

[48] Benjamini O, Jain P, Konoplev SN, et al. CD4(-)/CD8(-) variant of T-cell large granular lymphocytic leukemia or hepatosplenic T-cell lymphoma: a clinicopathologic dilemma. *Clin Lymphoma Myeloma Leuk.* 2013;13(5):610-613.

[49] Karasawa M, Mitsui T, Isoda A, et al. TCR Vbeta repertoire analysis in CD56+ CD16(dim/-) T-cell large granular lymphocyte leukaemia: association with CD4 single and CD4/CD8 double positive phenotypes. *Br J Haematol.* 2003;123(4):613-620.

[50] Olteanu H, Karandikar NJ, Eshoa C, Kroft SH. Laboratory findings in CD4(+) large granular lymphocytoses. *Int J Lab Hematol.* 2010;32(1 Pt 1):e9-16.

[51] Emile JF, Gaulard P. CD56 lymphomas. *Am J Surg Pathol.* 1996;20(2):252-253.

[52] Gorczyca W, Weisberger J, Liu Z, et al. An approach to diagnosis of T-cell lymphoproliferative disorders by flow cytometry. *Cytometry.* 2002;50(3):177-190.

[53] Qiu ZY, Shen WY, Fan L, et al. Assessment of clonality in T-cell large granular lymphocytic leukemia: flow cytometric T cell receptor Vbeta repertoire and T cell receptor gene rearrangement. *Leuk Lymphoma.* 2015;56(2):324-331.

[54] Morice WG, Kimlinger T, Katzmann JA, et al. Flow cytometric assessment of TCR-Vbeta expression in the evaluation of peripheral blood involvement by T-cell lymphoproliferative disorders: a comparison with conventional T-cell

immunophenotyping and molecular genetic techniques. *Am J Clin Pathol.* 2004;121(3):373-383.

[55] Feng B, Jorgensen JL, Hu Y, Medeiros LJ, Wang SA. TCR-Vbeta flow cytometric analysis of peripheral blood for assessing clonality and disease burden in patients with T cell large granular lymphocyte leukaemia. *J Clin Pathol.* 2010;63(2):141-146.

[56] Voskoboinik I, Smyth MJ, Trapani JA. Perforin-mediated target-cell death and immune homeostasis. *Nat Rev Immunol.* 2006;6(12):940-952.

[57] Liu CC, Young LH, Young JD. Lymphocyte-mediated cytolysis and disease. *N Engl J Med.* 1996;335(22):1651-1659.

[58] Bolitho P, Voskoboinik I, Trapani JA, Smyth MJ. Apoptosis induced by the lymphocyte effector molecule perforin. *Curr Opin Immunol.* 2007;19(3):339-347.

[59] McAlinden A, Liang L, Mukudai Y, Imamura T, Sandell LJ. Nuclear protein TIA-1 regulates COL2A1 alternative splicing and interacts with precursor mRNA and genomic DNA. *J Biol Chem.* 2007;282(33):24444-24454.

[60] Anderson P, Nagler-Anderson C, O'Brien C, et al. A monoclonal antibody reactive with a 15-kDa cytoplasmic granule-associated protein defines a subpopulation of CD8+ T lymphocytes. *J Immunol.* 1990;144(2):574-582.

[61] Oshimi K, Shinkai Y, Okumura K, Oshimi Y, Mizoguchi H. Perforin gene expression in granular lymphocyte proliferative disorders. *Blood.* 1990;75(3):704-708.

[62] Shi Y, Wang E. Hepatosplenic T-Cell Lymphoma: A Clinicopathologic Review With an Emphasis on Diagnostic Differentiation From Other T-Cell/Natural Killer-Cell Neoplasms. *Arch Pathol Lab Med.* 2015;139(9):1173-1180.

[63] Gaulard P, Jaffe ES, Krenacs L, Macon WR. Hepatosplenic T-cell lymphoma. In: Swerdlow SH, Campo E, Jaffe ES, Pileri SA, Thiele J, Vardiman JW, eds. *WHO classificationof tumours of haematopoietic and lymphoid tissue.* Lyon, France: WHO presss; 2008:292-293.

[64] Vega F, Medeiros LJ, Gaulard P. Hepatosplenic and other gammadelta T-cell lymphomas. *Am J Clin Pathol.* 2007;127(6):869-880.

[65] Evans HL, Burks E, Viswanatha D, Larson RS. Utility of immunohistochemistry in bone marrow evaluation of T-lineage large granular lymphocyte leukemia. *Hum Pathol.* 2000;31(10):1266-1273.

[66] Langerak AW, van Den Beemd R, Wolvers-Tettero IL, et al. Molecular and flow cytometric analysis of the Vbeta repertoire for clonality assessment in mature TCRalphabeta T-cell proliferations. *Blood.* 2001;98(1):165-173.

[67] van den Beemd R, Boor PP, van Lochem EG, et al. Flow cytometric analysis of the Vbeta repertoire in healthy controls. *Cytometry.* 2000;40(4):336-345.

[68] Behlke MA, Spinella DG, Chou HS, Sha W, Hartl DL, Loh DY. T-cell receptor beta-chain expression: dependence on relatively few variable region genes. *Science.* 1985;229(4713):566-570.

[69] Qu Y, Huang Y, Liu D, et al. High-Throughput Analysis of the T Cell Receptor Beta Chain Repertoire in PBMCs from Chronic Hepatitis B Patients with HBeAg Seroconversion. *Can J Infect Dis Med Microbiol.* 2016;2016:8594107.

[70] Tse E, Kwong YL. Diagnosis and management of extranodal NK/T cell lymphoma nasal type. *Expert Rev Hematol.* 2016;9(9):861-871.

[71] Iqbal J, Weisenburger DD, Chowdhury A, et al. Natural killer cell lymphoma shares strikingly similar molecular features with a group of non-hepatosplenic gammadelta T-cell lymphoma and is highly sensitive to a novel aurora kinase A inhibitor in vitro. *Leukemia.* 2011;25(2):348-358.

[72] Koo GC, Tan SY, Tang T, et al. Janus kinase 3-activating mutations identified in natural killer/T-cell lymphoma. *Cancer Discov.* 2012;2(7):591-597.

[73] Kucuk C, Jiang B, Hu X, et al. Activating mutations of STAT5B and STAT3 in lymphomas derived from gammadelta-T or NK cells. *Nat Commun.* 2015;6:6025.

[74] Lee S, Park HY, Kang SY, et al. Genetic alterations of JAK/STAT cascade and histone modification in extranodal NK/T-cell lymphoma nasal type. *Oncotarget.* 2015;6(19):17764-17776.

[75] Rajala HL, Porkka K, Maciejewski JP, Loughran TP, Jr., Mustjoki S. Uncovering the pathogenesis of large granular lymphocytic leukemia-novel STAT3 and STAT5b mutations. *Ann Med.* 2014;46(3):114-122.

[76] Rajala HL, Eldfors S, Kuusanmaki H, et al. Discovery of somatic STAT5b mutations in large granular lymphocytic leukemia. *Blood.* 2013;121(22):4541-4550.

[77] Koskela HL, Eldfors S, Ellonen P, et al. Somatic STAT3 mutations in large granular lymphocytic leukemia. *N Engl J Med.* 2012;366(20):1905-1913.

[78] Epling-Burnette PK, Liu JH, Catlett-Falcone R, et al. Inhibition of STAT3 signaling leads to apoptosis of leukemic large granular lymphocytes and decreased Mcl-1 expression. *J Clin Invest.* 2001;107(3):351-362.

[79] Andersson EI, Rajala HL, Eldfors S, et al. Novel somatic mutations in large granular lymphocytic leukemia affecting the STAT-pathway and T-cell activation. *Blood Cancer J.* 2013;3:e168.

[80] Loughran TP, Jr., Zickl L, Olson TL, et al. Immunosuppressive therapy of LGL leukemia: prospective multicenter phase II study by the Eastern Cooperative Oncology Group (E5998). *Leukemia.* 2015;29(4):886-894.

[81] Gentile TC, Uner AH, Hutchison RE, et al. CD3+, CD56+ aggressive variant of large granular lymphocyte leukemia. *Blood.* 1994;84(7):2315-2321.

[82] Wong KF, Chan JC, Liu HS, Man C, Kwong YL. Chromosomal abnormalities in T-cell large granular lymphocyte leukaemia: report of two cases and review of the literature. *Br J Haematol.* 2002;116(3):598-600.

[83] Pittman S, Morilla R, Catovsky D. Chronic T-cell leukemias. II. Cytogenetic studies. *Leuk Res.* 1982;6(1):33-42.

[84] Brito-Babapulle V, Matutes E, Parreira L, Catovsky D. Abnormalities of chromosome 7q and Tac expression in T cell leukemias. *Blood.* 1986;67(2):516-521.

[85] Mohty M, Faucher C, Vey N, et al. Features of large granular lymphocytes (LGL) expansion following allogeneic stem cell transplantation: a long-term analysis. *Leukemia.* 2002;16(10):2129-2133.

[86] Gentile TC, Hadlock KG, Uner AH, et al. Large granular lymphocyte leukaemia occurring after renal transplantation. *Br J Haematol.* 1998;101(3):507-512.

[87] Mohty M, Faucher C, Vey N, et al. High rate of secondary viral and bacterial infections in patients undergoing allogeneic bone marrow mini-transplantation. *Bone Marrow Transplant.* 2000;26(3):251-255.

[88] Semenzato G, Pandolfi F, Chisesi T, et al. The lymphoproliferative disease of granular lymphocytes. A heterogeneous disorder ranging from indolent to aggressive conditions. *Cancer.* 1987;60(12):2971-2978.

[89] Oshimi K, Yamada O, Kaneko T, et al. Laboratory findings and clinical courses of 33 patients with granular lymphocyte-proliferative disorders. *Leukemia.* 1993;7(6):782-788.

[90] Rossi D, Franceschetti S, Capello D, et al. Transient monoclonal expansion of CD8+/CD57+ T-cell large granular lymphocytes after primary cytomegalovirus infection. *Am J Hematol.* 2007;82(12):1103-1105.

[91] Roden AC, Morice WG, Hanson CA. Immunophenotypic attributes of benign peripheral blood gammadelta T cells and conditions associated with their increase. *Arch Pathol Lab Med.* 2008;132(11):1774-1780.

[92] Poullot E, Zambello R, Leblanc F, et al. Chronic natural killer lymphoproliferative disorders: characteristics of an international cohort of 70 patients. *Ann Oncol.* 2014;25(10):2030-2035.

[93] Villamor N, Morice WG, Chan WC, Foucar K. *Chronic lymphoproliferative disorders of NK cells.* 2008.

[94] Nash R, McSweeney P, Zambello R, Semenzato G, Loughran TP, Jr. Clonal studies of CD3- lymphoproliferative disease of granular lymphocytes. *Blood.* 1993;81(9):2363-2368.

[95] Lima M, Almeida J, Montero AG, et al. Clinicobiological, immunophenotypic, and molecular characteristics of monoclonal CD56-/+dim chronic natural killer cell large granular lymphocytosis. *Am J Pathol.* 2004;165(4):1117-1127.

[96] Kelly A, Richards SJ, Sivakumaran M, et al. Clonality of CD3 negative large granular lymphocyte proliferations determined by PCR based X-inactivation studies. *J Clin Pathol.* 1994;47(5):399-404.

[97] Perry AM, Diebold J, Nathwani BN, et al. Non-Hodgkin lymphoma in the developing world: review of 4539 cases from the International Non-Hodgkin Lymphoma Classification Project. *Haematologica.* 2016;101(10):1244-1250.

[98] Chan JKC, Quintanilla-Martinez L, Ferry JA. Extranodal NK/T-cell lymphoma, nasal type. In: Swerdlow SH, Campo E, Harris NL, eds. *WHO classification of tumours of Haematopoietic and lymphoid tissues.* Lyon, France: IARA press; 2008:285-288.

[99] Chan JK, Tsang WY, Lau WH, et al. Aggressive T/natural killer cell lymphoma presenting as testicular tumor. *Cancer.* 1996;77(6):1198-1205.

[100] Chan JK, Sin VC, Ng CS, Lau WH. Cutaneous relapse of nasal T-cell lymphoma clinically mimicking erythema multiforme. *Pathology.* 1989;21(3):164-168.

[101] Chan JK, Sin VC, Wong KF, et al. Nonnasal lymphoma expressing the natural killer cell marker CD56: a clinicopathologic study of 49 cases of an uncommon aggressive neoplasm. *Blood.* 1997;89(12):4501-4513.

[102] Chan WK, Au WY, Wong CY, et al. Metabolic activity measured by F-18 FDG PET in natural killer-cell lymphoma compared to aggressive B- and T-cell lymphomas. *Clin Nucl Med.* 2010;35(8):571-575.

[103] Pongpruttipan T, Sukpanichnant S, Assanasen T, et al. Extranodal NK/T-cell lymphoma, nasal type, includes cases of natural killer cell and alphabeta, gammadelta, and alphabeta/gammadelta T-cell origin: a comprehensive clinicopathologic and phenotypic study. *Am J Surg Pathol.* 2012;36(4):481-499.

[104] Jhuang JY, Chang ST, Weng SF, et al. Extranodal natural killer/T-cell lymphoma, nasal type in Taiwan: a relatively higher frequency of T-cell lineage and poor survival for extranasal tumors. *Hum Pathol.* 2015;46(2):313-321.

[105] Emile JF, Boulland ML, Haioun C, et al. CD5-CD56+ T-cell receptor silent peripheral T-cell lymphomas are natural killer cell lymphomas. *Blood.* 1996;87(4):1466-1473.

[106] Vasquez J, Serrano M, Lopez L, Pacheco C, Quintana S. Predictors of survival of natural killer/T-cell lymphoma, nasal type, in a non-Asian population: a single cancer centre experience. *Ecancermedicalscience.* 2016;10:688.

[107] Chim CS, Ma SY, Au WY, et al. Primary nasal natural killer cell lymphoma: long-term treatment outcome and relationship with the International Prognostic Index. *Blood.* 2004;103(1):216-221.

[108] Lee J, Suh C, Park YH, et al. Extranodal natural killer T-cell lymphoma, nasal-type: a prognostic model from a retrospective multicenter study. *J Clin Oncol.* 2006;24(4):612-618.

[109] Kim BS, Kim TY, Kim CW, et al. Therapeutic outcome of extranodal NK/T-cell lymphoma initially treated with chemotherapy--result of chemotherapy in NK/T-cell lymphoma. *Acta Oncol.* 2003;42(7):779-783.

[110] Au WY, Pang A, Choy C, Chim CS, Kwong YL. Quantification of circulating Epstein-Barr virus (EBV) DNA in the diagnosis and monitoring of natural killer cell and EBV-positive lymphomas in immunocompetent patients. *Blood.* 2004;104(1):243-249.

[111] Kwong YL, Pang AW, Leung AY, Chim CS, Tse E. Quantification of circulating Epstein-Barr virus DNA in NK/T-cell lymphoma treated with the SMILE protocol: diagnostic and prognostic significance. *Leukemia.* 2014;28(4):865-870.

[112] Kanakry JA, Hegde AM, Durand CM, et al. The clinical significance of EBV DNA in the plasma and peripheral blood mononuclear cells of patients with or without EBV diseases. *Blood.* 2016;127(16):2007-2017.

[113] Kim SJ, Choi JY, Hyun SH, et al. Risk stratification on the basis of Deauville score on PET-CT and the presence of Epstein-Barr virus DNA after completion of primary treatment for extranodal natural killer/T-cell lymphoma, nasal type: a multicentre, retrospective analysis. *Lancet Haematol.* 2015;2(2):e66-74.

[114] Nakashima Y, Tagawa H, Suzuki R, et al. Genome-wide array-based comparative genomic hybridization of natural killer cell lymphoma/leukemia: different genomic alteration patterns of aggressive NK-cell leukemia and extranodal Nk/T-cell lymphoma, nasal type. *Genes Chromosomes Cancer.* 2005;44(3):247-255.

[115] Siu LL, Wong KF, Chan JK, Kwong YL. Comparative genomic hybridization analysis of natural killer cell lymphoma/leukemia. Recognition of consistent patterns of genetic alterations. *Am J Pathol.* 1999;155(5):1419-1425.

[116] Suzuki R. Treatment of advanced extranodal NK/T cell lymphoma, nasal-type and aggressive NK-cell leukemia. *Int J Hematol.* 2010;92(5):697-701.

[117] Kwong YL. Natural killer-cell malignancies: diagnosis and treatment. *Leukemia.* 2005;19(12):2186-2194.

[118] Cheuk W, Chan JKC. NK-cell neoplasm. In: Jaffe ESea, ed. *Hematopathology.* Lyon, France: Saunders/Elsevier; 2011:473-491.

[119] Kwong YL. The diagnosis and management of extranodal NK/T-cell lymphoma, nasal-type and aggressive NK-cell leukemia. *J Clin Exp Hematop.* 2011;51(1):21-28.

[120] Kwong YL, Anderson BO, Advani R, et al. Management of T-cell and natural-killer-cell neoplasms in Asia: consensus statement from the Asian Oncology Summit 2009. *Lancet Oncol.* 2009;10(11):1093-1101.

[121] Li Y, Wei J, Mao X, et al. Flow Cytometric Immunophenotyping Is Sensitive for the Early Diagnosis of De Novo Aggressive Natural Killer Cell Leukemia (ANKL): A Multicenter Retrospective Analysis. *PLoS One.* 2016;11(8):e0158827.

[122] de Mel S, Li JB, Abid MB, et al. The utility of flow cytometry in differentiating NK/T cell lymphoma from indolent and reactive NK cell proliferations. *Cytometry B Clin Cytom.* 2017.

[123] Jaffe ES, Arber DA, Campo E, Harris NL, Quintanilla-Martinez L. *Hematopathology.* Philadelphia, PA: Elsevier; 2017.

[124] Vose J, Armitage J, Weisenburger D, International TCLP. International peripheral T-cell and natural killer/T-cell lymphoma study: pathology findings and clinical outcomes. *J Clin Oncol.* 2008;26(25):4124-4130.

[125] Hastrup N, Ralfkiaer E, Pallesen G. Aberrant phenotypes in peripheral T cell lymphomas. *J Clin Pathol.* 1989;42(4):398-402.

[126] Went P, Agostinelli C, Gallamini A, et al. Marker expression in peripheral T-cell lymphoma: a proposed clinical-pathologic prognostic score. *J Clin Oncol.* 2006;24(16):2472-2479.

[127] Asano N, Suzuki R, Kagami Y, et al. Clinicopathologic and prognostic significance of cytotoxic molecule expression in nodal peripheral T-cell lymphoma, unspecified. *Am J Surg Pathol.* 2005;29(10):1284-1293.

[128] Suchi T, Lennert K, Tu LY, et al. Histopathology and immunohistochemistry of peripheral T cell lymphomas: a proposal for their classification. *J Clin Pathol.* 1987;40(9):995-1015.

[129] Siegert W, Nerl C, Engelhard M, et al. Peripheral T-cell non-Hodgkin's lymphomas of low malignancy: prospective study of 25 patients with pleomorphic small cell lymphoma, lymphoepitheloid cell (Lennert's) lymphoma and T-zone lymphoma. The Kiel Lymphoma Study Group. *Br J Haematol.* 1994;87(3):529-534.

[130] Zhang L, Van den Bergh M, Sokol L. CD4-Positive T-Cell Large Granular Lymphocytosis Mimicking Sezary Syndrome in a Patient With Mycosis Fungoides. *Cancer Control.* 2017;24(2):207-212.

[131] Hidalgo Lopez JE, Yabe M, Carballo-Zarate AA, et al. Donor-Derived T-Cell Large Granular Lymphocytic Leukemia in a Patient With Peripheral T-Cell Lymphoma. *J Natl Compr Canc Netw.* 2016;14(8):939-944.

[132] Chen YH, Peterson L. Differential diagnosis of CD4-/CD8- gammadelta T-cell large granular lymphocytic leukemia and hepatosplenic T-cell lymphoma. *Am J Clin Pathol.* 2012;137(3):496-497.

[133] Feldman AL, Law M, Grogg KL, et al. Incidence of TCR and TCL1 gene translocations and isochromosome 7q in peripheral T-cell lymphomas using fluorescence in situ hybridization. *Am J Clin Pathol.* 2008;130(2):178-185.

[134] Wang CC, Tien HF, Lin MT, et al. Consistent presence of isochromosome 7q in hepatosplenic T gamma/delta lymphoma: a new cytogenetic-clinicopathologic entity. *Genes Chromosomes Cancer.* 1995;12(3):161-164.

[135] Weidmann E. Hepatosplenic T cell lymphoma. A review on 45 cases since the first report describing the disease as a distinct lymphoma entity in 1990. *Leukemia*. 2000;14(6):991-997.

[136] Saggini A, Saraceno R, Anemona L, Chimenti S, Di Stefani A. Mycosis fungoides in the setting of T-cell large granular lymphocyte proliferative disorder. *Acta Derm Venereol*. 2012;92(3):288-289.

[137] Pagano L, Valentini CG, Grammatico S, Pulsoni A. Blastic plasmacytoid dendritic cell neoplasm: diagnostic criteria and therapeutical approaches. *Br J Haematol*. 2016;174(2):188-202.

[138] Facchetti F, Vermi W, Mason D, Colonna M. The plasmacytoid monocyte/interferon producing cells. *Virchows Arch*. 2003;443(6):703-717.

[139] Falcone U, Sibai H, Deotare U. A critical review of treatment modalities for blastic plasmacytoid dendritic cell neoplasm. *Crit Rev Oncol Hematol*. 2016;107:156-162.

In: Benign and Malignant Disorders ...
Editors: Ling Zhang and Lubomir Sokol
ISBN: 978-1-53612-999-1
© 2018 Nova Science Publishers, Inc.

Chapter 7

CHRONIC LYMPHOPROLIFERATIVE DISORDER OF NATUAL KILLER CELLS: AN ENTITY FALLING TO A BENIGN OR MALIGNANT PROCESS

Prerna Rastogi[1], Rawan Faramand[2], Lubomir Sokol[2] and Ling Zhang[3]

[1]Department of Pathology- University of Iowa Hospitals and Clinics,
Iowa City, IA, US
[2]Division of Hematology-Oncology, H Lee Moffitt Cancer Center, Tampa, FL, US
[3]Department of Hematopathology and Laboratory Medicine,
H Lee Moffitt Cancer Center, Tampa, FL, US

ABSTRACT

Chronic lymphoproliferative disorder of natural killer (NK) cells (CLPD-NK) is characterized by an abnormal or sustained proliferation of NK cells (absolute NK cell count $>=2 \times 10^9$/L), for more than 6 to 12 months without a clearly identified etiology. It is an indolent disorder and listed as a provisional entity which is included in the 2008 and recently revised World Health Organization Classification of Lymphoid Neoplasms. CLPD-NK displays an immunophenotype similar to normal reactive NK cells, positive for cytoplasmic CD3, CD16, and dim CD56, which can be identified by flow cytometry or immunohistochemical study. The NK cell proliferation is usually characterized by expression of a restricted pattern or loss of killer-cell immunoglobulin-like receptors (KIRs), and variable density of surface CD94. The etiology of CLPD-NK is largely unknown. However, it is hypothesized that chronic antigen stimulation or autoimmunity could be implicated in the pathogenesis of this disorder. Recently, mutations in *STAT3* SH2 domain were identified in approximately 30% of the patients with CLPD-NK. While the majority of patients with CLPD-NK are asymptomatic, a subset of patients develops cytopenias, splenomegaly, and autoimmune disorders during the course of the disease and requires immunosuppressive therapy. This chapter will briefly discuss normal NK cell biology, epidemiology, etiology, clinical features, and therapeutic approaches of CLPD-NK.

1. INTRODUCTION

Natural killer (NK) cells are an important part of the innate immune system that primarily serves to eliminate virally infected and tumorigenic cells [1, 2]. They contain potent cytotoxic proteins which are stored in lysosomes and are secreted externally upon activation, resulting in cell lysis by forming pores in the target cells. NK cell function is mediated through ligand-receptor interaction and is regulated by a complex interplay of activating and inhibitory receptors [34]. NK cells can be divided into two subtypes based on their location and surface density expression of CD56 antigen. $CD56^{bright}$ cells are found in lymphoid tissues while $CD56^{dim}$ cells are found in circulating in peripheral blood [5, 6]. These subsets differ in their cytolytic activity; the immature $CD56^{bright}$ subset have limited cytolytic function while the more mature $CD56^{dim}$ cells act primarily as cytotoxic cells [5.6]. It is thought that the $CD56^{dim}$ cells arise from $CD56^{bright}$ cells and acquire cytolytic activity during maturation [5, 6]. In addition to density of surface CD56, several surface markers are used to determine NK cell phenotype, namely CD94, KIR, CD16, perforin, and CD57. The expression density varies between early and late stage of NK cell maturation [5, 8]. Clinical studies in healthy adults show that a subset of dim CD56 positive/CD16 positive NK cells is also positive for CD57 while their $CD56^{bright}$ NK cell counterparts reveal an absence of this antigen [9, 10]. Furthermore, study by Lopez-Verges et al. suggests that CD57 can be used as marker of terminally differentiated NK cells, as previously described in CD8 positive cytotoxic T lymphocytes (Figure 1) [9, 10, 11]. The surface density expression of CD94, a type II integral membrane protein that belongs to the C-type lectin superfamily, also plays a role in differentiating between NK cell subsets [5, 12]. The function of CD94 is to interact with the NKG2 family including NKG2A, B, C, E, and H, but not NKG2D [13]. The heterodimerization of CD94/NKG2 is via HLA-E ligand [13].

KIRs play a critical role in binding HLA class I molecules as their ligands. The consequence of KIRs binding with HLA class I molecules is to produce inhibitory signals that will protect healthy cells expressing HLA class I molecules from NK-cell-mediated cytolysis [14]. Virally infected cells and tumor cell downregulate major histocompatibility complex (MHC) class I expression and are thus targets for NK cell mediated killing [4, 14]. In addition, transformed cells can induce expression of the MHC class I chain-related (MIC) molecule A and B(MICA, and MICB), UL16 binding proteins (ULBPs) among others which are recognized by the NK cell activating receptor NKG2D and result in target cell killing [15-17]. However, if transformed cells or tumor cells do not express MICA, MICB, or ULBP, they will be able to evade recognition by NK cells.

NKp46, a member of natural cytotoxicity receptors (NCR) class, plays a key role in the destruction of virally-infected and malignant cells. Influenza hemagglutinin binds to NKp46, and activates the killing machinery [18]. Recent data showed that internalized intact influenza virion and free hemagglutinin protein in NK cells could downregulate the T-cell receptor zeta chain via the lysosomal pathway and further decrease NK cell cytotoxicity mediated by NKp46 and NKp30 which leads to viral transmission [19]. Finally it is also well recognized that NK cells express the low-affinity IgG receptor CD16, which can activate antibody-dependent cell-mediated cytotoxicity [20].

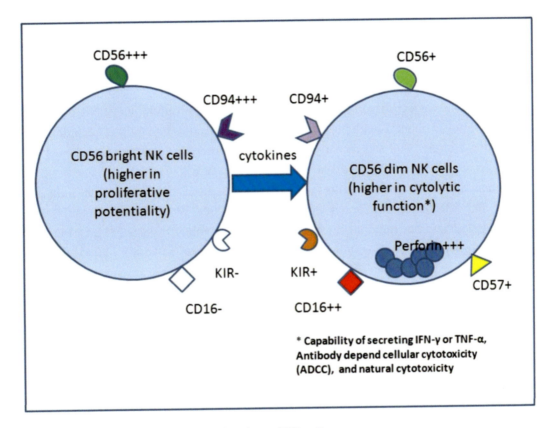

Figure 1. Surface markers and potential functions of NK-cells.

Figure 1 legend: After exposure to cytokines, the CD56^{bright} NK cells homing in secondary lymphoid tissue will progress to their mature stage, characterized by CD56^{dim} expression. These mature NK cells are enriched for perforin positive cytotoxic granules and are able to produce interferon gamma (INF gamma) and tumor necrosis factor beta (TNF β), resulting in cell lysis of tumor cells or virally infected cells. During the process of maturation of NK cells, there is a trend to have decreased CD94 expression and acquire KIR, CD16 and perforin expression. CD57 expression occurs at later stages. CD56^{dim} NK cells, a representative of terminally differentiated NK cells, exhibit relatively high cytolytic activity and gradual loss of their proliferative potential. Between the aforementioned CD56^{bright} and CD56^{dim} NK cells, intermediate stage of NK cells show different levels of surface CD94, KIR, CD56, and CD16 expression (not depicted in the Figure 1), which, however, does not deviate from the trend of development.

Secondary NK cell lymphocytosis is an immune surveillance mechanism which can be seen in reactive situations such as viral infections, autoimmune disorders, vasculitis, or post splenectomy. It may also be associated with solid tumors and hematologic neoplasms such as non-Hodgkin lymphoma [21, 22]. It is critical to differentiate between reactive and neoplastic proliferation of NK cells in clinical practice. Prior to the 2008 WHO classification of lymphoid neoplasms, several terms were used for description of CLPD-NK, namely chronic NK-cell lymphocytosis, chronic NK-large granular lymphocyte (LGL) lymphoproliferative disorder, NK-cell large granular lymphocyte proliferative disorder, NK-cell LGL lymphocytosis, indolent large granular NK-cell lymphoproliferative disorder and indolent leukemia of NK cells [23]. Additionally another term employed clinically was "large granular lymphocytic leukemia of NK-cell lineage (LGL-NK)" which was used previously to include abnormal NK proliferations with more an aggressive clinical course [24, 25].

CLPD-NK is characterized as an abnormal or sustained proliferation of NK cells for more than 6 to 12 months without a clearly identified etiology [26-32]. According to early studies and the 2008 and recently revised WHO criteria an absolute LGL count >2 × 10^9 /L is required to make the diagnosis [33]. However, a lower count (range, 0.4-2 × 10^9//L) may also be compatible with the diagnosis [28, 30-32]. It is usually an indolent disorder and listed as a provisional entity under the 2008 World Health Organization (WHO) classification of tumors of hematopoietic and lymphoid tissues [23]. CLPD-NK is a separate entity from T-cell large granular lymphocytic leukemia (T-LGLL) and aggressive NK cell leukemia. This is based on its unique phenotype, absence of episomal EBV and indolent clinical features. Generally, CLPD-NK is defined by increased circulating NK cells with surface CD3 negative (sCD3-), cytoplasmic CD3 epsilon positive, CD16 positive, CD56 dim positive that can be detected by flow cytometry [23]. Cytotoxic granules (TIA1, granzyme B and M) are identified [23]. Additionally, the increased cell numbers should be sustained for 6 months to 1 year and there should be no identifiable or explainable etiology such as a viral infection [23].

The diagnosis of CLPD-NK can be challenging as most laboratories possess limited ability to fully immunophenotype NK-cells. The clonal origin of NK cells is very difficult to determine since T cell receptor (TCR) genes are in the germinal configuration in NK cells. Evaluation of NK-cell receptors is not routinely used in clinical practice to confirm malignant origin of NK cell population [23]. Recent studies have suggested that malignant T-LGLs are derived from T-memory cytotoxic T-cells. T-LGLL, with indolent clinical features, is commonly associated with a variable degree of cytopenias. CLPD-NK is now regarded to be a counterpart to T-LGLL[23]. However, in contrast to T-LGLL, cytopenias can be seen with CLPD-NK but are not a part of the definition for the entity.

2. EPIDEMIOLOGY AND ETIOLOGY

The accurate incidence and prevalence of CLPD-NK is unknown due to rarity of this disease. Poullot et al. reported the largest cohort of patients with CLPD-NK [29]. In their retrospective series of 70 patients, the median age at diagnosis was reported in the sixth decade with age ranging from 23–82 years. It is slightly more common in males with a male to female ratio of 1.4. Interestingly, in a few of these patients there was a history of preceding malignant diagnosis ranging from solid neoplasm to hematologic malignancies Importantly, in contrast to aggressive NK cell leukemia, CLPD-NK does not appear to be related to a specific ethnicity and has no familial predisposition [29]. By definition CLPD-NK has no demonstrable association with EBV [33].

While the exact etiology of CLPD-NK is unknown, it is thought to be attributed to antigen stimulation or autoimmunity, as seen in T-LGLL [34]. In a series of French patients, human T cell lymphotropic virus (HTLV) I/II was not detected [35]. However, antibodies to HTLV-1 envelope proteins p21 and p24 have been demonstrated by serology in up to 30% of T-LGLL patients [36]. Similar results were seen in a series of 15 patients with CLPD-NK in which sera from 11 patients reacted with the recombinant HTLV envelope protein p21E and 10 of the 15 sera reacted with the epitope BA21. These studies suggest that exposure to a protein containing homology to BA21 may play an important role in the pathogenesis of this disease [37]. In the absence of any HTLV 1/2l DNA, NK-cells expressing KIR can expand, particularly after cytomegalovirus (CMV) infection, thereby suggesting a role for viral mediated expansion of NK cell, although by conventional definition active viral infections were exclusion factors for diagnosis of CLPD-NK [38].

3. MORPHOLOGY AND IMMUNOPHENOTYPE

The neoplastic NK cells in CLPD-NK usually exhibit normal large granular lymphocyte cell morphology which cannot be reliably distinguished from those in T-LGLL or a subset of aggressive NK cell leukemia. They are characterized by 15-20 micrometer size, round to oval nuclei, smooth to slightly irregular nuclear contour, and condensed chromatin, with inconspicuous nucleoli and an abundant light blue cytoplasm containing reddish cytotoxic granules

Bone marrow findings of NK cell proliferations are subtle and may also be accompanied with T-LGLL. Intra-sinusoidal cytotoxic marrow infiltration may be detected in 75% or more of T-LGLL and CLPD-NK cases, when using immunohistochemical stains for T and NK cells [41]. True cases of CLPD-NK that fulfill the criteria mentioned in the definition by Morice II W et al. may be exceedingly rare [24]. Phenotypically, the proliferative subpopulation of NK -cells is surface CD3 negative, myeloperoxidase negative and has germline configuration of TCR and immunoglobulin (Ig) genes [23, 42]. They may express T-associated markers such as CD2, CD7, and CD8. Uniformly aberrant expression of CD8 in CLPD-NK has not uncommonly reported, as well decreased or loss of CD2 and CD7 expression [43, 44], NK cell markers e.g., CD16, CD56, and CD57 are variably expressed upon the predominance of mature stage [43, 44] (Figure 2). In addition, expression of other activating and inhibitory receptors has also been reported including NKG2D, Ly49 or KIR, and CD94-NKG2 heterodimers [45]. The NKG2D activating receptors recognize ligands expressed by bacteria or virally infected cells and signal downstream to activate NK-cell cytotoxicity and the production of cytokines. The inhibitory CD94/NKG2 binds to HLA-E, and KIR binds to HLA-B. This complex inhibits NK-cell activity. Of the aforementioned two subtypes of NK cells, the CD56^{bright} NK cell subset has dim CD16, bright NKp46, dim to negative KIR expression while the CD56^{dim} NK cell subpopulation demonstrates dim NKp46 and bright CD16 expression respectively, along with expression of KIR that is characteristic for cytotoxic effector cells [6].

There may also be altered expression of NK cell-associated receptors (NKR) that recognize I MHC- class I antigens, either showing restricted KIR isoform, commonly activating receptor, or loss of KIR on NK cells [34, 43, 46]. Flow cytometric immunophenotyping is somewhat limited in its extent by relying on identifying CD16-positive, surface CD3-negative cells with diminished expression of CD56 for CLPD-NK. In particular there are aberrancies in KIR and/or CD94 expression [4, 42]. These markers are not commonly used in most laboratories and thus KIR testing is not feasible for clinical practice at this time. Diagnosis of CLPD-NK should therefore be carefully rendered only after repeat studies.

Additional studies for finding surrogate markers have also been attempted. Barcena et al. [47] investigated 60 patients expressing CD56^{dim} NK cells in peripheral blood, which were subcategorized into three groups: 23 cases were clonal [33], 14 were polyclonal [48], and 37 cases did not have definite clonality [31, 39, 40]. When compared with 10 healthy individuals, clonal NK cell group showed higher expression of CD2, CD94, and HLA-DR and weaker expression of CD7, CD11b, and CD38, along with restricted KIR expression (CD158a, CD158b and CD161). Uniform expression of CD94^{high+} and HLA-DR^{high+} was only found in the clonal NK group, suggesting that these antigens could be good surrogate markers for malignant NK cell population although both clonal and polyclonal CLPD-NK shared overlapping immunophenotype [47]. Additional phenotypic study from de Mel et al. [49] elaborated that flow cytometry was able to differentiate NK/T cell lymphoma from CLPD-NK as well as reactive NK cell proliferation. In the study authors indicated that in contrast to NK/T cell lymphoma with CD56 $^{bright+}$, CD16 $^{dim+}$, CD2+, CD7+, CD94+, HLADR+, CD25+, CD26+, and CD57-, the NK cells in CLPD-NK and reactive NK lymphocytosis exhibited CD56+ or dim, CD16+, CD57+ and dim CD94 + [49].

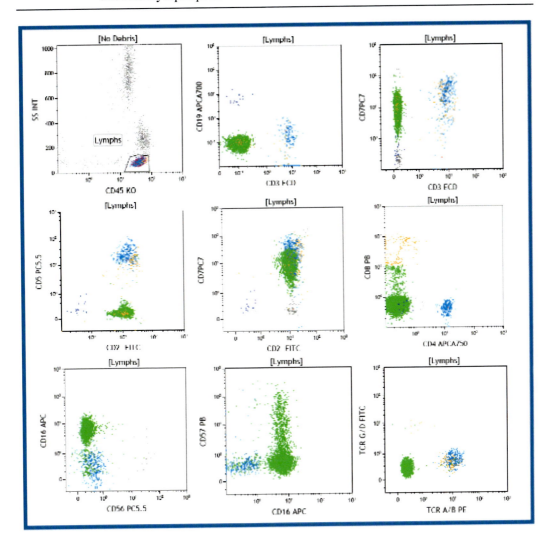

Figure 2. Immunophenotyping by flow cytometry on a patient with CLPD-NK.

Figure 2 legend: The flow cytometric analysis gating on small lymphocytes harvested from a 77 year old man reveals a distinct population (in green) of surface CD3(-)/CD19(-) cell population. The cells are phenotypically positive for CD2, CD7, CD16, CD57 (very small subset) and negative for CD5, CD4, CD8, CD56, TCR αβ and TCR γδ, consistent with NK cell origin. The NK cell population accounts for 91.5% of the gated lymphocytes with the calculated absolute NK cell count of 5.474 x 10^9/L in the patient.

The clonal nature of NK-cell proliferations may help differentiate malignant from benign NK-cell proliferation. There have been infrequent reports on assessment of human androgen receptor-X chromosome (HUMARA) assay that is limited to female patients [50]. In addition NK-cell proliferations also have an abnormal methylation pattern of the KIR genes promoters and may lack at least one or more inhibitory KIR receptor in a study published by Morice and collagues [44, 51].

4. Clinical Presentation and Diagnosis

CLPD-NK is frequently diagnosed in asymptomatic patients manifesting with peripheral blood lymphocytosis and can be associated with or without cytopenias. Peripheral blood reveals an increase in circulating mature NK-cells. Patient presentation is variable with approximately half of the patients asymptomatic at the time of diagnosis. In the largest series of CLPD-NK patients, a variable degree of splenomegaly was observed in 30% of patients [27]. Approximately 24% of the patients had autoimmune diseases and 15% of them had autoimmune cytopenias [27]. Increased NK cells have also been reported in patients with plasma cell dyscrasia and Hodgkin lymphoma [23, 52]. NK cell proliferations are more commonly associated with solid tumors and at presentation the degree of neutropenia is also significantly lower compared to T-LGLL. Similar to T-LGLL, overt lymphadenopathy is uncommon [23, 25].

In a study by Morice et al., CLPD-NK cases from the Mayo Clinic and the Medical College of Wisconsin were reviewed over a period of nine years. Patients were further categorized into three groups based on the expression of CD56. In this analysis, the subgroup of patients with CD56 partial positive or CD56 negative expression were more likely to have neutropenia and anemia [45]. Thrombocytopenia was uncommon among all groups as in consensus with the report by the Poullot group [27, 45]. Splenomegaly was uncommon and was present in 6 of the cases. In the larger series reported by the Poullot group, splenomegaly was an independent poor survival prognostic factor [27, 45].

Overall, CLPD-NK is a clinically indolent disease with an aggressive course rarely reported. Recently, a retrospective analysis of clinicopathological features defined major and minor diagnostic criteria for diagnosis of CLPD-NK summarized in Table 1. Although, these criteria can be helpful in clinical practice, it will be necessary to validate it prospectively on independent cohort of patients.

A clinical-pathological approach utilizing clinical presentation, morphology, immunophenotype, and genotype is needed for a definitive diagnosis of NK cell neoplasms, regardless of whether they are benign or malignant. Of these methods, flow cytometry can be easily employed to identify benign vs. malignant NK cell proliferation by using a combination of monoclonal antibodies discussed above. Using cytomorphology alone, it is very difficult if not impossible to distinguish various NK cell populations. Presence of episomal EBV, in conjunction with acute or aggressive clinical presentations, is indicative of a distinct malignant proliferation and therefore excludes diagnosis of CLPD-NK.

Table 1. Clinical and laboratory characteristics identified in patients with CLPD-NK [24]

Major or Minor diagnostic criteria*	Morphology and Laboratory Tests	Common Features	Uncommon Features
Major	Flow cytometric findings	CD16-positive, CD3-negative NK cells composing >50% of the total peripheral blood or bone marrow lymphocytes	• Loss of CD56 expression • Uniform CD8 expression (>75% of cells positive), may be dim • Loss of CD2 expression • Bright, uniform CD94 expression with or without NKG2A • Uniform expression or complete loss of one or more of the KIRs CD158a, CD158b, and CD158e
	Bone marrow findings and splenic infiltration	Intra-sinusoidal bone marrow or splenic infiltration by cytotoxic lymphocytes positive for CD8 and one or more of the cytotoxic markers TIA-1, granzyme B, granzyme M, or perforin	
	Mutation profile	*STAT-3* gene mutation	
Minor	Absolute count of NK cell in PB	>2x 10^9/L or >80% of total lymphocytes	
	Duration of NK lymphocytosis	Unexplained persistence for >6 months	
	Cytopenia	Unexplained neutropenia (<1.8x 10^9/L,) and/ or anemia (<10 g/dL)	
	Flow cytometry	Diminished CD7 expression	

*Diagnosis will be made if 3 major criteria or 2 major + 2 minor criteria are met.

Theoretically, any low grade lymphoid proliferation should include CLPD-NK in the differential diagnosis. However it is most critical to distinguish CLPD-NK from aggressive NK cell leukemia or leukemic phase of extranodal NK cell lymphoma since the treatment and prognosis is drastically different. In addition it is also necessary to distinguish T-cell neoplasms, myelomonocytic neoplasms, and myeloid neoplasms with CD56 expression and blastic plasmacytoid dendritic neoplasm (CD4/CD56 positive) from true NK cell neoplasms.

A prognostic model to predict the outcome is challenging to develop given the rarity of this disorder. Ultimately, a multi-institutional collaborative effort would be necessary to predict and validate prognostic system for this disorder.

5. MOLECULAR AND GENETIC ABERRATIONS

CLPD-NK has not been associated with any recurrent cytogenetic abnormality which makes it challenging to distinguish between reactive and malignant proliferations. Signal transducer and activator of transcription-3 (STAT-3) protein is a member of the JAK/STAT family. When overexpressed, it can promote survival of the neoplastic T clone [38]. Epling-Burnette et al. reported constitutive up-regulation of *STAT3* in majority of patients with LGL leukemia suggesting that JAK/STAT pathway could play an important role in pathogenesis of LGL leukemia [54]. More recently somatic mutations of *STAT3* have been identified in 30-70% of patients suggesting that this mutation playas very important role in both T-LGLL and CLPD-NK [55, 56]. Jerez et al. showed mutations to be primarily located in the domain of *STAT3* (at Src homology 2 (SH2) domain, residues 585-688) which mediates dimerization [56]. Inhibition of *STAT3* caused apoptosis of leukemic NK and cytotoxic T cells but was not deemed to be very specific [56]. However, the analysis of KIR expression revealed a restricted pattern in a half of the patients with CLPD-NK when compared to a healthy control population suggesting that the expression pattern of KIRs could be useful markers in differential diagnosis of CLPD-NK [56]. In a series of 12 patients with CLPD-NK, there was a constitutive activation of extracellular-regulated kinase (ERK) [57]. It was also found that Ras was constitutively active in patient NK cells which could serve as a targeted therapeutic target [57].

6. PATHOGENESIS

It has been previously shown that malignant LGLs can arise either from T- (85%) or NK cells (15%) and may often be underdiagnosed in the setting of an overlap with a reactive or indolent clonal proliferation. The WHO classification of hematopoietic and lymphoid tumors lists T and NK-cell disorders as two different diseases, relying primarily on the different lineage markers of T and NK cells. NK- and T-cell proliferations have essentially similar clinical presentations of cytopenias and associated co-morbidities. Cytomorphologic features of both entities appear very similar. Gazatto C. et al. have recently examined a series of CLPD-NK and report the presence of monoclonal T-cell populations in up to 48% of cases [58]. They propose that monoclonal populations might be present even during the entire natural history of CLPD-NK. This phenomenon could be explained by a driver mutation in common T/NK cell progenitor or strong antigenic stimulation capable of sustaining both T and NK-cell proliferations. In some patients, the T-cell population may eventually dominate leading to the shift from CLPD-NK to T-LGLL [58]. NK cells with activating KIR may be more successful in clonal expansion, while those with inhibitory KIRs may be suppressed [58]. Cytokines including interleukins (IL-2 and IL-15) can sustain both NK and T-cell proliferation and are routinely up-regulated in inflammatory response [59].

7. TREATMENT

Since CLPD-NK is an indolent disease, the majority of patients do not require treatment. In those patients with severe cytopenias or symptoms, immunosuppressive therapy with low dose oral methotrexate, cyclosporine A or cyclophosphamide is considered to be treatment of choice. This is based on extrapolation of data from patients with T-LGLL as there is limited data on the treatment of CPDNK due to its rarity. Thus, the treatment algorithm follows therapeutic recommendations for the more common T-LGLL (NCCN guidelines for NHL) [23, 51]. In patients with T-LGLL, the responders to methotrexate and cyclosporine A are usually recommended continuing therapy indefinitely due to a high risk of relapse after discontinuation [28, 60]. Treatment with oral cyclophosphamide is not usually extended over 12 months due to increased risk of therapy related secondary malignancies such as myelodysplastic syndromes and acute myeloid leukemia.

As previously described in other chapters, LGL leukemia was shown to have a constitutive activation of the ERK/RAS pathway. Thus, a phase 2 study using the RAS Farnesyl transferase inhibitor Tipifarnib was designed and enrolled 8 patients. While there were no hematologic responses observed, one patient with LGLL and pulmonary arterial hypertension had significant improved in the pulmonary hypertension [26, 40]. Since NK cells express CD52, it was reported that treatment with alemtuzumab, a monoclonal antibody directed against CD52, was successful in one patient with CLPD-NK who failed treatment with methotrexate and steroids. This was only reported in one patient so further studies are encouraged to determine the most effective therapy in patients with CLPD-NK who require treatment.

REFERENCES

[1] Moretta A, Bottino C, Mingari MC, Biassoni R, Moretta L. What is a natural killer cell? *Nat Immunol.* 2002;3(1):6-8.

[2] Vivier E, Tomasello E, Baratin M, Walzer T, Ugolini S. Functions of natural killer cells. *Nat Immunol.* 2008;9(5):503-510.

[3] Lanier LL. On guard--activating NK cell receptors. *Nat Immunol.* 2001;2(1):23-27.

[4] Lanier LL. NK cell recognition. *Annu Rev Immunol.* 2005;23:225-274.

[5] Moretta L. Dissecting CD56dim human NK cells. *Blood.* 2010;116(19):3689-3691.

[6] Romagnani C, Juelke K, Falco M, et al. CD56 bright CD16- killer Ig-like receptor-NK cells display longer telomeres and acquire features of CD56dim NK cells upon activation. *J Immunol.* 2007;178(8):4947-4955.

[7] Fauriat C, Long EO, Ljunggren HG, Bryceson YT. Regulation of human NK-cell cytokine and chemokine production by target cell recognition. *Blood.* 2010;115(11):2167-2176.

[8] Yu J, Mao HC, Wei M, et al. CD94 surface density identifies a functional intermediary between the CD56 bright and CD56dim human NK-cell subsets. *Blood.* 2010;115(2):274-281.

[9] Bjorkstrom NK, Riese P, Heuts F, et al. Expression patterns of NKG2A, KIR, and CD57 define a process of CD56dim NK-cell differentiation uncoupled from NK-cell education. *Blood.* 2010;116(19):3853-3864.

[10] Strioga M, Pasukoniene V, Characiejus D. CD8+ CD28- and CD8+ CD57+ T cells and their role in health and disease. *Immunology.* 2011;134(1):17-32.

[11] Lopez-Verges S, Milush JM, Pandey S, et al. CD57 defines a functionally distinct population of mature NK cells in the human CD56dimCD16+ NK-cell subset. *Blood.* 2010;116(19):3865-3874.

[12] Chang C, Rodriguez A, Carretero M, Lopez-Botet M, Phillips JH, Lanier LL. Molecular characterization of human CD94: a type II membrane glycoprotein related to the C-type lectin superfamily. *Eur J Immunol.* 1995;25(9):2433-2437.

[13] Borrego F, Masilamani M, Marusina AI, Tang X, Coligan JE. The CD94/NKG2 family of receptors: from molecules and cells to clinical relevance. *Immunol Res.* 2006;35(3):263-278.

[14] Parham P. MHC class I molecules and KIRs in human history, health and survival. *Nat Rev Immunol.* 2005;5(3):201-214.

[15] Moretta L, Moretta A. Killer immunoglobulin-like receptors. *Curr Opin Immunol.* 2004;16(5):626-633.

[16] Bahram S, Inoko H, Shiina T, Radosavljevic M. MIC and other NKG2D ligands: from none to too many. *Curr Opin Immunol.* 2005;17(5):505-509.

[17] Cosman D, Mullberg J, Sutherland CL, et al. ULBPs, novel MHC class I-related molecules, bind to CMV glycoprotein UL16 and stimulate NK cytotoxicity through the NKG2D receptor. *Immunity*. 2001;14(2):123-133.

[18] Arnon TI, Achdout H, Lieberman N, et al. The mechanisms controlling the recognition of tumor- and virus-infected cells by NKp46. *Blood*. 2004;103(2):664-672.

[19] Mao H, Tu W, Liu Y, et al. Inhibition of human natural killer cell activity by influenza virions and hemagglutinin. *J Virol*. 2010;84(9):4148-4157.

[20] Seidel UJ, Schlegel P, Lang P. Natural killer cell mediated antibody-dependent cellular cytotoxicity in tumor immunotherapy with therapeutic antibodies. *Front Immunol*. 2013;4:76.

[21] Costello RT, Sivori S, Marcenaro E, et al. Defective expression and function of natural killer cell-triggering receptors in patients with acute myeloid leukemia. *Blood*. 2002;99(10):3661-3667.

[22] Rey J, Veuillen C, Vey N, Bouabdallah R, Olive D. Natural killer and gammadelta T cells in haematological malignancies: enhancing the immune effectors. *Trends Mol Med*. 2009;15(6):275-284.

[23] Villamore N, Morice W, Chan W, Foucar K. Chronic lymphoproliferative disorders of NK cells. In: Swerdlow S, Campo E, Harris N, et al., eds. *WHO Classification of Tumours of Hematopoietic and Lymphoid Tissue*: WHO press; 20048:274.

[24] Morice II W. T-Cell and NK-Cell Large Granular Lymphocyte Proliferations. In: Jaffe E, Arber D, Campo E, Harris N, Quintanilla-Martinez L, eds. *Hematopathology*: Elsevier; 2015:599.

[25] Jamieson AM, Isnard P, Dorfman JR, Coles MC, Raulet DH. Turnover and proliferation of NK cells in steady state and lymphopenic conditions. *J Immunol*. 2004;172(2):864-870.

[26] Loughran TP, Jr. Clonal diseases of large granular lymphocytes. *Blood*. 1993;82(1):1-14.

[27] Tefferi A, Li CY, Witzig TE, Dhodapkar MV, Okuno SH, Phyliky RL. Chronic natural killer cell lymphocytosis: a descriptive clinical study. *Blood*. 1994;84(8):2721-2725.

[28] Lamy T, Loughran TP, Jr. How I treat LGL leukemia. *Blood*. 2011;117(10):2764-2774.

[29] Poullot E, Zambello R, Leblanc F, et al. Chronic natural killer lymphoproliferative disorders: characteristics of an international cohort of 70 patients. *Ann Oncol*. 2014;25(10):2030-2035.

[30] Semenzato G, Zambello R, Starkebaum G, Oshimi K, Loughran TP, Jr. The lymphoproliferative disease of granular lymphocytes: updated criteria for diagnosis. *Blood*. 1997;89(1):256-260.

[31] Bareau B, Rey J, Hamidou M, et al. Analysis of a French cohort of patients with large granular lymphocyte leukemia: a report on 229 cases. *Haematologica.* 2010;95(9):1534-1541.

[32] Mohan SR, Maciejewski JP. Diagnosis and therapy of neutropenia in large granular lymphocyte leukemia. *Curr Opin Hematol.* 2009;16(1):27-34.

[33] Pandolfi F, Loughran TP, Jr., Starkebaum G, et al. Clinical course and prognosis of the lymphoproliferative disease of granular lymphocytes. A multicenter study. *Cancer.* 1990;65(2):341-348.

[34] Hoffmann T, De Libero G, Colonna M, et al. Natural killer-type receptors for HLA class I antigens are clonally expressed in lymphoproliferative disorders of natural killer and T-cell type. *Br J Haematol.* 2000;110(3):525-536.

[35] Fouchard N, Flageul B, Bagot M, et al. Lack of evidence of HTLV-I/II infection in T CD8 malignant or reactive lymphoproliferative disorders in France: a serological and/or molecular study of 169 cases. *Leukemia.* 1995;9(12):2087-2092.

[36] Sokol L, Agrawal D, Loughran TP, Jr. Characterization of HTLV envelope seroreactivity in large granular lymphocyte leukemia. *Leuk Res.* 2005;29(4):381-387.

[37] Loughran TP, Jr., Hadlock KG, Yang Q, et al. Seroreactivity to an envelope protein of human T-cell leukemia/lymphoma virus in patients with CD3- (natural killer) lymphoproliferative disease of granular lymphocytes. *Blood.* 1997;90(5):1977-1981.

[38] Teramo A, Gattazzo C, Passeri F, et al. Intrinsic and extrinsic mechanisms contribute to maintain the JAK/STAT pathway aberrantly activated in T-type large granular lymphocyte leukemia. *Blood.* 2013;121(19):3843-3854, S3841.

[39] Ishihara S, Ohshima K, Tokura Y, et al. Hypersensitivity to mosquito bites conceals clonal lymphoproliferation of Epstein-Barr viral DNA-positive natural killer cells. *Jpn J Cancer Res.* 1997;88(1):82-87.

[40] Ishihara S, Okada S, Wakiguchi H, Kurashige T, Hirai K, Kawa-Ha K. Clonal lymphoproliferation following chronic active Epstein-Barr virus infection and hypersensitivity to mosquito bites. *Am J Hematol.* 1997;54(4):276-281.

[41] Morice WG, Kurtin PJ, Tefferi A, Hanson CA. Distinct bone marrow findings in T-cell granular lymphocytic leukemia revealed by paraffin section immunoperoxidase stains for CD8, TIA-1, and granzyme B. *Blood.* 2002;99(1):268-274.

[42] Anfossi N, Andre P, Guia S, et al. Human NK cell education by inhibitory receptors for MHC class I. *Immunity.* 2006;25(2):331-342.

[43] Morice WG, Kurtin PJ, Leibson PJ, Tefferi A, Hanson CA. Demonstration of aberrant T-cell and natural killer-cell antigen expression in all cases of granular lymphocytic leukaemia. *Br J Haematol.* 2003;120(6):1026-1036.

[44] Morice WG. The immunophenotypic attributes of NK cells and NK-cell lineage lymphoproliferative disorders. *Am J Clin Pathol.* 2007;127(6):881-886.

[45] Ham MF, Ko YH. Natural killer cell neoplasm: biology and pathology. *Int J Hematol.* 2010;92(5):681-689.

[46] Epling-Burnette PK, Painter JS, Chaurasia P, et al. Dysregulated NK receptor expression in patients with lymphoproliferative disease of granular lymphocytes. *Blood.* 2004;103(9):3431-3439.

[47] Barcena P, Jara-Acevedo M, Tabernero MD, et al. Phenotypic profile of expanded NK cells in chronic lymphoproliferative disorders: a surrogate marker for NK-cell clonality. *Oncotarget.* 2015;6(40):42938-42951.

[48] Epling-Burnette PK, Sokol L, Chen X, et al. Clinical improvement by farnesyltransferase inhibition in NK large granular lymphocyte leukemia associated with imbalanced NK receptor signaling. *Blood.* 2008;112(12):4694-4698.

[49] de Mel S, Li JB, Abid MB, et al. The utility of flow cytometry in differentiating NK/T cell lymphoma from indolent and reactive NK cell proliferations. *Cytometry B Clin Cytom.* 2017.

[50] Boudewijns M, van Dongen JJ, Langerak AW. The human androgen receptor X-chromosome inactivation assay for clonality diagnostics of natural killer cell proliferations. *J Mol Diagn.* 2007;9(3):337-344.

[51] Morice WG, Jevremovic D, Olteanu H, et al. Chronic lymphoproliferative disorder of natural killer cells: a distinct entity with subtypes correlating with normal natural killer cell subsets. *Leukemia.* 2010;24(4):881-884.

[52] Morice WG, Leibson PJ, Tefferi A. Natural killer cells and the syndrome of chronic natural killer cell lymphocytosis. *Leuk Lymphoma.* 2001;41(3-4):277-284.

[53] Gattazzo C, Teramo A, Miorin M, et al. Lack of expression of inhibitory KIR3DL1 receptor in patients with natural killer cell-type lymphoproliferative disease of granular lymphocytes. *Haematologica.* 2010;95(10):1722-1729.

[54] Epling-Burnette PK, Liu JH, Catlett-Falcone R, et al. Inhibition of STAT3 signaling leads to apoptosis of leukemic large granular lymphocytes and decreased Mcl-1 expression. *J Clin Invest.* 2001;107(3):351-362.

[55] Koskela HL, Eldfors S, Ellonen P, et al. Somatic STAT3 mutations in large granular lymphocytic leukemia. *N Engl J Med.* 2012;366(20):1905-1913.

[56] Jerez A, Clemente MJ, Makishima H, et al. STAT3 mutations unify the pathogenesis of chronic lymphoproliferative disorders of NK cells and T-cell large granular lymphocyte leukemia. *Blood.* 2012;120(15):3048-3057.

[57] Epling-Burnette PK, Bai F, Wei S, et al. ERK couples chronic survival of NK cells to constitutively activated Ras in lymphoproliferative disease of granular lymphocytes (LDGL). *Oncogene.* 2004;23(57):9220-9229.

[58] Gattazzo C, Teramo A, Passeri F, et al. Detection of monoclonal T populations in patients with KIR-restricted chronic lymphoproliferative disorder of NK cells. *Haematologica.* 2014;99(12):1826-1833.

[59] Zambello R, Facco M, Trentin L, et al. Interleukin-15 triggers the proliferation and cytotoxicity of granular lymphocytes in patients with lymphoproliferative disease of granular lymphocytes. *Blood.* 1997;89(1):201-211.

[60] Lamy T, Loughran TP, Jr. Clinical features of large granular lymphocyte leukemia. *Semin Hematol.* 2003;40(3):185-195.

In: Benign and Malignant Disorders …
Editors: Ling Zhang and Lubomir Sokol

ISBN: 978-1-53612-999-1
© 2018 Nova Science Publishers, Inc.

Chapter 8

T-CELL LARGE GRANULAR LYMPHOCYTIC LEUKEMIA: CONVENTIONAL TREATMENT APPROACHES AND NOVEL STRATEGIES

Magali Van den Bergh and Lubomir Sokol
Department of Hematology and Oncology,
H. Lee Moffitt Cancer Center & Research Institute, Tampa, FL, US

ABSTRACT

Large granular lymphocytic leukemia (LGLL) is an indolent lymphoproliferative disorder characterized by the clonal expansion of large granular lymphocytes (LGL) of either T-cell or NK-cell origin. Clinical features of LGLL characteristically consist of neutropenia, anemia, and/or rheumatoid arthritis. Cytopenias, symptomatic autoimmune diseases, and recurrent infections are the most common indications to start treatment. Up to forty percent of patients remain asymptomatic and can be observed. The majority of patients will require treatment, which may pose a challenge upon clinicians as no standard front-line therapy has been established based on randomized or larger prospective clinical trials. The mainstay of treatment of LGLL consists of single-agent immunosuppressive therapy, including methotrexate, cyclophosphamide, and cyclosporine A. In case of failure of first-line agent, a trial of another immunosuppressive agent is typically applied. Purine analogs such as pentostatin and fludarabine have a role in more aggressive and symptomatic disease. In the relapsed or refractory setting, clinical trials with novel agents should be offered to eligible patients. No curative therapeutic modalities are available and novel treatment options are needed. Most patients have an indolent disease course while infrequently fatalities may occur due to infections in the setting of severe neutropenia or rarely due to aggressive disease. The prognosis is favorable with median overall survival greater than 10 years. This chapter discusses the indications to initiate treatment, distinct treatment modalities, experimental therapies, response criteria, and prognosis in patients with LGLL.

1. INTRODUCTION

Large granular lymphocytic leukemia (LGLL) is a rare, indolent malignancy arising from aberrant proliferations of mature, post-thymic LGLs of cytotoxic T-cell or natural killer (NK)-cell origin. Malignant LGLs typically circulate in the peripheral blood, infiltrate bone marrow and spleen and less frequently involve liver. LGLL occurs in all age groups, usually presents in the sixth decade of life with the mean age at diagnosis of 61 years [1]. It affects males and females equally. Although its exact incidence is unknown, LGLL is estimated to affect one in one million subjects in the United States. Chronic antigenic stimulation with putative autoantigens is hypothesized to contribute to its pathogenesis, as suggested by its terminal effector memory phenotype [2]. Viruses have also been postulated to play a role in the pathogenesis of LGLL; however, no specific virus has been identified as a definite causative pathogen. LGLL can be unrecognized for prolonged time periods due to its indolent nature. Over time LGLL can manifest itself with neutropenia resulting in recurrent mucocutaneous infections, anemia, thrombocytopenia or symptomatic splenomegaly. The association between LGLL and autoimmune conditions is well-known and is often a clue in establishing the diagnosis [3]. Rheumatoid arthritis is by far the most common autoimmune disorder described in LGLL, followed by Sjögren syndrome and autoimmune cytopenias. Bone marrow failure disorders such as myelodysplastic syndromes, aplastic anemia, and paroxysmal nocturnal hemoglobinuria have been described in patients with LGLL [3]. T-cell LGLL has been reported to be the most common cause of secondary pure red cell aplasia in the United States, so the threshold for laboratory testing for LGLL should be low in this patient population in the appropriate clinical context. Increased rates of solid tumors and secondary hematological malignancies have been reported in the setting of LGLL, particularly monoclonal gammopathy of unknown significance (MGUS) and B-cell lymphoproliferative disorders [3-5]. Over sixty percent of patients with LGLL will require systemic therapy during the course of their disease due to development of cytopenias, symptomatic splenomegaly, exacerbations of autoimmune disorders, recurrent infections or systemic B-symptoms. As large randomized, prospective trials are absent, no standard first line treatment in LGLL has been established. The mainstay of treatment is immunosuppressive therapy. The moderate success of immunosuppressive agents can be partly explained by underlying molecular mechanisms involving platelet-derived growth factor (PDGF) and Interleukin-15 (IL-15) in the pathogenesis of LGLL. PDGF and IL-15 play a pivotal role in leukemic LGL cell survival by means of dysregulation of apoptosis and inhibition of activation-induced cell death [6-10]. More recently, *STAT3 up-regulation* has been identified to be a key driver of proliferation of LGLL. Activating somatic mutations of *STAT3* and *STAT5b* have been described in approximately forty percent of LGLL patients [11]. More recent data using whole-exome sequencing in LGLL revealed an average of 20 somatic mutations per patient establishing LGLL as a true malignant clonal disorder [12].

2. INDICATIONS FOR TREATMENT

Indications for treatment of T-cell and NK-cell LGLL are identical and include hemoglobin less than 10 g/dL in the absence of other causes, red blood cell transfusion dependence, absolute neutrophil count (ANC) less than 0.5×10^9/L, mild to moderate neutropenia with recurrent infections, or platelet count less than 50×10^9/L. Other indications to start systemic treatment include symptomatic splenomegaly, pulmonary hypertension, or systemic B-symptoms. Importantly, absolute LGL count is not linear with disease progression and in itself is not a prognostic marker; hence absolute LGL count should not guide treatment. The main aim of treatment is to correct the cytopenias and this can be achieved in the setting of a persistent LGL clone.

3. FIRST-LINE TREATMENT

3.1. Immunosuppressive Agents: Methotrexate, Cyclophosphamide, and Cyclosporine A

Although therapy of patients with LGLL is mostly based on retrospective studies and few prospective clinical trials, accepted first-line therapy includes low-dose methotrexate (MTX) +/- corticosteroids, cyclophosphamide (Cy) +/- corticosteroids, or cyclosporine A (CSA). Patients who achieve a partial response (PR) or complete response (CR) to MTX or CSA after four months of treatment should continue their treatment until progression of disease. CR and PR are defined according to the National Comprehensive Cancer Network (NCCN) treatment guidelines (see section on response criteria). The duration of Cy administration, however, should be limited to less than 12 months due to increased risk of secondary malignancies. Of note, CR refers to hematological CR as the existing studies evaluated responses in the peripheral blood and not in the bone marrow.

The efficacy of methotrexate in LGLL was first described by Loughran et al. who reported a response in 5 out of 10 patients [13]. MTX was administered at a dose of 10 mg/m² orally weekly. In several studies, overall response rate (ORR) ranged from 55% to 65% and CR rate from 11% to 21%. Median duration of response was variable with sustained responses up to 21 months [14, 15]. Time to response was up to 4 months, hence a trial of at least 4 months was warranted prior to changing to a different agent. The Eastern Cooperative Oncology Group conducted a phase II prospective study

(ECOG 5998) evaluating the efficacy of oral MTX in a first stage with non-responders switching to oral Cy. MTX was administered at a dose of 10 mg/m² weekly for up to 1 year and prednisolone was added during the initial 4 weeks of treatment to accelerate the response. Patients who did not achieve PR or CR were switched to oral cyclophosphamide 100mg daily for up to 1 year. Results of this prospective analysis showed an ORR to MTX of 38%. MTX non-responders switched to Cy revealed the ORR of 64%. Interestingly, the median overall survival (OS) and progression free survival (PFS) were more favorable for patients presenting with neutropenia compared to those with anemia (OS and PFS not reached versus 69 months and 29 months, respectively). ORR of 100% was seen in patients with *STAT3* Y640F mutations treated with methotrexate, suggesting that this particular mutation could predict a response to MTX therapy [11]. Table 1 shows a summary of results of MTX therapy in patients with LGL leukemia based on various retrospective studies.

The moderate efficacy of Cy in the treatment of LGLL was incidentally found when pure red cell aplasia patients with concomitant T-cell LGLL were treated with Cy. Subsequently, multiple large registries evaluated response rates to Cy in T-cell and NK-cell LGLL and reported an ORR ranging from 52% to 71% with a CR from 29% to 47% and a mean duration of response up to 31 months [14-16]. The median time to response was 4 months. Cy is given at a dose of 50 to100 mg orally daily. No significant differences were found between patients with T-cell versus NK-cell LGLL or between LGLL patients presenting with anemia versus neutropenia. Overall, treatment with Cy is well tolerated without a significant toxicity profile [17]. The main concern with long-term therapy with an alkylating agent such as Cy is the eventual development of secondary hematological malignancies, in particular, myelodysplastic syndromes (MDS) or acute myeloid leukemia (AML). Hence, the duration of Cy administration is limited to 12 months. Currently, a prospective trial comparing first-line therapy with MTX versus Cy is ongoing in France (ClinicalTrials.gov Identifier: NCT01976182). Table 2 shows a summary of results for Cy therapy in patients with LGLL based on several retrospective studies.

Cyclosporine A (CSA) is an alternative first-line immunomodulatory therapy effective in LGLL. CSA is typically administered at a dose of 3 to 10 mg/kg orally daily or 100 to 150 mg orally daily. Dosing is titrated based on renal function and hematologic responses rather than the serum drug levels. The ORR to CSA in LGLL ranges from 21% to 61% with a CR rate from 4% to 17% and a mean duration of response up to 12 months [14-16]. CSA is fairly well tolerated, although particularly elderly patients on long-term immunosuppression should be monitored for the development of secondary malignancies. Up to date, there are no prospective randomized clinical trials comparing CSA to other immunosuppressive agents in the first-line setting. Table 3 shows a summary of results for CSA therapy in patients with LGLL based on various retrospective studies.

3.2. Steroids

The addition of steroids during the first month of immunosuppressive therapy can aid in the resolution of constitutional symptoms and accelerate the improvement in cytopenias. Prednisone is typically administered at a dose of 1 mg/kg orally daily for the first month with tapering off by the end of the second month of treatment [11, 16, 18].

3.3. Hematopoietic Growth Factors: Granulocyte Colony-Stimulating Factor and Erythropoietin

Granulocyte colony-stimulating factor (G-CSF) as a monotherapy in the setting of LGLL with neutropenia has minimal efficacy. G-CSF can cause a transient increase in the neutrophil count; however the response is not lasting. G-CSF can accelerate splenomegaly and activate arthritic pains [19].

There is limited evidence of the benefit of erythropoietin (EPO) as a therapeutic agent in LGLL. It has been used concomitantly with CSA in the treatment of LGLL manifesting with anemia. The French registry encountered 7 LGLL patients treated with EPO of which 2 were responders [14].

Table 1. Various studies evaluating outcomes with methotrexate (MTX) therapy in patients with LGLL

Patients treated with MTX(n)	ORR(%)	CR(%)	PR(%)	TTR(weeks)	DOR(months)	Reference
10	60	50	10	2-12	12-108	[13]
2	100	NR	NR	NR	NR	[39]
4	100	67	33	8-12	NR	[40]
7	85	14	71	3-6	NR	[41]
8	38	NR	NR	NR	NR	[42]
62	55	21	34	4-12	12-60	[14]
3	66	33	33	NR	NR	[21]
96	55	21	34			Total

ORR: overall response rate, CR: complete response, PR: partial response, TTR: time to response, DOR: duration of response, NR: not reached.

Table 2. Studies evaluating outcomes with cyclophosphamide (Cy) therapy in patients with LGLL

Patients treated with Cy (n)	ORR(%)	CR(%)	PR(%)	TTR(weeks)	DOR(months)	Reference
16	69	NR	NR	NR	NR	[39]
9	65	NR	NR	NR	NR	[43]
4	33	33	0	4	NR	[41]
8	75	NR	NR	1	NR	[44]
16	44	NR	NR	NR	NR	[42]
32	66	NR	NR	NR	NR	[14]
85	61	-	-			Total

ORR: overall response rate, CR: complete response, PR: partial response, TTR: time to response, DOR: duration of response, NR: not reached.

Table 3. Studies evaluating outcomes with cyclosporine A (CSA) therapy in patients with LGLL

Patients treated with CSA(n)	ORR(%)	CR(%)	PR(%)	TTR(weeks)	DOR(months)	Reference
3	100	NR	NR	2-8	NR	[45]
5	100	NR	NR	3-9	NR	[46]
25	56	NR	NR	9	NR	[47]
23	78	NR	NR	2-60	NR	[41]
9	40	NR	NR	4-60	NR	[48]
5	44	NR	NR	2	NR	[44]
23	61	NR	NR	NR		[42]
10	70	NR	NR	11	NR	[49]
6	50	NR	NR	NR	NR	[14]
24	21	NR	NR	12-24	NR	[21]
123	56					Total

ORR: overall response rate, CR: complete response, PR: partial response, TTR: time to response, DOR: duration of response, NR: not reached.

4. TREATMENT OF RELAPSED OR REFRACTORY DISEASE

If disease is progressive or refractory to successive trials of the different first line therapies, other options can be explored. Second-line options include a clinical trial, purine analogs, alemtuzumab, splenectomy, or under certain circumstances a hematopoietic stem cell transplant [11, 19]. Table 4 shows a summary of results for various second-line therapies in patients with LGLL. Figure 1 displays a treatment algorithm for LGLL.

4.1. Purine Nucleoside Analogs: Pentostatin and Fludarabine

Chemotherapy in the form of purine nucleoside analogs has been effective as reported in a few case series of patients with LGLL. It is reserved for individuals with more aggressive disease, as demonstrated by symptomatic splenomegaly, extensive bone marrow infiltration, highly elevated lymphocyte counts, or evidence of widespread disease. Pentostatin has been reported effective in isolated case reports and a few case series of T-cell LGLL patients [20-22]. Pentostatin is administered at a dose of 4 mg/m^2 every 2 weeks for a total of 8 to 10 cycles. One series described an ORR of 75% while another series showed a CR of 40% [21, 22]. A case series involving 9 Chinese patients as well as 2 single case reports described the effective use of fludarabine-based treatment in patients with T-LGLL [23-25]. Fludarabine can be utilized as a single agent or in combination with mitoxantrone and dexamethasone. The Chinese case series reported an ORR in 100% with a CR in 5 out of 9 individuals [23].

4.2. Alemtuzumab

Alemtuzumab is a humanized monoclonal antibody that binds the CD52 membrane protein of lymphocytes and monocytes. It has shown efficacy in several hematologic disorders including chronic lymphocytic leukemia, T-cell prolymphocytic leukemia, MDS and aplastic anemia. As LGLLs strongly express membrane CD52, alemtuzumab was evaluated in this patient population [26]. Following documented responses in an isolated case report and a small case series, a prospective phase 2 single-arm clinical trial using alemtuzumab in T-LGLL was opened at the National Health Institute. Out of 25 participants, 24 had received prior immunomodulatory therapy. Alemtuzumab was given intravenously at a dose of 10 mg daily for a total of 10 consecutive days. ORR at the 3-month mark was 56% and CR was 36%. Responses were durable in 9 of the 25 patients, although they did not enter molecular remission as the T-cell clone persisted in the peripheral circulation. Overall treatment was well tolerated without significant side effects. *STAT3* mutations were identified in 50% of the tested patients and its presence did not have any significant prognostic value and was not predictive of response to alemtuzumab therapy [27].

4.3. Splenectomy

Splenectomy has been utilized as a treatment for LGLL in the setting of neutropenia, hemolytic anemia, or symptomatic splenomegaly. Lamy et al. reviewed the literature of splenectomy as a treatment modality in LGLL and found that a total of 31 out of 55 patients (56%) responded [16]. However, the most recently in the second largest retrospective study a less promising response rate of 4 out of 13 patients (31%) was observed [14].

4.4. Hematopoietic Stem Cell Transplant

Data from hematopoietic stem cell transplant (SCT) in LGLL are very limited due to the indolent nature of the disease. Few patients with aggressive, refractory disease have been managed successfully with either an autologous or an allogeneic SCT. A retrospective analysis from the European bone marrow transplantation registry identified 10 patients treated with an allogeneic SCT of which half were in CR at 30 months while the other half died. They reported 5 patients treated with an autologous SCT of which 2 were in CR at 30 months while the remainder died [28]. Stem cell transplantation is not indicated in LGLL with the exception of very aggressive disease refractory to multiple lines of treatment or in patients with overlap bone marrow failure syndromes such as LGLL with MDS or LGLL with aplastic anemia [19].

5. EXPERIMENTAL THERAPIES

5.1. Monoclonal Antibodies: Siplizumab and Hu-MiK-Beta 1

Siplizumab is a humanized monoclonal antibody that binds the CD2 antigen expressed on T-cell and NK-cell lymphocytes. Experimental studies and pre-clinical models have shown efficacy of siplizumab in adult T-cell leukemia/lymphoma. Based on these results, a single center phase 1 dose-escalating trial was conducted on a few dozen patients, including 7 individuals with T-cell LGLL. However, due to the emergence of Epstein-Barr virus (EBV)-associated lymphoproliferative disorders in several patients, the study was terminated early [29].

Hu-MiK-Beta 1 is a humanized monoclonal antibody directed at the shared IL-2/IL-15Rβ subunit (CD122). Both the IL-2 and IL-15 receptors play an integral role in the proliferation and survival of LGL leukemic cells [30-32]. Hu-MiK-Beta1 was studied in a single agent open-label phase I trial in patients with either treatment-naïve or immunosuppressive agent-refractory LGLL. Out of the 9 patients enrolled, only 3 had a transient rise in absolute neutrophil counts. Despite treatment, all patients had stable disease. No major toxicity was observed [31]. Table 5 displays a summary of outcomes and toxicities of LGLL patients treated with monoclonal antibodies.

Table 4. Summary of results for second-line agents in patients with LGL leukemia

Second-line agent	Patients (n)	ORR	DOR	Reference
Alemtuzumab	24 (10 case reports)	14/24 (58%)	6-24 months	[16]
Purine Analog	38 (11 case reports)	30/38 (79%)	3-40 months	[16]
Splenectomy	55 (8 case reports and case series)	31/55 (56%)	3-40 months	[16]
Stem cell transplant (SCT)	15 (1 case series with 10 allogeneic and 5 autologous SCT)	7/15 (47%)	47% in CR at 30 months	[28]

ORR: overall response rate, DOR: duration of response, CR: complete response.

5.2. Farnesyltransferase Inhibitor: Tipifarnib

Tipifarnib is a small molecule that inhibits one of three prenylases, farnesyltransferase (FT). FT transfers the 15-carbon farnesyl group to several hundred cellular polypeptides, including small guanosine triphosphate-binding proteins of the Ras, Rho, and Rheb families. Since the *Ras-Mek1-ERK* pathway is constitutively activated in LGLL and supports malignant cell survival, the inhibition of this pathway using FT inhibitor was a basis for novel targeted therapy. The efficacy of tipifarnib was studied in several early clinical trials targeting different cancers and leukemias. A case report describing a refractory NK-cell LGLL patient responding favorably to tipifarnib paved the path for a NCI phase 2 clinical trial evaluating activity of tipifarnib in T-cell LGLL. Eight patients with relapsed or refractory LGLL were enrolled; however none of the subjects achieved a hematological response (Table 5) [33].

5.3. *JAK3*-Specific Inhibitor: Tofacitinib

As the *JAK-STAT* pathway is constitutively activated in LGLL, enabling leukemic cell proliferation and survival, inhibitors of this pathway may pose a potential novel targeted therapeutic option for LGLL patients. Recently, gain-of-function mutations in *STAT3* and *STAT5b* genes were identified in about 40% of patients with T-LGLL. Even thought several *STAT3* inhibitors have been tested in various malignant disorders, clinical trials with these agents have not be conducted in patients with LGLL, yet [11, 18]. Tofacitinib is a JAK3-specific inhibitor that has proven activity in refractory rheumatoid arthritis and has been FDA-approved for this indication [34]. A clinical trial evaluating tofacitinib showed a hematological response in 6 out of 9 refractory T-cell LGLL patients. In addition, an *in vitro* analysis of *STAT3* mutant individuals showed greater drug sensitivity compared to *STAT3* wild-type cells. Large, prospective trials are needed to confirm these preliminary findings [35]. Phase 1/2 clinical trials evaluating *STAT3* inhibitors in multiple cancers are underway. Pimozide, a *STAT5* inhibitor, is currently under development and may be an alternative novel therapeutic agent for T-cell LGLL, particularly those with *STAT5b* mutations who tend to have a more aggressive disease course [19].

5.4. Proteasome Inhibitor: Bortezomib

The *NF-kB* pathway is another activated pathway in T-cell LGLL that prevents apoptosis independently of *STAT3* activation. Bortezomib is a proteasome inhibitor that downregulates the *NF-kB* signaling and is approved for treatment of multiple myeloma and relapsed mantle cell lymphoma based on results of several studies. *In vitro* studies have shown activity of bortezomib in LGLL by means of inducing apoptosis of leukemic cells, however, no clinical trials of bortezomib have been conducted in LGLL so far [19].

6. RESPONSE CRITERIA

Treatment should be continued for at least 4 months to assess for response to therapy, granted its toxicity is not limiting the duration of therapy. There are no uniform response criteria and several large studies have utilized slightly different response criteria. The NCCN guidelines follow the criteria documented in the French registry as follows; a complete response (CR) is defined as recovery of peripheral blood counts to hemoglobin > 12 g/dL, absolute neutrophil count > 1.5 x 10^9/L, platelet count > 150 x 10^9/L, resolution of lymphocytosis with absolute lymphocyte count < 4 x 10^9/L, and normalization of circulating LGL counts with absolute LGL count < 0.5 x 10^9/L. Partial response (PR) is defined as hemoglobin > 8 g/dL, absolute neutrophil count > 0.5 x 10^9/L, platelet count > 50 x 10^9/L, and absence of transfusions (Table 6) [14].

Table 5. Summary of outcomes and toxicities with experimental therapies in LGLL

Experimental agent	Patients (n)	ORR	Toxicity	Reference
Phase 2: Tipifarnib (Zarnestra)	8	0/8 (0%)	Significant myelotoxicity	[33]
Phase 1: Hu-MiK-beta-1 (anti-CD122)	9	No major hematologic response	No significant toxicity	[31, 32]
Phase 1: Siplizumab (anti-CD2)	7	Study was terminated due to toxicity	EBV-related lymphoproliferative disorder in 2/7 patients	[29]

ORR: overall response rate, EBV: Epstein-Barr virus.

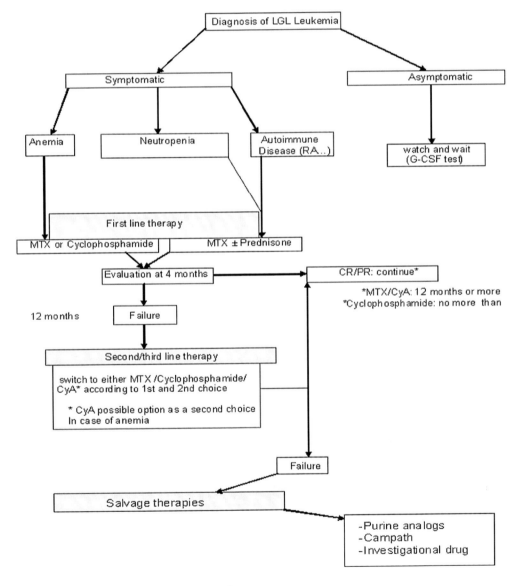

Figure 1. Treatment algorithm for LGLL [16].

Table 6. Response criteria in LGLL per NCCN guidelines [13, 18]

Response	Hemoglobin	ANC	Platelets	Other
CR	> 12 g/dL	> 1.5 x 10^9/L	> 150 x 10^9/L	Lymphocytes < 4 x 10^9/L LGL count < 0.5 x 10^9/L
PR	> 8 g/dL	> 0.5 x 10^9/L	> 50 x 10^9/L	Absence of transfusions

ANC: absolute neutrophil count, CR: Complete Response, PR: Partial Response.

Loughran et al. described slightly less strict response criteria with CR defined as hemoglobin > 11 g/dL, absolute neutrophil count > 1.5 x 10^9/L, platelet count > 100 x 10^9/L, resolution of lymphocytosis with absolute lymphocyte count < 4 x 10^9/L, and normalization of circulating LGL counts. Partial response (PR) is defined as improvement in hematologic parameters in the absence of CR with 1) ANC > 0.5 x 10^9/L, as long as this represented 50% increase; 2) improvement in ANC > 50% over baseline; 3) increase in hemoglobin by > 1g/dL for at least four months duration; and 4) decrease in monthly transfusion requirements of > 50% for at least four months duration. Loughran et al. described progressive disease as worsening of hematologic parameters in patients previously achieving CR or PR. No response is defined as lack of CR or PR. Complete molecular remission is attained when the T cell clone is absent upon repeating T cell receptor gene rearrangement studies [11].

7. PROGNOSIS

The prognosis of patients with LGLL is variable, with a few patients demonstrating rapid progression while the majority remains relatively asymptomatic and survive for years to even decades. Two large registry studies showed a 5-year OS ranging from 75% to 89% and a 10-year OS of 63% [14, 15]. In the French series, the mortality rate was 6.6%. The most common causes of death include infections and sepsis and only rarely aggressive disease progression leads to a fatal outcome [14]. Prolonged immunosuppressive therapy is a potential risk factor for transformation into a high-grade large T-cell lymphoma, although this is rather an extremely rare event [36]. Patients with mutant *STAT5b* LGLL tend to have a more aggressive course of disease with increased refractoriness to immunosuppressive agents compared to patients with wild-type *STAT5b* [37].

To date, there is no validated prognostic system in place. A multivariate analysis of 286 T-cell LGLL patients at Mayo Clinic identified that anemia (hemoglobin <12 g/dL), severe neutropenia (absolute neutrophil count <0.1 × 10^9/L), and lymphopenia (absolute lymphocyte count < 1 × 10^9/L) were independent risk factors portraying worse prognosis in T-cell LGLL [38]. In this study, a prognostic scoring system was developed based on the three identified risk factors (anemia, severe neutropenia, and lymphopenia). Each risk factor was assigned 1 point and median overall survival was found to be 105, 55, and 5 months for a total score of 0, 1, and 2 or more points, respectively (Table 7) [39]. This prognostic scoring system excluded NK-cell LGLL patients and has not been validated prospectively or retrospectively, yet.

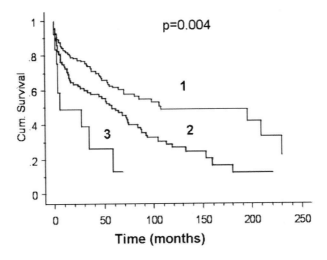

Figure 2. Overall survival in T-cell LGLL patients with according to number of cytopenias [38].

Table 7. T-cell LGLL prognostication system [7, 37]

Number of Cytopenias*	T-cell LGLL Median Overall Survival
0	105 months
1	55 months
2-3	5 months

* Cytopenias are defined as hemoglobin<12 g/dL, absolute neutrophil count <0.1 x 10^9/L and absolute lymphocyte count <1 x 10^9/L.

8. SUMMARY

In summary, LGLL is a rare, indolent lymphoproliferative disorder. The most common indication for starting therapy is cytopenia. Therapeutic recommendations are based mainly on retrospective, single institutional studies, as randomized clinical trials are absent. Efficacy of immunosuppressive therapy with methotrexate, cyclophosphamide, and cyclosporine A with or without steroids is comparable. Therapy with alemtuzumab, purine analogs, and splenectomy are salvage options. Novel therapies with inhibitors of activated *STAT3/STAT5b* pathways are underway and will hopefully reveal higher response rates and an improved duration of responses.

REFERENCES

[1] Rose, MG; Berliner, N. T-cell large granular lymphocyte leukemia and related disorders. *Oncologist.*, 2004, 9(3), 247-58.

[2] Yang, J; Epling-Burnette, PK; Painter, JS; et al. Antigen activation and impaired Fas-induced death-inducing signaling complex formation in T-large-granular lymphocyte leukemia. *Blood.*, 2008, 111(3), 1610–1616.

[3] Isenalumhe, L; Van den Bergh, M; Wang, E; et al. Frequency of additional malignancies in patients with large granular lymphocytic leukemia (LGLL): A single institutional experience. *J Clin Oncol.*, 2017, 35(8 Supplement), 7542.

[4] Viny, AD; Maciejewski, JP. High rate of both hematopoietic and solid tumors associated with large granular lymphocyte leukemia. *Leuk Lymphoma.*, 2015, 56(2), 503–504.

[5] Van den Bergh, M; Isenalumhe, L; Wang, E; et al. A single institution analysis of patients with dual diagnosis of T-cell large granular lymphocytic leukemia and either a plasma cell and/or a B-cell lymphoproliferative disorder. *Clin Lymphoma Myeloma Leuk.*, 2016, 16 (2 Supplement), 117.

[6] Zhang, R; Shah, MV; Yang, J; et al. Network model of survival signaling in large granular lymphocyte leukemia. *Proc Natl Acad Sci USA.*, 2008, 105(42), 16308–16313.

[7] Shah, MV; Zhang, R; Irby, R; et al. Molecular profiling of LGL leukemia reveals role of sphingolipid signaling in survival of cytotoxic lymphocytes. *Blood.*, 2008, 112(3), 770–781.

[8] Epling-Burnette, PK; Liu, JH; Catlett-Falcone, R; et al. Inhibition of STAT3 signaling leads to apoptosis of leukemic large granular lymphocytes and decreased Mcl-1 expression. *J Clin Invest.*, 2001, 107(3), 351–362.

[9] Schade, AE; Powers, JJ; Wlodarski, MW; et al. Phosphatidylinositol-3-phosphate kinase pathway activation protects leukemic large granular lymphocytes from undergoing homeostatic apoptosis. *Blood.*, 2006, *107*(12), 4834–4840.

[10] Yang, J; Liu, X; Nyland, SB; et al. Platelet-derived growth factor mediates survival of leukemic large granular lymphocytes via an autocrine regulatory pathway. *Blood.*, 2010, 115(1), 51–60.

[11] Loughran, TP; Jr. Zickl, L; Olson, TL; et al. Immunosuppressive therapy of LGL leukemia: prospective multicenter phase II study by the Eastern Cooperative Oncology Group (E5998). *Leukemia.*, 2015, 29(4), 886–894.

[12] Coppe, A; Andersson, EI; Binatti, A; et al. Genomic landscape characterization of large granular lymphocyte leukemia with a systems genetics approach. *Leukemia.*, 2017, 31, 1243–1246.

[13] Loughran, TP; Jr. Kidd, PG; Starkebaum, G. Treatment of large granular lymphocyte leukemia with oral low-dose methotrexate. *Blood.*, 1994, 84, 2164–2170.

[14] Bareau, B; Rey, J; Hamidou, M; et al. Analysis of a French cohort of patients with large granular lymphocyte leukemia: a report on 229 cases. *Haematologica.*, 2010, 95(9), 1534–1541.

[15] Van den Bergh, M; Isenalumhe, L; Wang, E; et al. A single institutional experience of 261 patients with large granular lymphocytic leukemia (LGLL). *J Clin Oncol.*, 2017, 35(15 Supplement), 7555.

[16] Lamy, T; Loughran, Jr. TP. How I treat LGL Leukemia. *Blood.*, 2011, 117, 2764-2774.

[17] Moignet, A; Hasanali, Z; Zambello, R; et al. Cyclophosphamide as a first-line therapy in LGL leukemia. *Leukemia.*, 2014, 28(5), 1134–1136

[18] Van den Bergh, M; Sokol, L. T-Cell Large Granular Lymphocytic Leukemia. In: Sallman DA, Chaudhury A, Nguyen J, Zhang L, List AF (editors). *Handbook of Hematologic Malignancies.* 1st edition. New York, NY: Springer Publishing Company, 2017. Chapter 23, pp. 137-141. ISBN: 9781620700945.

[19] Matutes, E. Large granular lymphocytic leukemia. Current diagnostic and therapeutic approaches and novel treatment options. *Expert Review of Hematology.*, 2017, 10(3), 251-258.

[20] Tsirigotis, P; Venetis, E; Kapsimali, V; et al. 2-deoxycoformycin in the treatment of T-large granular lymphocyte leukemia. *Leuk Res.*, 2003, 27, 865–867.

[21] Fortune, AF; Kelly, K; Sargent, J; et al. Large granular lymphocyte leukemia: natural history and response to treatment. *Leuk Lymphoma.*, 2010, 51, 839–845.

[22] Mercieca, J; Matutes, E; Dearden, C; et al. The role of pentostatin in the treatment of T-cell malignancies: analysis of response rate in 145 patients according to disease subtype. *J Clin Oncol.*, 1994, 12(12), 2588–2593.

[23] Ma, SY; Au, WY; Chim, CS; et al. Fludarabine, mitoxantrone and dexamethasone in the treatment of indolent B- and T-cell lymphoid malignancies in Chinese patients. *Br J Haematol.*, 2004, 124(6), 754–761.

[24] Sternberg, A; Eagleton, H; Pillai, N; et al. Neutropenia and anaemia associated with T-cell large granular lymphocyte leukemia responds to fludarabine with minimal toxicity. *Br J Haematol.*, 2003, 120, 699–701.

[25] Tse, E; Chan, JC; Pang, A; et al. Fludarabine, mitoxantrone and dexamethasone as first-line treatment for T-cell large granular lymphocyte leukemia. *Leukemia.*, 2007, 21, 2225–2226.

[26] Osuji, N; Del Giudice, I; Matutes, E; et al. CD52 expression in T-cell large granular lymphocyte leukemia–implications for treatment with alemtuzumab. *Leuk Lymphoma.*, 2005, 46, 723–727.

[27] Dumitriu, B; Ito, S; Feng, X; et al. Alemtuzumab in T-cell large granular lymphocytic leukaemia: interim results from a single-arm, open-label, phase 2 study. *Lancet Haematol.*, 2016, 3(1), e22–9.

[28] Marchand, T; Lamy, T; Finel, H; et al. Hematopoietic stem cell transplantation for T-cell large granular lymphocyte leukemia: a retrospective study of the European Society for Blood and Marrow Transplantation. *Leukemia.*, 2016, 30(5), 1201–1204.

[29] O'Mahony, D; Morris, JC; Stetler-Stevenson, M; et al. EBV related lymphoproliferative disease complicating therapy with the antiCD2 monoclonal antibody, siplizumab, in patients with T-cell malignancies. *Clin Cancer Res.*, 2009, 15, 2514–2522.

[30] Hodge, DL; Yang, J; Buschman, MD; et al. Interleukin-15 enhances proteasomal degradation of bid in normal lymphocytes: implications for large granular lymphocyte leukemias. *Cancer Res.*, 2009, 69(9), 3986–3994.

[31] Morris, JC; Janik, JE; White, JD; et al. Preclinical and phase I clinical trial of blockade of IL-15 using Mikbeta1 monoclonal antibody in T cell large granular lymphocyte leukemia. *Proc Natl Acad Sci USA.*, 2006, 103(2), 401–406.

[32] Waldmann, TA; Conlon, KC; Stewart, DM; et al. Phase 1 trial of IL-15 *trans* presentation blockade using humanized Mik-Beta-1 mAb in patients with T-cell large granular lymphocytic leukemia. *Blood.*, 2013, 121, 476-484.

[33] Epling-Burnette, PK; Sokol, L; Chen, X; et al. Clinical improvement by farnesyltransferase inhibition in NK large granular lymphocyte leukemia associated with imbalanced NK receptor signaling. *Blood.*, 2008, 112, 4694–4698.

[34] Wallenstein, GV; Kanik, KS; Wilkinson, B; et al. Effects of the oral Janus kinase inhibitor tofacitinib on patient-reported outcomes in patients with active rheumatoid arthritis: results of two Phase 2 randomised controlled trials. *Clin Exp Rheumatol.*, 2016, 34 (3), 430–442.

[35] Bilori, B; Thota, S; Clemente, MJ; et al. Tofacitinib as a novel salvage therapy for refractory T-cell large granular lymphocytic leukemia. *Leukemia.*, 2015, 29(12), 2427–2429.

[36] Matutes, E; Wotherspoon, AC; Parker, NE; et al. Transformation of T-cell large granular lymphocyte leukemia into a high-grade large T-cell lymphoma. *Br J Haematol.*, 2001, 115, 801–806.

[37] Rajala, HL; Eldfors, S; Kuusanmäki, H; et al. Discovery of somatic STAT5b mutations in large granular lymphocytic leukemia. *Blood.*, 2013, 121(22), 4541–4550.

[38] Nowakowski, GS; Morice, WG; Zent, CS; et al. Initial Presentation and Prognostic Factors in 286 Patients with T-Cell Large Granular Lymphocyte Leukemia. *Blood.*, 2006, 108, 300.

[39] Dhodakpar, MV; Li, CY; Lust, JA; et al. Clinical spectrum of clonal proliferations of T-large granular lymphocytes: a T-cell clonopathy of undetermined significance? *Blood.*, 1994, 84(5), 1620–1627.

[40] Hamidou, M; Lamy, T. Large granular lymphocyte proliferations: clinical and pathogenic aspects. *Rev Med Interne.*, 2001, 22(5), 452–459.

[41] Osuji, N; Matutes, E; Tjonnfjord, G; et al. T-cell large granular lymphocyte leukemia: a report on the treatment of 29 patients and a review of the literature.*Cancer.*, 2006, 107(3), 570–578.

[42] Mohan, SR; Maciejewski, JP. Diagnosis and therapy of neutropenia in large granular lymphocyte leukemia. *Curr Opin Hematol.*, 2009, 16(1), 27–34.

[43] Go, RS; Li, CY; Tefferi, A; et al. Acquired pure red cell aplasia associated with lymphoproliferative disease of granular T lymphocytes. *Blood.*, 2001, 98(2), 483–485.

[44] Fujishima, N; Sawada, K; Hirokawa, M; et al. Long-term responses and outcomes following immunosuppressive therapy in large granular lymphocyte leukemia-associated pure red cell aplasia: a Nationwide Cohort Study in Japan for the PRCA Collaborative Study Group. *Haematologica.*, 2008, 93(10), 1555–1559.

[45] Bible, KC; Tefferi, A. Cyclosporine A alleviates severe anaemia associated with refractory large granular lymphocytic leukaemia and chronic natural killer cell lymphocytosis. *Br J Haematol.*, 1996, 93(2), 406–408.

[46] Sood, R; Stewart, CC; Aplan, PD; et al. Neutropenia associated with T-cell large granular lymphocyte leukemia: long-term response to cyclosporine therapy despite persistence of abnormal cells. *Blood.*, 1998, 91(9), 3372–3378.

[47] Battiwalla, M; Melenhorst, J; Saunthararajah, Y; et al. HLA-DR4 predicts haematological response to cyclosporine in T-large granular lymphocyte lymphoproliferative disorders. *Br J Haematol.*, 2003, 123(3), 449–453.

[48] Aribi, A; Huh, Y; Keating, M; et al. T-cell large granular lymphocytic (T-LGL) leukemia: experience in a single institution over 8 years. *Leuk Res.*, 2007, 31(7), 939–945.

[49] Pawarode, A; Wallace, PK; Ford, LA; et al. Long-term safety and efficacy of cyclosporin A therapy for T-cell large granular lymphocyte leukemia. *Leuk Lymphoma.*, 2010, 51(2), 338–341.

In: Benign and Malignant Disorders …
Editors: Ling Zhang and Lubomir Sokol

ISBN: 978-1-53612-999-1
© 2018 Nova Science Publishers, Inc.

Chapter 9

EXTRANODAL NK/T-CELL LYMPHOMA, NASAL TYPE-DIAGNOSTIC APPROACHES

Stefanie Grewe[1], Carolina Domiguez[1] and Haipeng Shao[2,]*

[1]Department of Pathology and Cell Biology, University of South Florida Morsani College of Medicine, Tampa, FL, US

[2]Department of Hematopathology and Laboratory Medicine, H. Lee Moffitt Cancer Center and Research Institute, Tampa, FL, US

ABSTRACT

Extranodal natural killer/T cell lymphoma, nasal type (ENKTL) is an Epstein-Barr virus (EBV) associated highly aggressive lymphoma with a characteristic racial and geographical distribution, most commonly occurring in East Asia. The most frequent site of involvement is the nasal cavity, but dissemination to other sites such as skin and the gastrointestinal tract is common. Diagnosis of ENKTL requires a thorough clinical evaluation, histological and phenotypic examination, and molecular cytogenetic analysis. Histologically, ENKTL shows characteristic angiocentric and angiodestructive growth patterns associated with necrosis and ulceration. The lymphoma cells show the phenotype of activated NK-cells with expression of cytoplasmic CD3ε, CD56 and cytotoxic markers, and are nearly always positive for EBV by Epstein-Barr encoding region (EBER) in situ hybridization. ENKTL typically demonstrates complex chromosomal abnormalities with frequent deletion of the chromosome 6q21-25, where multiple potential tumor suppressor genes such as *PRDM1* have been identified. Combined radiotherapy and chemotherapy is standard for the treatment of localized early stage disease. ENKTL responds poorly to anthracycline-based chemotherapy. Combination chemotherapy with regimens incorporating L-asparaginase and non-multidrug resistance (MDR)-dependent drugs is the mainstay therapy for advanced stage and relapsed disease.

---

[*] Corresponding Author: E-mail: Haipeng.shao@moffitt.org; Tel: 813-745-2672; Fax: 813-745-1708.

Three clinical prognostication models are based on the international prognostic index (IPI), the Korean prognostic index (KPI), and the NK prognostic index.

1. INTRODUCTION

Extranodal natural killer/T cell lymphoma, nasal type (ENKTL) is a rare and well-defined highly aggressive extranodal non-Hodgkin lymphoma [1, 2], which is most frequently found in the nasal cavity and upper aerodigestive tract (nasopharynx, paranasal sinuses, and palate) [3, 4]. The neoplastic proliferation is characterized histologically by angioinvasion, angiodestruction, prominent necrosis, and strong association with the Epstein-Barr virus (EBV) [1, 3]. Since the first description by McBride in 1897 [5], it has been referred to by a variety of names, such as lethal midline granuloma, granuloma gangrenescens, polymorphic reticulosis, midline malignant reticulosis, idiopathic midline destructive disease, and Stewart's granuloma *et al.* because of the disease's common clinical presentation as malignant destructive lesions involving the midline facial structures as well as a lack of understanding of the nature of malignant cells. It was considered a type of malignant lymphoma due to the presence of large atypical lymphoid cells in many cases and frequent dissemination [6]. The application of immunohistochemical studies first suggested that it was a T-cell lymphoma because the atypical lymphoid cells were immunoreactive for polyclonal antibodies directed against human T-cells [7, 8]. But subsequent studies demonstrated rare clonal T-cell receptor gene rearrangement and positive immunoreactivity for NK cell marker CD56 [9, 10]. Later, the neoplastic cells were shown to have cytologic features of large granular lymphocytes with ample cytoplasm and large cytoplasmic azurophilic granules, characteristic of NK cells or cytotoxic T-cells [11]. The accumulating data indicated that it is a lymphoma of activated NK cells [12-14]. Therefore, the terminology of this entity evolved from "angiocentric lymphoma" proposed by the revised European-American classification of lymphoid neoplasms (REAL) in 1994 [15], to "nasal or nasal-type T/NK-cell lymphoma" by a joint workshop of the University of Hong Kong and the Society for Hematopathology [16]. The current designation of "extranodal NK/T-cell lymphoma, nasal type" was eventually adopted and the diagnostic criteria defined by the 3rd and 4th editions of the World Health Organization (WHO) Classification of tumors of haematopoietic and lymphoid tissues [17, 18].

2. EPIDEMIOLOGY

ENKTL most commonly affects adults in the fourth to fifth decade of life with a male to female ratio of ~2-3:1 [19-22]. Rare cases in children and adolescents have been reported [3]. It has a strong ethnic and geographic predilection. It is more common in Far East Asia (namely China, Japan, Korea, and Hong Kong) and Central and South America (especially Peru), representing approximately 7-10% of non-Hodgkin lymphomas compared to North America and Europe, where it accounts for approximately 1-1.5% of all non-Hodgkin lymphomas [20, 23-32]. The frequency of ENKTL per 100,000 patients ranges from 8 to 40.8 in Japan, Korea and China, as compared to 4 in United Kingdom [33-35]. The frequency rate varies even in East Asia countries, with the rate 5 times higher in Korea than that in Japan. In the sinonasal tract, ENKTL is the most common type of lymphoma in Asia and Latin America, while B-cell lymphomas are more common in Western countries [8, 29, 36-40]. ENKTL in the United States occurs most frequently in ethnic groups from areas of high frequency (Asia and Latin America), but less commonly in native American populations [41]. The incidence of ENKTL is persistently higher in Asian immigrants in North America, suggesting a genetic predisposition [42]. Since the 1990s, there is a decreased frequency of ENKTL in Korea but not in Japan. The frequency rate per 100,000 outpatients of ears, nose and throat (ENT) clinics in Korea had decreased from 40 to 20 between the periods of 1977–1989 and 1990–1996, while there were no significant changes in Japan during the period studied [43]. In contrast, a few studies suggested an increased incidence rate of ENKTL in Indian population [44, 45].

3. ETIOLOGY

3.1. EBV Infection

EBV, genetic and environmental factors appear to play causative roles in the development of ENKTL. The etiologic role of EBV infection is inferred from the nearly ubiquitous presence of EBV in nearly all cases of ENKTL [29, 30, 41, 46-56], with rare exceptions [57]. In children and young adults, ENKTL can develop after chronic active EBV infection [58, 59]. EBV infection of lymphocytes could result in latent infection, in which 11 viral genes are expressed, including EBV nuclear antigens (*EBNA*) 1, 2, 3A, 3B, 3C and 5, latent proteins (*LMP*) 1, 2A and 2B, and small non-coding RNAs (*EBER* 1 and 2). The EBNA-2 protein is a major transcriptional activator regulating viral latent genes and cellular gene expression. EBNA 2 has two antigenically different alleles, EBNA 2A and EBNA 2B, with approximately 50% amino acid homology [60]. EBV is classified as type 1 and type 2 (formerly known as type A and B) based on presence of either EBNA 2A or EBNA 2B allele. EBV type 1 has a higher transforming efficiency and is more frequently detected in Caucasian and Asian healthy individuals, while EBV type 2 is relatively more prevalent in Africa and often seen in lymphoma of immunocompromised individuals [61-66]. There is a geographic difference of EBV types in ENKTL. Nearly all cases of ENKTL in Asia have type 1 EBV [51, 67-70], while variable proportions of type 2 EBV are detected in cases of Western countries and Latin America [1, 30, 71-73].

3.2. Pesticides

The use of pesticides has been identified as a risk factor for the development of ENKTL. A familial case of ENKTL involving a father and one of his children was reported in which they frequently used large amounts of pesticides in a greenhouse [74]. Pesticides have also been associated with increased risk of developing non-Hodgkin lymphoma [75, 76]. An epidemiological study demonstrated that life-style and environmental factors related to exposure to pesticides and chemical solvents might be risk factors for NK-T cell lymphoma (NKTCL) [77]. In this multi-centers study of patients in Japan, Korea and China, the odds ratio (OR) of NKTCL was 4.15 (95% confidence interval (CI), 1.74-9.87) for farmers, 2.81 (95% CI, 1.49-5.29) for producers of crops, 4.01 (95% CI, 1.99-8.09) for pesticide users, 11.65 (95% CI, 1.17-115.82) for residents near garbage burning plants, and 2.95 (95% CI, 1.25-6.95) for former drinkers. The ORs for crop producers, who minimized the exposure to pesticides with the use of gloves and glasses, and sprinkling downwind at the time of pesticide use, were 3.30 (95% CI, 1.28-8.54), 1.18 (95% CI, 0.11-12.13) and 2.20 (95% CI, 0.88-5.53), respectively, which were lower than that of producers who did not take these precautions.

3.3. Human Immunodeficiency Virus (HIV) Infection

ENKTL has been reported in patients with HIV infection and in transplant recipients, suggesting immunosuppression as a risk factor for the development of ENKTL [78-83].

3.4. Genetic Factor

Genetic risks of ENKTL have recently been studied with genome-wide association study (GWAS) [84]. An early genetic typing study showed significant lower frequency of the HLA-A*0201 allele in patients with ENKTL [85]. However, the association between HLA-A*0201 and risk of ENKTL was not confirmed by the genome-wide association study (GWAS) [84]. The GWAS identified a strong association between HLA-DPB1 amino acids and susceptibility to ENKTL [84]. Single-nucleotide polymorphisms (SNPs) rs9277378 (located in HLA-DPB1) had the strongest association with ENKTL susceptibility (odds ratio [OR] 1·84 [95% CI 1·61-2·11]). Four aminoacid residues

(Gly84-Gly85-Pro86-Met87) in near-complete linkage disequilibrium at the edge of the peptide-binding groove of HLA-DPB1 likely account for most of the association between the rs9277378*A risk allele and NKTCL susceptibility (OR 2·38, p value for haplotype 2·32 × 10(-14)). This association was distinct from MHC associations with Epstein-Barr virus infection. HLA-DPB1 is the β1 subunit of the HLA-DP heterodimer, and participates in extracellular antigen presentation to CD4-positive T-cell lymphocytes [86]. The four amino acid residues at 84–87 form one of the key hydrophobic anchor pockets within the peptide-binding groove, and are important for antigen presentation [87]. The association of SNPs at these key amino acid residues with risk of ENKTL suggesting antigen recognition and processing and lymphoma cell clearance play a role in the development of ENKTL.

4. CLINICAL PRESENTATIONS

ENKTLs are nearly universally extranodal [88]. The clinical presentation varies according to the site(s) of involvement. Approximately 80% cases of ENKTL present locally in the upper aerodigestive tract (nasal cavity, nasopharynx, paranasal sinuses, and palate) with nasal cavity the most frequent site of involvement [1, 17, 21, 24, 89]. Extranasal sites of involvement include skin [90, 91], gastrointestinal (GI) tract [92, 93], testis [94, 95, 96], soft tissue [97], liver, spleen, bone marrow [98] and brain [99]. The skin and GI tract are the most common extranasal sites of involvement [24, 100]. Rare case of breast ENKTL associated with saline implant has been reported [101].

Destructive lesions in the nasal cavity can destroy the cavity floor leading to the characteristic mid-line hard-palate perforation. Clinically, symptoms of upper aerodigestive tract involvement include nasal congestion, epistaxis, dysphagia, facial edema, sinus headache, and purulent rhinorrhea. B symptoms such as fever, malaise, and weight loss are common. Nasal ENKTL may show dissemination to extranasal sites, such as skin, gastrointestinal tract, testis, salivary glands, and soft tissues. Primary extranasal ENKTL shows more adverse clinical features such as high stage, elevated lactate dehydrogenase (LDH), bulky disease, and poor performance status, and is more likely to show anemia and thrombocytopenia [24]. But imaging studies with positron emission tomography/computed tomography (PET/CT) has demonstrated that most if not all cases of extranasal ENKTL have occult primary nasal disease [102-105], even in cases without apparent nasal lesions. Therefore, many of the extranasal ENKTL likely represent disseminated nasal ENKTL. A strict criteria of extranasal ENKTL should requires demonstration of absence of nasal disease by random nasopharyngeal biopsies and PET/CT [106]. With current era of L-asparaginase–based chemotherapy, primary sites of involvement are no longer an independent prognostic factor [107]. Some ENKTL may be complicated by hemophagocytic syndrome/hemophagocytic lymphohistiocytosis (HLH) at disease presentation or at the terminal phase of the disease [108-110]. ENKTL shows high response rate to chemotherapy/radiotherapy, but relapse rate is high up to 77% [111-114]. A few cases (<5%) show more indolent clinical course characterized by repeated relapse or progression and long-term survival, and relatively low Ki-67 proliferation index [115, 116].

Patients with cutaneous ENKTL present with subcutaneous mass, erythematous or violaceous nodules, ulcerative lesion, cellulitis or abscess-like lesion [90, 117-119]. The skin lesions are more often multiple or generalized than solitary. They are predominantly located throughout the extremities and trunk, especially the lower extremities [90, 117, 120]. Patients with primary cutaneous ENKTL often present with low stage disease (stage I or II) [90, 117, 121], but elevated LDH, lymphadenopathy, visceral and bone marrow involvement can be seen [117, 121]. B-symptoms are uncommon. Cases with IPI score >2 are often secondary cutaneous involvement by nasal ENKTL rather than primary cutaneous ENKTL. Rare cases of primary cutaneous ENKTL may have long waxing and waning clinical course, or spontaneous regression [122, 123].

Patients with ENKTL in the GI tract are predominantly middle aged male. The GI tract lesions most commonly manifest as abdominal pain, GI bleeding and bowel perforation [92, 93, 124]. Fever and B symptoms are frequent. The most commonly involved GI sites are the small intestine, especially ileum, jejunum and cecum. More than 60% of the patients present with advanced stage disease. The prognosis is dismal with OS of less than a year. The patients often died of disease progression and sepsis. ENKTL in testis and other sites usually presents with mass lesion [95].

5. MORPHOLOGIC AND IMMUNOPHENOTYPIC FEATURES

ENKTL shows characteristic morphological features regardless of the site of involvement. The ENKTL cells show a diffuse infiltrate with a characteristic angiocentric and angiodestructive growth pattern [3]. The angiocentric pattern is defined as accentuation of lymphoma cells around blood vessels. Angiodestructive pattern is defined as invasion of blood vessel wall with fibrinoid necrosis and fragmentation of the elastic lamina. Zonal coagulation necrosis with ghosts of lymphoma cells and karyorrhexis is common. ENKTL has a broad spectrum of cell sizes with variable cytologic atypia, including small, medium, large, or pleomorphic cells or a mixture of small and large cells [3, 19]. The small lymphoma cells usually show more irregular nuclei and pale cytoplasm, but may be difficult to distinguish from benign background small mature lymphocytes. The medium lymphoma cells often have irregular or folded nuclei, granular chromatin, inconspicuous nucleoli and moderate pale cytoplasm. Vesicular nuclei and prominent nucleoli are mostly seen in the large cells [2]. Pleomorphic cells demonstrate hyperlobated or anaplastic nuclei. There are usually variably numbers of background inflammatory cells such as small mature lymphocytes, plasma cells, histiocytes, neutrophils and less commonly eosinophils. Occasionally the prominent presence of background inflammatory cells may resemble an inflammatory process. The vascular destruction and luminal microthrombi are also present in areas not infiltrated by lymphoma cells. Mitotic figures are usually easily identified and apoptotic bodies are frequent [125]. The underlying normal structures such as submucosal glands are destructed, and the overlying epithelium can exhibit pseudoepitheliomatous hyperplasia in some instances [3]. In small biopsies, not all the characteristic histologic features may be present, due to sampling variation.

In the skin, there is a dense perivascular, periadnexal, or diffuse lymphomatous infiltrate in the mid and deep dermis. Epidermal involvement is variable [90, 117, 126, 127]. Angiocentric and angiodestructive growth is prominent in approximately 40-60% of the cases [21, 91, 117, 126]. Tumor necrosis is commonly seen [90, 117, 121, 126]. In cases with predominantly subcutaneous involvement, the lymphoma cells surround deep subcutaneous adipocytes mimicking panniculitis [117, 128]. Florid pseudoepitheliomatous hyperplasia of the overlying epithelium may be present as in nasal lesions [129].

In the GI tract, there is lymphomatous infiltrate in the lamina propria associated with necrosis and deep ulceration [92, 93]. The crypt epithelium shows infiltrate by lymphoma cells. In the testis, ENKTL shows dense infiltrate of interstitium with atrophic or infiltrated seminiferous tubules, often associated with necrosis and vascular destruction [130]. In other tissues, the underlying structures are destroyed by the lymphomatous infiltrate, and the characteristic angiocentric and angiodestructive pattern is often seen.

ENKTL demonstrates a distinctive immunophenotype of activated NK-cells. The lymphoma cells are nearly always positive for cytoplasmic CD3ε, CD56, CD2, and cytotoxic markers (TIA1, granzyme B and perforin), and negative for surface CD3 [3, 19, 101, 131-133]. The pan-T cell antigen CD5 is typically negative, and CD7 is variably expressed. The lymphoma cells are usually double negative for CD4 and CD8, but CD8 can be expressed in a small subset of cases. CD30 is positive in up to 40% of cases, usually patchy and not intense, and present in the large cells [21, 24, 57, 134, 135]. The other NK-cell associated antigens CD16 and CD57 are usually negative. CD25 expression can be seen in some cases [125]. Fas (CD95) and Fas ligand (CD178) are commonly expressed [136, 137]. NK-cell receptor (NKR) molecules (CD94, NKG2A) are expressed by most ENKTL, while killer inhibitory receptors (KIR) are only expressed in some cases [138, 139]. The proliferative rate by Ki-67 immunostaining is usually high (>50%), even in cases with mostly small lymphoma cells. While most cases of ENKTL are of NK-cell lineage, approximately 11-18% of the cases are of T-cell lineage based on expression of αβ-TCR or γδ-TCR and presence of clonal T-cell gene rearrangements [125, 140]. Occasional CD56-negative nasal lymphomas but otherwise with positive CD3ε, cytotoxic markers, and EBV should still be classified as ENKTL.

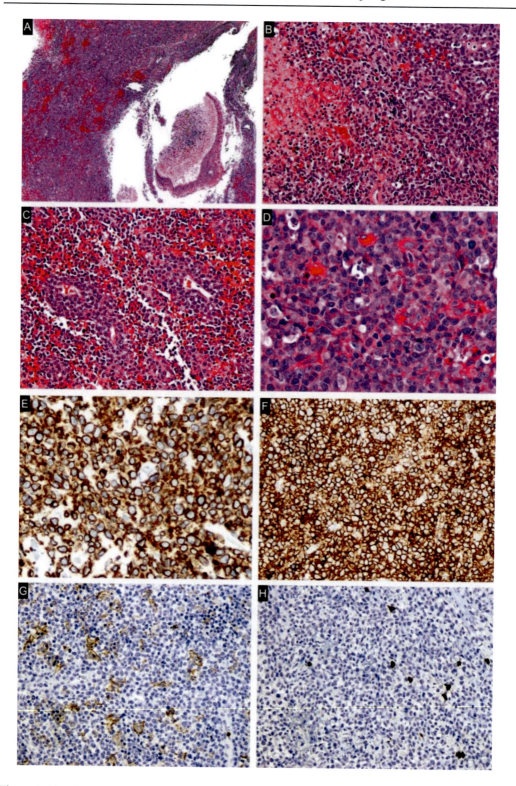

Figure 1. (Continued).

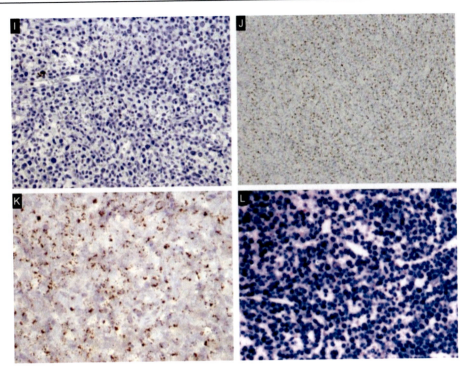

Figure 1. Extranodal NK/T-cell lymphoma, nasal type. The nasal biopsy shows extensive atypical lymphoid infiltrate (A), with tissue necrosis (B) and angiocentric growth pattern (C). The lymphoma cells are medium to large with irregular nuclei, and mitotic figures (D). The lymphoma cells are positive for CD3 (cytoplasmic staining, E), CD56 (F), and negative for CD4 (G), CD8 (H) and CD5 (I). They are positive for cytotoxic markers, TIA1 (J) and granzyme B (K). In situ hybridization for EBV-encoded RNA (EBER) shows numerous EBV positive lymphoma cells (L).

6. DIFFERENTIAL DIAGNOSIS

Establishing the diagnosis of ENKTL can be challenging especially with small biopsies or at unusual locations. The differential diagnosis varies depending on the anatomic sites of the lesions.

6.1. Nasal and Systemic Disease

6.1A. Herpes Simplex Infection of Nasopharynx
Herpes simplex virus (HSV) infection of the nasopharynx may present as a mass lesion. There is a dense lymphoid infiltrate associated with necrosis, and CD56 positive lymphocytes can be seen [141]. It does not exhibit vascular invasion or vascular destruction [141]. The identification of characteristic HSV viral inclusions in cells and absence of EBV will establish the diagnosis of HSV infection.

6.1B. Granulomatosis with Polyangiitis

Granulomatosis with polyangiitis (GPA), previously known as Wegener's granulomatosis (WG), is a rare vasculitis affecting predominantly small to medium sized blood vessels. It may show similar clinical symptoms as ENKTL, such as fever, facial pain, rhinorrhea, and epistaxis. It has a preferential involvement of the upper respiratory tract, lungs, and kidneys. GPA is characterized histologically by necrotizing vasculitis involving arteries and veins, necrosis, ulceration and mixed inflammatory infiltrate. GPA can be distinguished from ENKTL by positive anti-neutrophil cytoplasmic antibodies (c-ANCA), absence of cytologic atypia of the lymphocytes and negative EBV by EBER.

6.1C. Reactive Lymphoid Hyperplasia

Reactive lymphoid hyperplasia or inflammatory conditions can mimic ENKTL of the small cell type with necrosis and mildly atypical lymphocytes. Occasional EBV positive reactivated bystander small mature lymphocytes can be present. Helpful histologic features favoring ENKTL include more than occasional mitotic figures, angioinvasion and angiodestruction, destruction of underlying structures such as mucosal glands, presence of more atypical medium to large lymphoid cells with clear cytoplasm, strong positivity for CD56, and large numbers of EBV positive lymphoid cells by EBER.

6.1D. Chronic Active EBV Infection

Chronic active EBV infection is a rare disease commonly seen in Asian and South America [58]. It is usually seen in children and adolescence and often has a fatal course. Clinically it is characterized by chronic illness of >3 months, unremitting fever, cytopenia, lymphadenopathy and hepatosplenomegaly. High titers of anti–virus capsid antigen and anti–early antigen antibodies are present. Reduced levels of perforin are thought to contribute to the pathogenesis [142]. Histologically there are numerous EBV positive lymphocytes, and the EBV positive cells are mostly T cells. Chronic active EBV infection is distinguished from ENKTL by the protracted clinical course, no significant cytologic atypia of the lymphocytes, absence of CD56 positive cells, and no angiocentric and angiodestructive growth.

6.1E. Aggressive NK Cell Leukemia

Aggressive NK cell leukemia is an aggressive disease characterized by the leukemic infiltrate of EBV positive NK cells. More commonly seen in Asians, this lymphoproliferative disorder occurs predominantly in males. The phenotype is similar to that of ENKTL, with expression of cytoplasmic CD3ε, CD56, cytotoxic markers [143]. In contrast to ENKTL, aggressive NK cell leukemia show leukemic infiltrate of peripheral blood, less common involvement of the skin, high frequency involvement of bone marrow, liver and spleen, and frequent expression of CD16.

6.1F. Lymphomatoid Granulomatosis

Lymphomatoid granulomatosis is a rare EBV associated B-cell lymphoma that is characterized by its prominent pulmonary involvement [144]. The EBV positive cells are large B-cells admixed in the background of small benign T-cells.

6.1G. Diffuse Large B-Cell Lymphoma

Diffuse large B-cell lymphoma (DLBCL) can occur in the sinonasal tract with high predilection for the paranasal sinuses [145]. Histologically, DLBCL comprises large neoplastic cells positive for B-cell markers, such as CD20 and CD79a, and usually negative for EBV by EBER.

6.1H. Squamous Cell Carcinoma

Squamous cell carcinoma can enter into the differential diagnosis in cases of ENKTL with marked pseudoepitheliomatous hyperplasia. Squamous cell carcinoma is distinguished by presence of atypical epithelial cells with invasion and the lack of an atypical lymphoid infiltrate.

6.1I. Nasopharyngeal Carcinoma

Nasopharyngeal carcinoma commonly presents clinically with painless, unilateral cervical lymphadenopathy, epistaxis, nasal obstruction, and nasal discharge. Nasopharyngeal carcinoma and ENKTL are both rare and associated with EBV and have a higher incidence in the male population. Nasopharyngeal carcinoma histologically is composed of large neoplastic with prominent nucleoli and cystic changes. The neoplastic cells of nasopharyngeal carcinoma are strongly positive for pan-cytokeratin, high molecular weight cytokeratin, EBER, and EMA and negative for CK7 and CK20.

6.1J. Metastatic Neuroendocrine Tumor

Metastatic neuroendocrine tumor could mimic ENKTL by atypical cytology, expression of CD56, and involving nasal or extranasal site such as skin, GI *et al*. However, metastatic neuroendocrine tumors are usually positive for cytokeratin as well as markers indicating neuroendocrine differentiation e.g., synaptophysin, chromogranin and neuron-specific enolase. Merkel cell carcinoma shows characteristic "perinuclear dot-like pattern" of CK20 staining.

6.2. Skin Disease

6.2A. Benign Inflammatory Dermatosis

Inflammatory dermatoses are composed of a complex variety of inflammatory and immunologic processes in skin that are commonly seen in daily practice. However, given their variable histopathologic presentations, it could cause diagnostic challenge.

Cutaneous ENKTL can histologically mimic benign inflammatory dermatosis [146]. Such cases clinically present as erythematous to purpuric patches, facial swelling, or cellulitis-like swelling. Histologically they most commonly show nonspecific perivascular lymphocytic infiltrate and a small subset of cases show lupus erythematosus-like histological features, psoriasiform lichenoid reaction, or vasculitis-like features. The perivascular infiltrate involves the superficial and deep dermis and associated vasculopathy and panniculitic infiltrate are common. The lymphoma cells in these cases tend to be small sized lymphoid cells with mild cytologic atypia rather than the mainly medium to large sized atypical lymphoid cells [21, 91, 147]. The lymphoma cells in these cases are always positive for CD56 and EBER. It is important to keep cutaneous ENKTL in the differential diagnosis in cases with perivascular lymphocytic infiltration in the dermis and especially in cases associated with vasculopathy and/or panniculitic type infiltrate. A comprehensive panel of immunohistochemical stain including CD56 and EBER should be performed. The prognoses of these cases are similar to typical cutaneous ENKTL.

6.2B. Primary Cutaneous γδ T-Cell Lymphoma

Primary Cutaneous γδ T-cell Lymphoma (PCGD-TCL) may mimic cutaneous ENKTL clinically and pathologically. Patients with PCGD-TCL may present with patch and plaque lesions or deep dermal or subcutaneous nodules with ulcers and necrosis [148]. The lymphoma cells of PCGD-TCL may have a predominantly epidermotropic, dermal, or subcutaneous infiltrate [149]. Similar to cutaneous ENKTL, angiocentric and angiodestructive growth patterns are common [150]. The phenotype of PCGD-TCL is also similar to cutaneous ENKTL of the T-cell lineage. The lymphoma cells of PCGD-TCL are typically positive for CD2, CD3, CD56, TCRγ, and cytotoxic markers, and negative for CD4, CD5, CD8 and TCRβF1. EBER is critical in the differential diagnosis, as PCGD-TCL is negative for EBV [151]. The gene expression profiles of extranodal ENKTL and non-hepatosplenic γδ T-cell lymphoma show strikingly similarities, suggesting a common origin from a subset of γδ T cells [152].

6.2C. Subcutaneous Panniculitis-Like T-Cell Lymphoma

Cutaneous ENKTL with subcutaneous involvement and rimming around adipocytes may be confused with subcutaneous panniculitis-like T-cell lymphoma (SPTCL) [148]. SPTCL is an indolent $CD8^+$ T-cell lymphoma with exclusive infiltrate of the subcutaneous adipose tissue [17, 148]. Patients typically present with subcutaneous nodules or deep plaques involving the extremities or trunk. Histologically SPTCL cells infiltrate fat lobules with a panniculitis-like pattern with spare of the septa. There is no infiltrate of the epidermis and dermis. Rimming of the adipocytes by neoplastic $CD8^+$ cells is a characteristic finding. The SPTCL cells are αβ T-cells with expression of CD3, CD8, and cytotoxic markers and without expression of CD56 or EBV by EBER. Positive

TCR-βF1, negative CD56 and EBER allow easy differentiation of SPTCL from cutaneous ENKTL.

6.2D. Blastic Plasmacytoid Dendritic Cell Neoplasm

Blastic plasmacytoid dendritic cell neoplasm (BPDCN) shows characteristic high frequency of skin involvement. Patients often present with skin bruises, plaques or nodules. The cells are medium sized and blastoid with finely disperse chromatin. The infiltration pattern is leukemic and angiocentric/angiodestructive growth is rarely seen. The BPDCN cells are positive for CD4, CD56, BDCA2, CD123, TCL-1, and may show expression of CD7 but not cytotoxic markers. EBER and cytoplasmic CD3ε are consistently negative in BPDCN. Attention to the cytologic features and a comprehensive panel of immunohistochemical stains including CD3, EBER, CD123 and TCL-1 will establish the diagnosis.

6.2E. Mycosis Fungiodes

Rare cases of cutaneous ENKTL may show epidermotropism with Pautrier microabscesses, mimicking mycosis fungoides [148]. Mycosis fungoides typically shows expression of CD4 with loss of CD7 and negative EBER. CD56 expression is infrequent. A standard immunohistochemical workup for mycosis fungoides can easily distinguish cutaneous ENKTL from mycosis fungoides.

6.2F. Primary Cutaneous CD56-Positive Peripheral T-Cell Lymphoma

Rare cases of primary cutaneous CD56-positive peripheral T cell lymphoma (CD56$^+$ PC-PTCL) show equally aggressive clinical course as cutaneous ENKTL. Patients with CD56$^+$ PC-PTCL often present with ulcers, erythema, papules and subcutaneous nodules in the extremities and trunk [90]. CD56$^+$ PC-PTCL shows less frequent tumor necrosis, older age and lower frequency of CD16 and CD30 expression than cutaneous ENKTL. EBER is consistently negative in CD56$^+$ PC-PTCL, which would allow distinction between the two entities.

6.2G. Hydroa vacciniforme-Like Lymphoma

Hydroa vacciniforme-like lymphoma (HVLL) is similar to ENKTL in that it is an EBV positive disorder occurring in Asia, Central America, and South America. In contrast to ENKTL, it affects children and adolescents and rarely in adults. Patients present with papulovesicular cutaneous eruptions in sun-exposed areas that proceed to ulcers and scarring [153], and often accompanied by fever, lymphadenopathy or hepatosplenomegaly. Histologically it closely mimics ENKTL. There are numerous EBV positive lymphoid cells that are cytotoxic T-cells or less commonly NK cells with expression of CD56. Necrosis, angioinvasion and angiodestruction are frequently present. Unlike HVLL, cutaneous ENKTL usually presents with multiple or generalized skin lesions in sun-exposed and non-exposed areas. The neoplastic cells of ENKTL infiltrate both dermis and subcutis diffusely and often show more cytologic atypia.

6.2H. Mosquito-Bite Hypersensitivity

Mosquito-bite hypersensitivity is most commonly seen in Asian and South American populations [154]. It is most prevalent in children. Patients present with papulovesicular skin lesions with progression to ulceration and scarring due to bites from mosquito or other arthropods. Fever, lymphadenopathy and hepatosplenomegaly may develop in occasional cases. Histologically it is characterized by atypical EBV-infected lymphoid cells, usually cytotoxic T cells and occasionally NK cells, infiltrate the epidermis and subcutis. It shows overlapping histologic features with hydroa vacciniforme-like lymphoma and the distinction from ENKTL relies on the characteristic clinical presentation in children, and papulovesicular lesions in sun exposed areas and less cytologic atypia of the lymphocytes.

6.2I. Primary Cutaneous CD8 Positive Aggressive Epidermotropic Cytotoxic T-Cell Lymphoma

A subset of cutaneous ENKTL is positive for dim to moderate CD8, which could mimic primary cutaneous CD8 positive aggressive epidermotropic cytotoxic T-cell lymphoma. Both lymphomas manifest with skin ulceration, necrosis, hyperkeratotic plaques, and tissue destruction and immunophenotypically express cytotoxic markers. However, primary cutaneous CD8 positive aggressive epidermotropic cytotoxic T-cell lymphoma cells are positive for CD8 and TCRβF1 and negative for EBER. These tumor cells express surface CD3, rather than CD3ε that can be better detected using flow cytometric study.

6.3. Gastrointestinal Tract Disease

6.3A. Monomorphic Epitheliotropic Intestinal T-Cell Lymphoma

Monomorphic epitheliotropic intestinal T-cell lymphoma (MEITL), previously known as "enteropathy-associated T-cell lymphoma type II" shows similar racial and geographic distribution as ENKTL, with increased incidence in Asians and Hispanic populations. The MEITL cells are medium sized often with clear cytoplasm, and show prominent infiltrate of the intestinal crypt epithelium. There is usually no angiocentric and angiodestructive growth, and necrosis is often absent. They are positive for CD8 and CD56, and negative for CD5 and EBV by EBER. The cells are often γδ T-cells with expression of TCRγ, but some cases are of αβ T-cells with positive βF1. The distinction from GI ENKTL mostly relies on the demonstration of negative EBER.

6.3B. NK-Cell Enteropathy (Lymphomatoid Gastropathy)

NK-cell enteropathy is a benign and self-limiting NK-cell proliferation in the GI mucosa [155, 156]. It presents with small (about 1.0 cm) superficial edematous lesions and ulcers most often in the stomach, followed by the duodenum and small and large bowel. The lesions often show spontaneous resolution but can persist for years. Histologically it shows medium-sized atypical lymphoid cells infiltrating the mucosa and between the crypts. There is no angiocentric and angiodestruction growth. The lymphoid cells show typical NK-cell phenotype with expression of cytoplasmic CD3ε, CD2, CD7, CD56, and cytotoxic markers. They are negative for CD5 and EBER. The clinically small superficial lesions, absence of angioinvasion and angiodestruction and negative EBER will distinguish NK-cell enteropathy from ENKTL.

7. GENETICS AND MOLECULAR FEATURES

Cytogenetic studies, mainly with comparative genomic hybridization (CGH), showed complex chromosomal abnormalities but no specific chromosomal changes for ENKTL [157-161]. Deletion of the chromosome 6q21-25 appears to be the most common recurrent chromosomal abnormality. Other recurrent non-random chromosomal aberrations include losses at chromosomes 1p, 2p, 4q, 5p, 5q, 11q, 12q, 13q and 17p and gains of chromosomes 1p, 2q, 6p, 10q, 11q, 12q, 13q, 17q, 19p, 20q, and Xp. A study using loss of heterozygosity (LOH) and homozygosity mapping of deletion (HOMOD) analyses defined a distinct 3.0 Mb smallest region of overlapping (SRO) deletion on chromosome 6q25, and subsequent quantitative multiplex polymerase chain reaction analysis refined the putative tumor suppressor-gene-containing region to a 2.6 Mb interval between TIAM2 and SNX9 genes [162]. Combined gene expression profiling (GEP) and array-based comparative genomic hybridization analyses (aCGH) identified four known tumor suppressor genes, *PRDM1*, *ATG5*, *AIM1* and *HACE1* with decreased gene expression in the minimal common region of the frequently deleted 6q21 [163, 164]. Mutations resulted in truncated *PRDM1* and changes in conserved amino-acid sequences of AIM1, and hypermethylation of CpG islands at 5' resulted in low expression of *PRDM1* and AIM1 [163]. *PRDM1* is a transcriptional repressor that induces terminal differentiation of B-cells into plasma cells and regulates T-cell homeostasis and function [165, 166]. Inactivation due to mutations or suppression of *PRDM1* likely contributes to ENKTL pathogenesis through altered T-cell homeostasis [163, 166]. ATG5 is essential for autophagosome biogenesis and also a pro-apoptotic molecule after cleaved by calpain [167, 168]. In interferon-gamma induced cell death, ATG5 interacts with FADD (Fas-associated protein with death domain, a mediator of death receptor-dependent apoptosis) to trigger autophagic cell death. The truncated form of ATG5 translocates to mitochondria and inactivates Bcl-xL to promote apoptosis. The inactivated ATG5 may function to antagonize the apoptosis pathway in ENKTL. AIM1 (Absent In Melanoma-1) is a non-lens member of the beta-gamma-crystallin superfamily, and a tumor suppressor of malignant melanoma, possibly through interactions with the cytoskeleton [169]. HACE1 is frequently deleted in ENKTL and the remaining allele often has hypermethylation of CpG islands leading to low transcription [170]. HACE1 is a member of the HECT family of E3 ubiquitin ligases that ubiquitylate proteins for degradation by the 26S proteasome. HECT E3 also regulates the trafficking of many receptors, transporters and viral proteins [171]. HECT E3 is frequently downregulated in human tumors and may function as a tumor suppressor by inhibiting cell cycle progression via degradation of phosphorylated cyclin D1 [172]. Additional important potential tumor suppressor genes have also been mapped to 6q by GEP, including *FOXO3* [173], *PTPRK* [174] and *TNFAIP3* [152]. FOXO3 is a member of the forkhead family of proteins and down-regulated in ENKTL, re-expression of FOXO3 suppressed proliferation of the NK cell line [173]. PTPRK (receptor-type tyrosine-protein phosphatase κ) negatively regulates *STAT3* in NKTCL. Downregulation of PTPRK leads to *STAT3* activation. TNFAIP (tumor necrosis factor-α-induced protein) is an inhibitor of NF-κB, and downregulated in ENKTL. Genes in the AKT, Janus kinase-signal transducers and activators of transcription (JAK-STAT), and nuclear factor-kappa B pathways have been mapped to regions of recurrent copy number aberrations, including AKT3 at 1q44, IL6R at 1q21.3, CCL2 at 17q12, and TNFRSF21 at 6p12.3, and dysregulation of these pathways can be confirmed by nuclear expression of phosphorylated AKT, *STAT3*, and RelA in NKTCL [164].

GEP studies have shown overexpression of genes in angiogenesis (*ANGPT2, VEGFA, VEGFB, VEGFC, KDR*), growth factors and their receptors (*PDGFRA, PDGFB, PDGFC*, transforming growth factor-B2 [*TGF-B2*], TGF-B3), oncogenes (*MAFB, MET, MYC*), microenvironment especially macrophages (*CLU, CD68, CD163*), autophagy (*ATG3, ATG7*), cell-cycle control (*CCND1*), cell-to-cell interactions (*CDH1, ITGA7, ITGA9, ITGB4, VCAM1*), chemokines (*CX3CL1, CXCL9, CXCL10*), cytokines (*IL-8, IL-20, IL-33*), extracellular matrix interactions (*MMP11, MMP14, TIMP1, TIMP2, TIMP3*), innate immunity (*IL4I1, TLR4, TLR7, TLR8*), local invasion and metastasis (*COL1A1, COL1A2, FN1, LAMB1*), and genes induced by EBV (*CDH1, EBI3, BASP1, DNASE1L3, HCK, HLA-DQA1, IFI30, IFI44L, IFITM3, LGALS9, THRA, TNFRSF10D*) [164]. One study showed the molecular classifier for ENKTL composed of 84 genes with the majority of them expressed by the neoplastic cells [152]. Huang *et al.* demonstrated activation of pathways in apoptosis, cell adhesion, cell communication, extracellular matrix-receptor interaction, cell cycle (p27 regulation), cytokine-cytokine receptor interaction, as well as TGF-β, mitogen-activated protein kinase, WNT, and JAK-STAT signaling pathways by GEP [164]. Interestingly, NF-κB pathway genes were not found to be enriched in the ENKTL gene signature by Iqbal *et al.* [152]. The overexpression of genes related to angiogenesis may contribute to the angiocentric and angiodestructive growth in ENKTL. The angiogenesis gene *VEGFA* is a downstream target of *STAT3*, and its receptor VEGFR2 (KDR) is also upregulated in ENKTL. The activation of both VEGFA and its receptor leads to autocrine growth of vasculature.

P53 protein overexpression is present in up to 86% of ENKTL, and *TP53* gene mutation rate is up to 62% [175-179]. A key regulator of TP53 pathway, AURKA (the Aurora kinase A or ST6) was identified as highly expressed in ENKTL cells [152]. AURKA phosphorylates TP53 and induces its ubiquitination by MDM2 and subsequent proteasomal degradation [180]. Targeted inhibition of AURKA by small-molecular inhibitors can cause significant growth arrest in NK-cell lines [152]. Thus, p53 mediated pathways appear to play important roles in the pathogenesis of ENKTL. Early sequencing studies demonstrated mutations of *TP53* and *c-kit* genes in ENKTL with location-specific differences in frequencies in Asian countries [175, 177, 178, 181, 182] and Mexico [183]. The frequency of *TP53* mutations was high in Japan and Indonesia and low in Mexico, Korea, and North China. Transitions (G:C to A:T) were the predominant pattern of mutations in Asian countries but not in Mexico [183]. Despite the presence of *TP53* mutation, ENKTL is not characterized by genetic instability as evidenced by widespread microsatellite instability [184]. One study suggested that p53 overexpression is associated with large cell morphology, advanced stage and poor prognosis [183]. Mutations of the *c-Kit* are detected in 5-71% of cases [178, 179]. The frequency of *c-kit* mutations was significantly higher in China (71.4%) [181] than in Japan (15.5%) [177], Korea (11.9%) [177], northeast China (10%) [178], and Indonesia (11.1%) [182]. These early studies suggested that environmental and geneticfactors might contribute to the differences in mutation frequencies of key oncogenes.

Next generation sequencing (NGS)studies identified recurrent mutations in tumor suppressor genes (*TP53* and *MGA*), genes of JAK-STAT pathway (*JAK1, JAK3, STAT3* and *STAT5B*), epigenetic modifiers (*BCOR, MLL2, ARID1A, EP300, KMT2A/MLL* and *ASXL3*) and RNA helicase gene (*DDX3X*) [185-189]. The most frequently mutated genes are *STAT3, BCOR,* and *MLL2*. JAK/STAT pathway and histone modification related genes accounted for 55.9% and 38.2% of ENKTL, respectively. Therefore, the molecular genetic studies indicate essential role of JAK/STAT pathway and epigenetic dysregulation in the development of ENKTL. Deletions of *FAS* gene sequences and mutations of *FAS* gene are reported in approximately 50-60% of cases [190-192], which likely contribute to the resistance to apoptosis, despite frequent expression of FAS and FAS ligand (FasL) in ENKTL cells.

ENKTL cells exhibit latency II pattern of EBV viral gene expression, limited to EBNA1, LMP1, and LMP2 [193]. The cells infected by virus are primarily eliminated by host cytotoxic T-lymphocytes (CTL) in a MHC-class-I-restricted manner [194]. LMP-1 is an EBV antigen targeted by CTL to eliminate EBV infected cells [195]. Several mechanisms may contribute to the immune escape of ENKTL cells, including downregulation of the immunogenic EBV nuclear antigens by alternative promoter usage and preferential selection of the deletion genotype of LMP-1 [69, 193]. LMP1 contains two CTL-epitopes that are pan HLA A*02-restricted [196]. The lower frequency of HLA-A*0201 allele in patients with ENKTL compared with that of the normal population may provide an underlying genetic background for the development of ENKTL [85]. Expression of IL-10, an immunosuppressive cytokine, may also play a role [197]. The tissue necrosis and vascular damage characteristically associated with ENKTL are most likely caused by EBV-induced production of chemokines CXCL9 (Mig) and CXCL10 (IP10) [198].

The ENKTL cells show germline *TCR* and immunoglobingenes configuration in most cases. Approximately 10- 40% cases show clonal TCR generearrangements, most likely in cases of cytotoxic T cell origin.

8. PROGNOSTIC FACTORS

Patients with ENKTL need to be stratified based on prognostic factors for appropriate treatment. Retrospective studies of cases of ENKTL revealed a number of variables associated with poor survival, including high-presentation EBV DNA (> 6.1×10^7 copies/mL) [199], lymph node involvement [111], serum lactate dehydrogenase (LDH) level [111], paranasal extension [200-202], B-symptoms [200, 203] and extranasal disease [140]. Three clinical prognostic models had been used in patients treated with anthracycline-based regimens (cyclophosphamide, doxorubicin/Hydroxydanomycin, vincristine/Oncovin, prednisolone CHOP or CHOP-like chemotherapy): the international prognostic index (IPI), the Korean prognostic index (KPI), and NK prognostic index [24, 204]. The IPI was designed for diffuse large B-cell lymphoma to predict clinical outcome. While an early study showed that IPI was not applicable to ENKTL [205], a subsequent retrospective study validated the prognostic significance of IPI in ENKTL patients treated with radiotherapy only, anthracycline-containing chemotherapy plus consolidation radiotherapy, or non-anthracycline-containing chemotherapy plus radiotherapy [204]. In this study of 67 patients with ENKTL, most patients (84%) had stage I/II disease with an IPI score of 1 or less (52%). The IPI score had prognostic significance for the whole group with the 20-year OS significantly longer in patients with IPI $\leq$ 1 than in patients with IPI $\geq$ 2 (57.4% versus 27.6%, P = 0.012). In patients treated with chemotherapy/radiotherapy, the patients with IPI $\leq$ 1 had higher CR rate (76.7% versus 35.7%, P = .017), and longer 10-year OS (63.8% versus 26.8%, P = .003) over patients with IPI $\geq$ 2 [204]. The Korean prognostic score based on four prognostic factors: B symptoms, stage, lactate dehydrogenase (LDH), and lymph-node involvement effectively stratify ENKTL patients into four groups with more balanced distribution of patients and better prognostic discrimination as compared with the IPI: group 1 (no adverse factor); group 2 (one factor); group 3 (two factors); and group 4 (three or four factors) [206]. In a retrospectively analysis of 150 patients with ENKTL, an NK prognostic index was constructed based on four significant prognostic factors identified by multivariate analysis: non-nasal type, stage, performance status and numbers of extranodal involvement [207]. The four-year OS of patients with 0, 1, 2 and 3 or 4 adverse factors were 55%, 33%, 15% and 6%, respectively [207]. A recent study of 158 Chinese patients identified total protein (TP) < 60 g/L, fasting blood glucose (FBG) > 100 mg/dL, KPI score ≥ 2 as independent prognostic factors [208]. A new prognostic model composed of these prognostic factors stratified patients into group 1 (no adverse factors), group 2 (one adverse factor), and group 3 (two or three adverse factors) with 5-year OS of 88.9%, 35.6% and 12.7%, respectively (p < 0.001) [208].

When patients received chemotherapy with L-asparaginase containing regimens, only IPI but not the Korean prognostic index was the most significant factor impacting on outcome and survivals by multivariate analysis [107]. Studies had shown that the location of ENKTL had prognostic significance. Extranasal ENKTL was a significant factor affecting OS [140, 209, 210]. The median OS of patients with extranasal ENKTL was significantly shorter, 8.6 months versus 86.5 months in patients with nasal ENKTL [209]. Similarly, when ENKTL was subdivided into upper aerodigestive tract NK/T-cell lymphoma (UNKTL) and extra-upper aerodigestive tract NK/T-cell lymphoma (EUNKTL) groups, the EUNKTL group had advanced stage at diagnosis, higher LDH, higher IPI score, poorer performance and inferior response to the anthracycline-based chemotherapy, and inferior survival rate as compared to UNKTL group [211]. A recent multinational retrospective study of 527 patients examined newly diagnosed ENKTL treated with non-anthracycline-based chemotherapies with or without upfront concurrent chemo-radiotherapy or radiotherapy [212]. This study showed that age greater than 60 years, stage III or IV disease, distant lymph-node involvement, and non-nasal type disease were significantly associated with worse OS and PFS. A prognostic index of natural killer lymphoma (PINK) composed of these factors stratified ENKTL patients into low-risk (no risk factors), intermediate-risk (one risk factor), or high-risk (two or more risk factors) groups, with 3-year OS of 81% (95% CI 75–86), 62% (95% CI 55–70), and 25% (95% CI 20–34), respectively. A detectable EBV viral DNA titer was determined to be an independent prognostic factor for OS in 328 patients with available data on Epstein-Barr virus DNA. EBV viral DNA titer was added to PINK as the basis for another prognostic index (PINK-E). Similar to PINK, PINK-E stratified patients to low-risk (zero or one risk factor), intermediate-risk (two risk factors), and high-risk (three or more risk factors) groups with OS of 81% (95% CI 75–87%), 55% (95% CI 44–66), and 28% (95% CI 18–40%), respectively. Hence, PINK and PINK-E appear to be more appropriate prognostic models for ENKTL patients treated with contemporary non-anthracycline-based therapy.

A number of pathologic features have been evaluated for prognostic significance. The high proliferation index by immunohistochemical stain for Ki-67 is consistently associated with poor survival, although at different levels (>50%, ≥60 or ≥65%) according to different studies [21, 213, 214]. One study showed prognostic significance of Ki-67 at >50% in nasal disease, but not in extra nasal disease [24]. High level of plasma EBV DNA correlates with higher tumor load and a poorer prognosis [199, 215-218]. The prognostic significance of p53 overexpression, large cell cytology and CD30 expression is controversial [21, 24, 99, 134, 135, 175, 176, 183]. Expression of CD94/NKG2A is associated with better prognosis [219]. The lineage of ENKTL (NK or T-cells) does not have prognostic significance [132, 140]. Bone marrow involvement, CD25 expression, loss of expression of SERPINB9 (also known as PI9, a Granzyme B-specific serine protease inhibitor), and low apoptotic index are adverse prognostic factors [125, 220]. Negative EBV DNA after treatment is associated with favorable outcome [217, 221].

CONCLUSION

ENKTL has unique clinical and histologic characteristics. It occurs most frequently in the upper aerodigestive tract, but dissemination to other sites (skin, GI tract *et al.*) are common. Rare cases of ENKTL can develop as primary extranasal lymphoma, and usually have a more aggressive clinical course than the nasal disease. The histological findings may be variable, mimicking other T/NK-cell lymphomas/leukemia or reactive entities. The diagnosis can usually be confirmed by the typical immunophenotype of the lymphoma cells (positive for cytoplasmic CD3ε, CD56, cytotoxic markers, and diffuse and strong positivity for EBV by EBER). The patients with higher international prognostic index (IPI), the Korean prognostic index (KPI), and the NK prognostic index have a worse clinical outcome. ENKTL responds poorly to traditional anthracycline-based chemotherapy and requires L-asparaginase–based chemotherapy regimens and/or radiotherapy.

REFERENCES

[1] Gualco, G., P. Domeny-Duarte, L. Chioato, G. Barber, Y. Natkunam, and C. E. Bacchi. 2011. "Clinicopathologic and molecular features of 122 Brazilian cases of nodal and extranodal NK/T-cell lymphoma, nasal type, with EBV subtyping analysis." *Am J Surg Pathol* 35:1195-203. doi: 10.1097/PAS.0b013e31821ec4b5.

[2] Kluin, P. M., A. Feller, P. Gaulard, E. S. Jaffe, C. J. Meijer, H. K. Muller-Hermelink, and S. Pileri. 2001. "Peripheral T/NK-cell lymphoma: a report of the IXth Workshop of the European Association for Haematopathology." *Histopathology* 38:250-70.

[3] Huang, Y., J. Xie, Y. Ding, and X. Zhou. 2016. "Extranodal Natural Killer/T-Cell Lymphoma in Children and Adolescents: A Report of 17 Cases in China." *Am J Clin Pathol* 145:46-54. doi: 10.1093/ajcp/aqv010.

[4] Huang, Y. H., Q. L. Wu, Y. S. Zong, Y. F. Feng, and J. H. Hou. 2011. "Nasopharyngeal extranodal NK/T-cell lymphoma, nasal type: retrospective study of 18 consecutive cases in Guangzhou, China." *Int J Surg Pathol* 19:51-61. doi: 10.1177/1066896910388806.

[5] McBride, P. 1991. "Photographs of a case of rapid destruction of the nose and face. 1897." *J Laryngol Otol* 105:1120.

[6] Eichel, B. S., E. G. Harrison, Jr., K. D. Devine, P. W. Scanlon, and H. A. Brown. 1966. "Primary lymphoma of the nose including a relationship to lethal midline granuloma." *Am J Surg* 112:597-605.

[7] Ishii, Y., N. Yamanaka, K. Ogawa, Y. Yoshida, T. Takami, A. Matsuura, H. Isago, A. Kataura, and K. Kikuchi. 1982. "Nasal T-cell lymphoma as a type of so-called "lethal midline granuloma"." *Cancer* 50:2336-44.

[8] Chan, J. K., C. S. Ng, W. H. Lau, and S. T. Lo. 1987. "Most nasal/nasopharyngeal lymphomas are peripheral T-cell neoplasms." *Am J Surg Pathol* 11:418-29.

[9] Weiss, L. M., L. J. Picker, T. M. Grogan, R. A. Warnke, and J. Sklar. 1988. "Absence of clonal beta and gamma T-cell receptor gene rearrangements in a subset of peripheral T-cell lymphomas." *Am J Pathol* 130:436-42.

[10] Ng, C. S., J. K. Chan, and S. T. Lo. 1987. "Expression of natural killer cell markers in non-Hodgkin's lymphomas." *Hum Pathol* 18:1257-62.

[11] Aozasa, K., M. Ohsawa, Y. Tomita, S. Tagawa, and T. Yamamura. 1995. "Polymorphic reticulosis is a neoplasm of large granular lymphocytes with CD3+ phenotype." *Cancer* 75:894-901.

[12] Emile, J. F., M. L. Boulland, C. Haioun, P. Kanavaros, T. Petrella, M. H. Delfau-Larue, A. Bensussan, J. P. Farcet, and P. Gaulard. 1996. "CD5-CD56+ T-cell receptor silent peripheral T-cell lymphomas are natural killer cell lymphomas." *Blood* 87:1466-73.

[13] Suzumiya, J., M. Takeshita, N. Kimura, M. Kikuchi, T. Uchida, S. Hisano, Y. Eura, M. Kozuru, Y. Nomura, K. Tomita, and et al. 1994. "Expression of adult and fetal natural killer cell markers in sinonasal lymphomas." *Blood* 83:2255-60.

[14] Ohsawa, M., S. Nakatsuka, H. Kanno, H. Miwa, S. Kojya, Y. Harabuchi, W. I. Yang, and K. Aozasa. 1999. "Immunophenotypic and genotypic characterization of nasal lymphoma with polymorphic reticulosis morphology." *Int J Cancer* 81:865-70.

[15] Harris, N. L., E. S. Jaffe, H. Stein, P. M. Banks, J. K. Chan, M. L. Cleary, G. Delsol, C. De Wolf-Peeters, B. Falini, K. C. Gatter, and et al. 1994. "A revised European-American classification of lymphoid neoplasms: a proposal from the International Lymphoma Study Group." *Blood* 84:1361-92.

[16] Jaffe, E. S., J. K. Chan, I. J. Su, G. Frizzera, S. Mori, A. C. Feller, and F. C. Ho. 1996. "Report of the Workshop on Nasal and Related Extranodal Angiocentric T/Natural Killer Cell Lymphomas. Definitions, differential diagnosis, and epidemiology." *Am J Surg Pathol* 20:103-11.

[17] Swerdlow, S. H., E. Campo, N. L. Harris, E. S. Jaffe, S. A. Pileri, H. Stein, J. Thiele, and J. W. Vardiman. 2008. *WHO classification of tumours of haematopoietic and lymphoid tissues*. 4th ed. Lyon: IARC.

[18] Jaffe, E. S., N. L. Harris, H. Stein, and J. W. Vardiman. 2001. *World Health Organization Classification of Tumours: Pathology & genetics of tumours of haematopoietic and lymphoid tissues*. Lyon: IARC.

[19] Kuo, T. T., L. Y. Shih, and N. M. Tsang. 2004. "Nasal NK/T cell lymphoma in Taiwan: a clinicopathologic study of 22 cases, with analysis of histologic subtypes, Epstein-Barr virus LMP-1 gene association, and treatment modalities." *Int J Surg Pathol* 12:375-87.

[20] Au, W. Y., S. Y. Ma, C. S. Chim, C. Choy, F. Loong, A. K. Lie, C. C. Lam, A. Y. Leung, E. Tse, C. C. Yau, R. Liang, and Y. L. Kwong. 2005. "Clinicopathologic features and treatment outcome of mature T-cell and natural killer-cell lymphomas diagnosed according to the World Health Organization classification scheme: a single center experience of 10 years." *Ann Oncol* 16:206-14. doi: 10.1093/annonc/mdi037.

[21] Li, S., X. Feng, T. Li, S. Zhang, Z. Zuo, P. Lin, S. Konoplev, C. E. Bueso-Ramos, F. Vega, L. J. Medeiros, and C. C. Yin. 2013. "Extranodal NK/T-cell lymphoma, nasal type: a report of 73 cases at MD Anderson Cancer Center." *Am J Surg Pathol* 37:14-23. doi: 10.1097/PAS.0b013e31826731b5.

[22] Liang, X., and D. K. Graham. 2008. "Natural killer cell neoplasms." *Cancer* 112:1425-36. doi: 10.1002/cncr.23316.

[23] Yoon, S. O., C. Suh, D. H. Lee, H. S. Chi, C. J. Park, S. S. Jang, H. R. Shin, B. H. Park, and J. Huh. 2010. "Distribution of lymphoid neoplasms in the Republic of Korea: analysis of 5318 cases according to the World Health Organization classification." *Am J Hematol* 85:760-4. doi: 10.1002/ajh.21824.

[24] Au, W. Y., D. D. Weisenburger, T. Intragumtornchai, S. Nakamura, W. S. Kim, I. Sng, J. Vose, J. O. Armitage, R. Liang, and T. Cell Lymphoma Project International Peripheral. 2009. "Clinical differences between nasal and extranasal natural killer/T-cell lymphoma: a study of 136 cases from the International Peripheral T-Cell Lymphoma Project." *Blood* 113:3931-7. doi: 10.1182/blood-2008-10-185256.

[25] Anderson, J. R., J. O. Armitage, and D. D. Weisenburger. 1998. "Epidemiology of the non-Hodgkin's lymphomas: distributions of the major subtypes differ by geographic locations. Non-Hodgkin's Lymphoma Classification Project." *Ann Oncol* 9:717-20.

[26] Oshimi, K. 2007. "Progress in understanding and managing natural killer-cell malignancies." *Br J Haematol* 139:532-44. doi: 10.1111/j.1365-2141.2007.06835.x.

[27] Chen, C. Y., M. Yao, J. L. Tang, W. Tsay, C. C. Wang, W. C. Chou, I. J. Su, F. Y. Lee, M. C. Liu, and H. F. Tien. 2004. "Chromosomal abnormalities of 200 Chinese patients with non-Hodgkin's lymphoma in Taiwan: with special reference to T-cell lymphoma." *Ann Oncol* 15:1091-6. doi: 10.1093/annonc/mdh263.

[28] Ko, Y. H., C. W. Kim, C. S. Park, H. K. Jang, S. S. Lee, S. H. Kim, H. J. Ree, J. D. Lee, S. W. Kim, and J. R. Huh. 1998. "REAL classification of malignant lymphomas in the Republic of Korea: incidence of recently recognized entities and changes in clinicopathologic features. Hematolymphoreticular Study Group of the Korean Society of Pathologists. Revised European-American lymphoma." *Cancer* 83:806-12.

[29] Arber, D. A., L. M. Weiss, P. F. Albujar, Y. Y. Chen, and E. S. Jaffe. 1993. "Nasal lymphomas in Peru. High incidence of T-cell immunophenotype and Epstein-Barr virus infection." *Am J Surg Pathol* 17:392-9.

[30] Elenitoba-Johnson, K. S., A. Zarate-Osorno, A. Meneses, L. Krenacs, D. W. Kingma, M. Raffeld, and E. S. Jaffe. 1998. "Cytotoxic granular protein expression, Epstein-Barr virus strain type, and latent membrane protein-1 oncogene deletions in nasal T-lymphocyte/natural killer cell lymphomas from Mexico." *Mod Pathol* 11:754-61.

[31] 1997. "A clinical evaluation of the International Lymphoma Study Group classification of non-Hodgkin's lymphoma. The Non-Hodgkin's Lymphoma Classification Project." *Blood* 89:3909-18.

[32] Ho, F. C., D. Todd, S. L. Loke, R. P. Ng, and R. K. Khoo. 1984. "Clinico-pathological features of malignant lymphomas in 294 Hong Kong Chinese patients, retrospective study covering an eight-year period." *Int J Cancer* 34:143-8.

[33] Aozasa, K., M. Ohsawa, K. Tajima, R. Sasaki, H. Maeda, T. Matsunaga, and I. Friedmann. 1989. "Nation-wide study of lethal mid-line granuloma in Japan: frequencies of wegener's granulomatosis, polymorphic reticulosis, malignant lymphoma and other related conditions." *Int J Cancer* 44:63-6.

[34] Aozasa, K., W. J. Yang, Y. B. Lee, W. S. Pan, Y. F. Wy, K. Horiuchi, B. H. Hyun, and K. Tajima. 1992. "Lethal midline granuloma in Seoul (Korea) and Shanghai (China)." *Int J Cancer* 52:673-4.

[35] Kojya, S., T. Itokazu, N. Maeshiro, H. Esu, Y. Noda, K. Mishima, M. Ohsawa, and K. Aozasa. 1994. "Lethal midline granuloma in Okinawa with special emphasis on polymorphic reticulosis." *Jpn J Cancer Res* 85:384-8.

[36] Hatta, C., H. Ogasawara, J. Okita, A. Kubota, M. Ishida, and M. Sakagami. 2001. "Non-Hodgkin's malignant lymphoma of the sinonasal tract--treatment outcome for 53 patients according to REAL classification." *Auris Nasus Larynx* 28:55-60.

[37] Yamanaka, N., Y. Harabuchi, S. Sambe, F. Shido, F. Matsuda, A. Kataura, Y. Ishii, and K. Kikuchi. 1985. "Non-Hodgkin's lymphoma of Waldeyer's ring and nasal cavity. Clinical and immunologic aspects." *Cancer* 56:768-76.

[38] Calderon-Garciduenas, L., R. Delgado, A. Calderon-Garciduenas, A. Meneses, L. M. Ruiz, J. De La Garza, H. Acuna, A. Villarreal-Calderon, N. Raab-Traub, and R. Devlin. 2000. "Malignant neoplasms of the nasal cavity and paranasal sinuses: a series of 256 patients in Mexico City and Monterrey. Is air pollution the missing link?" *Otolaryngol Head Neck Surg* 122:499-508. doi: 10.1067/mhn.2000.103080.

[39] Kitamura, A., Y. Yamashita, Y. Hasegawa, H. Kojima, T. Nagasawa, and N. Mori. 2005. "Primary lymphoma arising in the nasal cavity among Japanese." *Histopathology* 47:523-32. doi: 10.1111/j.1365-2559.2005.02265.x.

[40] Wu, X. C., P. Andrews, V. W. Chen, and F. D. Groves. 2009. "Incidence of extranodal non-Hodgkin lymphomas among whites, blacks, and Asians/Pacific Islanders in the United States: anatomic site and histology differences." *Cancer Epidemiol* 33:337-46. doi: 10.1016/j.canep.2009.09.006.

[41] Gaal, K., N. C. Sun, A. M. Hernandez, and D. A. Arber. 2000. "Sinonasal NK/T-cell lymphomas in the United States." *Am J Surg Pathol* 24:1511-7.

[42] Au, W. Y., R. D. Gascoyne, R. D. Klasa, J. M. Connors, R. P. Gallagher, N. D. Le, F. Loong, C. K. Law, and R. Liang. 2005. "Incidence and spectrum of non-Hodgkin lymphoma in Chinese migrants to British Columbia." *Br J Haematol* 128:792-6. doi: 10.1111/j.1365-2141.2005.05387.x.

[43] Ohsawa, M., N. Shingu, H. Inohara, T. Kubo, W. I. Yang, J. H. Yoon, and K. Aozasa. 1999. "Chronological changes in incidences of polymorphic reticulosis in Korea and Japan." *Oncology* 56:202-7. doi: 11966.

[44] Sahni, C. S., and S. B. Desai. 2007. "Distribution and clinicopathologic characteristics of non-Hodgkin's lymphoma in India: a study of 935 cases using WHO classification of lymphoid neoplasms (2000)." *Leuk Lymphoma* 48:122-33. doi: 10.1080/10428190601043351.

[45] Naresh, K. N., V. Srinivas, and C. S. Soman. 2000. "Distribution of various subtypes of non-Hodgkin's lymphoma in India: a study of 2773 lymphomas using R.E.A.L. and WHO Classifications." *Ann Oncol* 11 Suppl 1:63-7.

[46] Harabuchi, Y., N. Yamanaka, A. Kataura, S. Imai, T. Kinoshita, F. Mizuno, and T. Osato. 1990. "Epstein-Barr virus in nasal T-cell lymphomas in patients with lethal midline granuloma." *Lancet* 335:128-30.

[47] Kanavaros, P., M. C. Lescs, J. Briere, M. Divine, F. Galateau, I. Joab, J. Bosq, J. P. Farcet, F. Reyes, and P. Gaulard. 1993. "Nasal T-cell lymphoma: a clinicopathologic entity associated with peculiar phenotype and with Epstein-Barr virus." *Blood* 81:2688-95.

[48] Mishima, K., K. Horiuchi, S. Kojya, H. Takahashi, M. Ohsawa, and K. Aozasa. 1994. "Epstein-Barr virus in patients with polymorphic reticulosis (lethal midline granuloma) from China and Japan." *Cancer* 73:3041-6.

[49] Chan, J. K., T. T. Yip, W. Y. Tsang, C. S. Ng, W. H. Lau, Y. F. Poon, C. C. Wong, and V. W. Ma. 1994. "Detection of Epstein-Barr viral RNA in malignant lymphomas of the upper aerodigestive tract." *Am J Surg Pathol* 18:938-46.

[50] Tomita, Y., M. Ohsawa, Y. Mishiro, T. Kubo, N. Maeshiro, S. Kojya, Y. Noda, and K. Aozasa. 1995. "The presence and subtype of Epstein-Barr virus in B and T cell lymphomas of the sino-nasal region from the Osaka and Okinawa districts of Japan." *Lab Invest* 73:190-6.

[51] Tomita, Y., M. Ohsawa, K. Qiu, M. Hashimoto, W. I. Yang, G. E. Kim, and K. Aozasa. 1997. "Epstein-Barr virus in lymphoproliferative diseases in the sino-nasal region: close association with CD56+ immunophenotype and polymorphic-reticulosis morphology." *Int J Cancer* 70:9-13.

[52] Jaffe, E. S. 1995. "Nasal and nasal-type T/NK cell lymphoma: a unique form of lymphoma associated with the Epstein-Barr virus." *Histopathology* 27:581-3.

[53] Ho, F. C., G. Srivastava, S. L. Loke, K. H. Fu, B. P. Leung, R. Liang, and D. Choy. 1990. "Presence of Epstein-Barr virus DNA in nasal lymphomas of B and 'T' cell type." *Hematol Oncol* 8:271-81.

[54] Kanavaros, P., J. Briere, M. C. Lescs, and P. Gaulard. 1996. "Epstein-Barr virus in non-Hodgkin's lymphomas of the upper respiratory tract: association with sinonasal localization and expression of NK and/or T-cell antigens by tumour cells." *J Pathol* 178:297-302. doi: 10.1002/(SICI)1096-9896(199603)178:3<297::AID-PATH469>3.0.CO;2-E.

[55] Tsang, W. Y., J. K. Chan, T. T. Yip, C. S. Ng, K. F. Wong, Y. F. Poon, and V. W. Ma. 1994. "In situ localization of Epstein-Barr virus encoded RNA in non-nasal/nasopharyngeal CD56-positive and CD56-negative T-cell lymphomas." *Hum Pathol* 25:758-65.

[56] van Gorp, J., L. Weiping, K. Jacobse, Y. H. Liu, F. Y. Li, R. A. De Weger, and G. Li. 1994. "Epstein-Barr virus in nasal T-cell lymphomas (polymorphic reticulosis/midline malignant reticulosis) in western China." *J Pathol* 173:81-7. doi: 10.1002/path.1711730203.

[57] Schwartz, E. J., H. Molina-Kirsch, S. Zhao, R. J. Marinelli, R. A. Warnke, and Y. Natkunam. 2008. "Immunohistochemical characterization of nasal-type extranodal NK/T-cell lymphoma using a tissue microarray: an analysis of 84 cases." *Am J Clin Pathol* 130:343-51. doi: 10.1309/V561QTM6854W4WAV.

[58] Ohshima, K., H. Kimura, T. Yoshino, C. W. Kim, Y. H. Ko, S. S. Lee, S. C. Peh, J. K. Chan, and Caebv Study Group. 2008. "Proposed categorization of pathological states of EBV-associated T/natural killer-cell lymphoproliferative disorder (LPD) in children and young adults: overlap with chronic active EBV infection and

infantile fulminant EBV T-LPD." *Pathol Int* 58:209-17. doi: 10.1111/j.1440-1827.2008.02213.x.

[59] Nitta, Y., K. Iwatsuki, H. Kimura, S. Kojima, T. Morishima, K. Tsuji, and T. Oono. 2005. "Fatal natural killer cell lymphoma arising in a patient with a crop of Epstein-Barr virus-associated disorders." *Eur J Dermatol* 15:503-6.

[60] Dambaugh, T., K. Hennessy, L. Chamnankit, and E. Kieff. 1984. "U2 region of Epstein-Barr virus DNA may encode Epstein-Barr nuclear antigen 2." *Proc Natl Acad Sci U S A* 81:7632-6.

[61] Apolloni, A., and T. B. Sculley. 1994. "Detection of A-type and B-type Epstein-Barr virus in throat washings and lymphocytes." *Virology* 202:978-81.

[62] Shim, Y. S., C. W. Kim, and W. K. Lee. 1998. "Sequence variation of EBNA2 of Epstein-Barr virus isolates from Korea." *Mol Cells* 8:226-32.

[63] Thorley-Lawson, D. A., and A. Gross. 2004. "Persistence of the Epstein-Barr virus and the origins of associated lymphomas." *N Engl J Med* 350:1328-37. doi: 10.1056/NEJMra032015.

[64] Correa, R. M., M. D. Fellner, L. V. Alonio, K. Durand, A. R. Teyssie, and M. A. Picconi. 2004. "Epstein-barr virus (EBV) in healthy carriers: Distribution of genotypes and 30 bp deletion in latent membrane protein-1 (LMP-1) oncogene." *J Med Virol* 73:583-8. doi: 10.1002/jmv.20129.

[65] Yao, Q. Y., R. J. Tierney, D. Croom-Carter, G. M. Cooper, C. J. Ellis, M. Rowe, and A. B. Rickinson. 1996. "Isolation of intertypic recombinants of Epstein-Barr virus from T-cell-immunocompromised individuals." *J Virol* 70:4895-903.

[66] Boyle, M. J., W. A. Sewell, T. B. Sculley, A. Apolloni, J. J. Turner, C. E. Swanson, R. Penny, and D. A. Cooper. 1991. "Subtypes of Epstein-Barr virus in human immunodeficiency virus-associated non-Hodgkin lymphoma." *Blood* 78:3004-11.

[67] Suzumiya, J., K. Ohshima, M. Takeshita, M. Kanda, C. Kawasaki, N. Kimura, K. Tamura, and M. Kikuchi. 1999. "Nasal lymphomas in Japan: a high prevalence of Epstein-Barr virus type A and deletion within the latent membrane protein gene." *Leuk Lymphoma* 35:567-78. doi: 10.1080/10428199909169621.

[68] Peh, S. C., K. Sandvej, and G. Pallesen. 1995. "Epstein-Barr virus (EBV) in Malaysian upper-aerodigestive-tract lymphoma: incidence and sub-type." *Int J Cancer* 61:327-32.

[69] Chiang, A. K., K. Y. Wong, A. C. Liang, and G. Srivastava. 1999. "Comparative analysis of Epstein-Barr virus gene polymorphisms in nasal T/NK-cell lymphomas and normal nasal tissues: implications on virus strain selection in malignancy." *Int J Cancer* 80:356-64.

[70] Pongpruttipan, T., T. Kummalue, A. Bedavanija, A. Khuhapinant, K. Ohshima, F. Arakawa, D. Niino, and S. Sukpanichnant. 2011. "Aberrant antigenic expression in extranodal NK/T-cell lymphoma: a multi-parameter study from Thailand." *Diagn Pathol* 6:79. doi: 10.1186/1746-1596-6-79.

[71] Borisch, B., I. Hennig, R. H. Laeng, E. R. Waelti, R. Kraft, and J. Laissue. 1993. "Association of the subtype 2 of the Epstein-Barr virus with T-cell non-Hodgkin's lymphoma of the midline granuloma type." *Blood* 82:858-64.

[72] Barrionuevo, C., M. Zaharia, M. T. Martinez, L. Taxa, O. Misad, A. Moscol, G. Sarria, I. Guerrero, L. Casanova, C. Flores, and E. A. Zevallos-Giampietri. 2007. "Extranodal NK/T-cell lymphoma, nasal type: study of clinicopathologic and prognosis factors in a series of 78 cases from Peru." *Appl Immunohistochem Mol Morphol* 15:38-44.

[73] Garcia-Cosio, M., A. Santon, M. C. Mendez, C. Rivas, C. Martin, and C. Bellas. 2003. "Nasopharyngeal/nasal type T/NK lymphomas: analysis of 14 cases and review of the literature." *Tumori* 89:278-84.

[74] Kojya, S., J. Matsumura, L. Ting, T. Hongyo, J. Inazawa, M. Kirihata, and K. Aozasa. 2001. "Familial nasal NK/T-cell lymphoma and pesticide use." *Am J Hematol* 66:145-7. doi: 10.1002/1096-8652(200102)66:2<145::AID-AJH1033>3.0.CO;2-V.

[75] Zahm, S. H., and A. Blair. 1992. "Pesticides and non-Hodgkin's lymphoma." *Cancer Res* 52:5485s-88s.

[76] Miligi, L., A. S. Costantini, V. Bolejack, A. Veraldi, A. Benvenuti, O. Nanni, V. Ramazzotti, R. Tumino, E. Stagnaro, S. Rodella, A. Fontana, C. Vindigni, and P. Vineis. 2003. "Non-Hodgkin's lymphoma, leukemia, and exposures in agriculture: results from the Italian multicenter case-control study." *Am J Ind Med* 44:627-36. doi: 10.1002/ajim.10289.

[77] Xu, J. X., Y. Hoshida, W. I. Yang, H. Inohara, T. Kubo, G. E. Kim, J. H. Yoon, S. Kojya, N. Bandoh, Y. Harabuchi, K. Tsutsumi, I. Koizuka, X. S. Jia, M. Kirihata, H. Tsukuma, and K. Aozasa. 2007. "Life-style and environmental factors in the development of nasal NK/T-cell lymphoma: a case-control study in East Asia." *Int J Cancer* 120:406-10. doi: 10.1002/ijc.22313.

[78] Kwong, Y. L., C. C. Lam, and T. M. Chan. 2000. "Post-transplantation lymphoproliferative disease of natural killer cell lineage: a clinicopathological and molecular analysis." *Br J Haematol* 110:197-202.

[79] Stadlmann, S., F. Fend, P. Moser, P. Obrist, R. Greil, and S. Dirnhofer. 2001. "Epstein-Barr virus-associated extranodal NK/T-cell lymphoma, nasal type of the hypopharynx, in a renal allograft recipient: case report and review of literature." *Hum Pathol* 32:1264-8.

[80] Hoshida, Y., T. Hongyo, S. Nakatsuka, M. Nishiu, T. Takakuwa, Y. Tomita, T. Nomura, and K. Aozasa. 2002. "Gene mutations in lymphoproliferative disorders of T and NK/T cell phenotypes developing in renal transplant patients." *Lab Invest* 82:257-64.

[81] Mizuno, H., J. Koya, Y. Fujioka, T. Ibaraki, F. Nakamura, A. Hayashi, A. Shinozaki-Ushiku, N. Akamatsu, K. Hasegawa, N. Kokudo, M. Fukuyama, and M.

Kurokawa. 2017. "Extranodal NK/T cell lymphoma in a living donor liver transplant recipient." *Ann Hematol*. doi: 10.1007/s00277-017-2969-y.

[82] Acosta, A. M., V. Alagiozian-Angelova, P. Kovarik, and M. Sekosan. 2016. "Post-transplant extranodal NK/T-cell lymphoma, nasal type with cutaneous and pulmonary involvement." *Pathology* 48:380-3. doi: 10.1016/j.pathol.2016.03.011.

[83] Manley, K., J. Dunning, M. Nelson, and M. Bower. 2012. "HIV-associated gastric natural killer/T-cell lymphoma." *Int J STD AIDS* 23:66-7. doi: 10.1258/ijsa.2009.009121.

[84] Li, Z., Y. Xia, L. N. Feng, J. R. Chen, H. M. Li, J. Cui, Q. Q. Cai, K. S. Sim, M. L. Nairismagi, Y. Laurensia, W. Y. Meah, W. S. Liu, Y. M. Guo, L. Z. Chen, Q. S. Feng, C. P. Pang, L. J. Chen, S. H. Chew, R. P. Ebstein, J. N. Foo, J. Liu, J. Ha, L. P. Khoo, S. T. Chin, Y. X. Zeng, T. Aung, B. Chowbay, C. P. Diong, F. Zhang, Y. H. Liu, T. Tang, M. Tao, R. Quek, F. Mohamad, S. Y. Tan, B. T. Teh, S. B. Ng, W. J. Chng, C. K. Ong, Y. Okada, S. Raychaudhuri, S. T. Lim, W. Tan, R. J. Peng, C. C. Khor, and J. X. Bei. 2016. "Genetic risk of extranodal natural killer T-cell lymphoma: a genome-wide association study." *Lancet Oncol* 17:1240-7. doi: 10.1016/S1470-2045(16)30148-6.

[85] Kanno, H., S. Kojya, T. Li, M. Ohsawa, S. Nakatsuka, M. Miyaguchi, Y. Harabuchi, and K. Aozasa. 2000. "Low frequency of HLA-A*0201 allele in patients with Epstein-Barr virus-positive nasal lymphomas with polymorphic reticulosis morphology." *Int J Cancer* 87:195-9.

[86] Klein, J., and A. Sato. 2000. "The HLA system. First of two parts." *N Engl J Med* 343:702-9. doi: 10.1056/NEJM200009073431006.

[87] Diaz, G., M. Amicosante, D. Jaraquemada, R. H. Butler, M. V. Guillen, M. Sanchez, C. Nombela, and J. Arroyo. 2003. "Functional analysis of HLA-DP polymorphism: a crucial role for DPbeta residues 9, 11, 35, 55, 56, 69 and 84-87 in T cell allorecognition and peptide binding." *Int Immunol* 15:565-76.

[88] Kwong, Y. L. 2005. "Natural killer-cell malignancies: diagnosis and treatment." *Leukemia* 19:2186-94. doi: 10.1038/sj.leu.2403955.

[89] Pagano, L., A. Gallamini, G. Trape, L. Fianchi, D. Mattei, G. Todeschini, A. Spadea, S. Cinieri, E. Iannitto, M. Martelli, A. Nosari, E. D. Bona, M. E. Tosti, M. C. Petti, P. Falcucci, M. Montanaro, A. Pulsoni, L. M. Larocca, G. Leone, and Linfomi Intergruppo Italiano. 2006. "NK/T-cell lymphomas 'nasal type': an Italian multicentric retrospective survey." *Ann Oncol* 17:794-800. doi: 10.1093/annonc/mdl015.

[90] Takata, K., M. E. Hong, P. Sitthinamsuwan, F. Loong, S. Y. Tan, J. Y. Liau, P. P. Hsieh, S. B. Ng, S. F. Yang, T. Pongpruttipan, S. Sukpanichnant, Y. L. Kwong, Y. Hyeh Ko, Y. T. Cho, W. J. Chng, T. Matsushita, T. Yoshino, and S. S. Chuang. 2015. "Primary cutaneous NK/T-cell lymphoma, nasal type and CD56-positive peripheral T-cell lymphoma: a cellular lineage and clinicopathologic study of 60

patients from Asia." *Am J Surg Pathol* 39:1-12. doi: 10.1097/PAS. 0000000000000312.

[91] Yu, J. B., Z. Zuo, Y. Tang, S. Zhao, Y. C. Zhang, C. F. Bi, W. Y. Wang, W. Y. Zhang, L. Wang, and W. P. Liu. 2009. "Extranodal nasal-type natural killer/T-cell lymphoma of the skin: a clinicopathologic study of 16 cases in China." *Hum Pathol* 40:807-16. doi: 10.1016/j.humpath.2008.08.020.

[92] Kim, S. J., H. A. Jung, S. S. Chuang, H. Hong, C. C. Guo, J. Cao, X. N. Hong, R. Suzuki, H. J. Kang, J. H. Won, W. J. Chng, Y. L. Kwong, C. Suh, Y. Q. Song, J. Zhu, K. Tay, S. T. Lim, J. Suzumiya, T. Y. Lin, W. S. Kim, and Group Asia Lymphoma Study. 2013. "Extranodal natural killer/T-cell lymphoma involving the gastrointestinal tract: analysis of clinical features and outcomes from the Asia Lymphoma Study Group." *J Hematol Oncol* 6:86. doi: 10.1186/1756-8722-6-86.

[93] Chim, C. S., W. Y. Au, T. W. Shek, J. Ho, C. Choy, S. K. Ma, H. M. Tung, R. Liang, and Y. L. Kwong. 2001. "Primary CD56 positive lymphomas of the gastrointestinal tract." *Cancer* 91:525-33.

[94] Au, W. Y., A. C. Chan, and Y. L. Kwong. 1998. "Scrotal skin ulcer in a patient with a previous tonsillectomy because of natural killer cell lymphoma." *Am J Dermatopathol* 20:582-5.

[95] Liang, D. N., Z. R. Yang, W. Y. Wang, S. Zhao, Q. P. Yang, Y. Tang, C. F. Bi, and W. P. Liu. 2012. "Extranodal nasal type natural killer/T-cell lymphoma of testis: report of seven cases with review of literature." *Leuk Lymphoma* 53:1117-23. doi: 10.3109/10428194.2011.645209.

[96] Ayadi, L., S. Makni, N. Toumi, S. Hammami, S. Charfi, M. Frikha, A. Khabir, and T. Boudawara. 2010. "Aggressive nasal-type natural killer/T-cell lymphoma associated with Epstein Barr virus presenting as testicular tumor." *Tunis Med* 88:196-8.

[97] Chim, C. S., W. Y. Au, C. Poon, G. C. Ooi, C. C. Lam, and Y. L. Kwong. 2002. "Primary natural killer cell lymphoma of skeletal muscle." *Histopathology* 41:371-4.

[98] Chang, S. E., S. Y. Lee, J. H. Choi, K. J. Sung, K. C. Moon, and J. K. Koh. 2002. "Cutaneous dissemination of nasal NK/T-cell lymphoma with bone marrow, liver and lung involvement." *Clin Exp Dermatol* 27:120-2.

[99] Ng, S. B., K. W. Lai, S. Murugaya, K. M. Lee, S. L. Loong, S. Fook-Chong, M. Tao, and I. Sng. 2004. "Nasal-type extranodal natural killer/T-cell lymphomas: a clinicopathologic and genotypic study of 42 cases in Singapore." *Mod Pathol* 17:1097-107. doi: 10.1038/modpathol.3800157.

[100] Chan, J. K., V. C. Sin, K. F. Wong, C. S. Ng, W. Y. Tsang, C. H. Chan, M. M. Cheung, and W. H. Lau. 1997. "Nonnasal lymphoma expressing the natural killer cell marker CD56: a clinicopathologic study of 49 cases of an uncommon aggressive neoplasm." *Blood* 89:4501-13.

[101] Aladily, T. N., B. N. Nathwani, R. N. Miranda, R. Kansal, C. C. Yin, R. Protzel, G. S. Takowsky, and L. J. Medeiros. 2012. "Extranodal NK/T-cell lymphoma, nasal type, arising in association with saline breast implant: expanding the spectrum of breast implant-associated lymphomas." *Am J Surg Pathol* 36:1729-34. doi: 10.1097/PAS.0b013e31826a006f.

[102] Chan, W. K., W. Y. Au, C. Y. Wong, R. Liang, A. Y. Leung, Y. L. Kwong, and P. L. Khong. 2010. "Metabolic activity measured by F-18 FDG PET in natural killer-cell lymphoma compared to aggressive B- and T-cell lymphomas." *Clin Nucl Med* 35:571-5. doi: 10.1097/RLU.0b013e3181e4dcbf.

[103] Khong, P. L., C. B. Pang, R. Liang, Y. L. Kwong, and W. Y. Au. 2008. "Fluorine-18 fluorodeoxyglucose positron emission tomography in mature T-cell and natural killer cell malignancies." *Ann Hematol* 87:613-21. doi: 10.1007/s00277-008-0494-8.

[104] Tse, E., R. Leung, P. L. Khong, W. H. Lau, and Y. L. Kwong. 2009. "Non-nasal natural killer cell lymphoma: not non-nasal after all." *Ann Hematol* 88:185-7. doi: 10.1007/s00277-008-0562-0.

[105] Tse, E., and Y. L. Kwong. 2012. "Practical management of natural killer/T-cell lymphoma." *Curr Opin Oncol* 24:480-6. doi: 10.1097/CCO.0b013e3283556142.

[106] Kwong, Y. L., B. O. Anderson, R. Advani, W. S. Kim, A. M. Levine, S. T. Lim, and Summit Asian Oncology. 2009. "Management of T-cell and natural-killer-cell neoplasms in Asia: consensus statement from the Asian Oncology Summit 2009." *Lancet Oncol* 10:1093-101. doi: 10.1016/S1470-2045(09)70265-7.

[107] Kwong, Y. L., W. S. Kim, S. T. Lim, S. J. Kim, T. Tang, E. Tse, A. Y. Leung, and C. S. Chim. 2012. "SMILE for natural killer/T-cell lymphoma: analysis of safety and efficacy from the Asia Lymphoma Study Group." *Blood* 120:2973-80. doi: 10.1182/blood-2012-05-431460.

[108] Ng, C. S., J. K. Chan, P. N. Cheng, and S. C. Szeto. 1986. "Nasal T-cell lymphoma associated with hemophagocytic syndrome." *Cancer* 58:67-71.

[109] Chubachi, A., H. Imai, S. Nishimura, M. Saitoh, and A. B. Miura. 1992. "Nasal T-cell lymphoma associated with hemophagocytic syndrome. Immunohistochemical and genotypic studies." *Arch Pathol Lab Med* 116:1209-12.

[110] Takahashi, N., I. Miura, A. Chubachi, A. B. Miura, and S. Nakamura. 2001. "A clinicopathological study of 20 patients with T/natural killer (NK)-cell lymphoma-associated hemophagocytic syndrome with special reference to nasal and nasal-type NK/T-cell lymphoma." *Int J Hematol* 74:303-8.

[111] You, J. Y., K. H. Chi, M. H. Yang, C. C. Chen, C. H. Ho, W. K. Chau, H. C. Hsu, J. P. Gau, C. H. Tzeng, J. H. Liu, P. M. Chen, and T. J. Chiou. 2004. "Radiation therapy versus chemotherapy as initial treatment for localized nasal natural killer (NK)/T-cell lymphoma: a single institute survey in Taiwan." *Ann Oncol* 15:618-25.

[112] Koom, W. S., E. J. Chung, W. I. Yang, S. J. Shim, C. O. Suh, J. K. Roh, J. H. Yoon, and G. E. Kim. 2004. "Angiocentric T-cell and NK/T-cell lymphomas: radiotherapeutic viewpoints." *Int J Radiat Oncol Biol Phys* 59:1127-37. doi: 10.1016/j.ijrobp.2003.12.006.

[113] Cheung, M. M., J. K. Chan, W. H. Lau, R. K. Ngan, and W. W. Foo. 2002. "Early stage nasal NK/T-cell lymphoma: clinical outcome, prognostic factors, and the effect of treatment modality." *Int J Radiat Oncol Biol Phys* 54:182-90.

[114] Kim, G. E., J. H. Cho, W. I. Yang, E. J. Chung, C. O. Suh, K. R. Park, W. P. Hong, I. Y. Park, J. S. Hahn, J. K. Roh, and B. S. Kim. 2000. "Angiocentric lymphoma of the head and neck: patterns of systemic failure after radiation treatment." *J Clin Oncol* 18:54-63. doi: 10.1200/JCO.2000.18.1.54.

[115] Jiang, Q. P., S. Y. Liu, Y. X. Yang, X. X. Tan, J. Peng, Z. T. Xiong, and Z. Li. 2012. "CD20-positive NK/T-cell lymphoma with indolent clinical course: report of case and review of literature." *Diagn Pathol* 7:133. doi: 10.1186/1746-1596-7-133.

[116] Kim, S. J., Y. Park, B. S. Kim, I. Kim, Y. H. Ko, and W. S. Kim. 2012. "Extranodal natural killer/T-cell lymphoma with long-term survival and repeated relapses: does it indicate the presence of indolent subtype?" *Korean J Hematol* 47:202-6. doi: 10.5045/kjh.2012.47.3.202.

[117] Lee, W. J., J. M. Jung, C. H. Won, S. E. Chang, J. H. Choi, K. Chan Moon, C. S. Park, J. Huh, and M. W. Lee. 2014. "Cutaneous extranodal natural killer/T-cell lymphoma: a comparative clinicohistopathologic and survival outcome analysis of 45 cases according to the primary tumor site." *J Am Acad Dermatol* 70:1002-9. doi: 10.1016/j.jaad.2013.12.023.

[118] Natkunam, Y., B. R. Smoller, J. L. Zehnder, R. F. Dorfman, and R. A. Warnke. 1999. "Aggressive cutaneous NK and NK-like T-cell lymphomas: clinicopathologic, immunohistochemical, and molecular analyses of 12 cases." *Am J Surg Pathol* 23:571-81.

[119] Miyamoto, T., T. Yoshino, T. Takehisa, Y. Hagari, and M. Mihara. 1998. "Cutaneous presentation of nasal/nasal type T/NK cell lymphoma: clinicopathological findings of four cases." *Br J Dermatol* 139:481-7.

[120] Qi, S. N., Y. X. Li, W. H. Wang, J. Jin, S. L. Wang, Y. P. Liu, Y. W. Song, H. Fang, H. Ren, N. N. Lu, Q. F. Liu, R. Y. Wu, X. M. Zhang, X. F. Liu, and Z. H. Yu. 2012. "The extent of cutaneous lesions predicts outcome in extranodal nasal-type natural killer/T-cell lymphoma of the upper aerodigestive tract with secondary cutaneous involvement." *Leuk Lymphoma* 53:855-61. doi: 10.3109/10428194.2011.634040.

[121] Berti, E., S. Recalcati, V. Girgenti, D. Fanoni, L. Venegoni, and P. Vezzoli. 2010. "Cutaneous extranodal NK/T-cell lymphoma: a clinicopathologic study of 5 patients with array-based comparative genomic hybridization." *Blood* 116:165-70. doi: 10.1182/blood-2009-11-252957.

[122] Isobe, Y., N. Aritaka, M. Sasaki, K. Oshimi, and K. Sugimoto. 2009. "Spontaneous regression of natural killer cell lymphoma." *J Clin Pathol* 62:647-50. doi: 10.1136/jcp.2008.062976.

[123] Chang, S. E., G. S. Yoon, J. Huh, J. H. Choi, K. J. Sung, K. C. Moon, and J. K. Koh. 2002. "Comparison of primary and secondary cutaneous CD56+ NK/T cell lymphomas." *Appl Immunohistochem Mol Morphol* 10:163-70.

[124] Jiang, M., X. Chen, Z. Yi, X. Zhang, B. Zhang, F. Luo, Y. Jiang, and L. Zou. 2013. "Prognostic characteristics of gastrointestinal tract NK/T-cell lymphoma: an analysis of 47 patients in China." *J Clin Gastroenterol* 47:e74-9. doi: 10.1097/MCG.0b013e31829e444f.

[125] Pongpruttipan, T., S. Sukpanichnant, T. Assanasen, P. Wannakrairot, P. Boonsakan, W. Kanoksil, K. Kayasut, W. Mitarnun, A. Khuhapinant, U. Bunworasate, T. Puavilai, A. Bedavanija, A. Garcia-Herrera, E. Campo, J. R. Cook, J. Choi, and S. H. Swerdlow. 2012. "Extranodal NK/T-cell lymphoma, nasal type, includes cases of natural killer cell and alphabeta, gammadelta, and alphabeta/gammadelta T-cell origin: a comprehensive clinicopathologic and phenotypic study." *Am J Surg Pathol* 36:481-99. doi: 10.1097/PAS. 0b013e31824433d8.

[126] Peck, T., and M. R. Wick. 2015. "Primary cutaneous natural killer/T-cell lymphoma of the nasal type: a report of 4 cases in North American patients." *Ann Diagn Pathol* 19:211-5. doi: 10.1016/j.anndiagpath.2015.04.003.

[127] Choi, Y. L., J. H. Park, J. H. Namkung, J. H. Lee, J. M. Yang, E. S. Lee, D. Y. Lee, K. T. Jang, and Y. H. Ko. 2009. "Extranodal NK/T-cell lymphoma with cutaneous involvement: 'nasal' vs. 'nasal-type' subgroups--a retrospective study of 18 patients." *Br J Dermatol* 160:333-7. doi: 10.1111/j.1365-2133.2008.08922.x.

[128] Yamashita, Y., T. Tsuzuki, A. Nakayama, M. Fujino, and N. Mori. 1999. "A case of natural killer/T cell lymphoma of the subcutis resembling subcutaneous panniculitis-like T cell lymphoma." *Pathol Int* 49:241-6.

[129] Swerdlow, Steven H., International Agency for Research on Cancer., and World Health Organization. 2008. *WHO classification of tumours of haematopoietic and lymphoid tissues*. 4th ed, *World Health Organization classification of tumours*. Lyon, France: International Agency for Research on Cancer.

[130] Chan, J. K., W. Y. Tsang, W. H. Lau, M. M. Cheung, W. F. Ng, W. C. Yuen, and C. S. Ng. 1996. "Aggressive T/natural killer cell lymphoma presenting as testicular tumor." *Cancer* 77:1198-205.

[131] Suzuki, R. 2012. "NK/T-cell lymphomas: pathobiology, prognosis and treatment paradigm." *Curr Oncol Rep* 14:395-402. doi: 10.1007/s11912-012-0245-9.

[132] Hong, M., T. Lee, S. Young Kang, S. J. Kim, W. Kim, and Y. H. Ko. 2016. "Nasal-type NK/T-cell lymphomas are more frequently T rather than NK lineage based on

T-cell receptor gene, RNA, and protein studies: lineage does not predict clinical behavior." *Mod Pathol* 29:430-43. doi: 10.1038/modpathol.2016.47.

[133] Yu, W. W., P. P. Hsieh, and S. S. Chuang. 2013. "Cutaneous EBV-positive gammadelta T-cell lymphoma vs. extranodal NK/T-cell lymphoma: a case report and literature review." *J Cutan Pathol* 40:310-6. doi: 10.1111/cup.12066.

[134] Li, P., L. Jiang, X. Zhang, J. Liu, and H. Wang. 2014. "CD30 expression is a novel prognostic indicator in extranodal natural killer/T-cell lymphoma, nasal type." *BMC Cancer* 14:890. doi: 10.1186/1471-2407-14-890.

[135] Kim, W. Y., S. J. Nam, S. Kim, T. M. Kim, D. S. Heo, C. W. Kim, and Y. K. Jeon. 2015. "Prognostic implications of CD30 expression in extranodal natural killer/T-cell lymphoma according to treatment modalities." *Leuk Lymphoma* 56:1778-86. doi: 10.3109/10428194.2014.974048.

[136] Ng, C. S., S. T. Lo, and J. K. Chan. 1999. "Peripheral T and putative natural killer cell lymphomas commonly coexpress CD95 and CD95 ligand." *Hum Pathol* 30:48-53.

[137] Ohshima, K., J. Suzumiya, K. Shimazaki, A. Kato, T. Tanaka, M. Kanda, and M. Kikuchi. 1997. "Nasal T/NK cell lymphomas commonly express perforin and Fas ligand: important mediators of tissue damage." *Histopathology* 31:444-50.

[138] Haedicke, W., F. C. Ho, A. Chott, L. Moretta, T. Rudiger, G. Ott, and H. K. Muller-Hermelink. 2000. "Expression of CD94/NKG2A and killer immunoglobulin-like receptors in NK cells and a subset of extranodal cytotoxic T-cell lymphomas." *Blood* 95:3628-30.

[139] Dukers, D. F., M. H. Vermeer, L. H. Jaspars, C. A. Sander, M. J. Flaig, W. Vos, R. Willemze, and C. J. Meijer. 2001. "Expression of killer cell inhibitory receptors is restricted to true NK cell lymphomas and a subset of intestinal enteropathy-type T cell lymphomas with a cytotoxic phenotype." *J Clin Pathol* 54:224-8.

[140] Jhuang, J. Y., S. T. Chang, S. F. Weng, S. T. Pan, P. Y. Chu, P. P. Hsieh, C. H. Wei, S. C. Chou, C. L. Koo, C. J. Chen, J. D. Hsu, and S. S. Chuang. 2015. "Extranodal natural killer/T-cell lymphoma, nasal type in Taiwan: a relatively higher frequency of T-cell lineage and poor survival for extranasal tumors." *Hum Pathol* 46:313-21. doi: 10.1016/j.humpath.2014.11.008.

[141] Taddesse-Heath, L., J. I. Feldman, G. A. Fahle, S. H. Fischer, L. Sorbara, M. Raffeld, and E. S. Jaffe. 2003. "Florid CD4+, CD56+ T-cell infiltrate associated with Herpes simplex infection simulating nasal NK-/T-cell lymphoma." *Mod Pathol* 16:166-72. doi: 10.1097/01.MP.0000051680.14007.D7.

[142] Katano, H., M. A. Ali, A. C. Patera, M. Catalfamo, E. S. Jaffe, H. Kimura, J. K. Dale, S. E. Straus, and J. I. Cohen. 2004. "Chronic active Epstein-Barr virus infection associated with mutations in perforin that impair its maturation." *Blood* 103:1244-52. doi: 10.1182/blood-2003-06-2171.

[143] Soliman, D. S., A. A. Sabbagh, H. E. Omri, F. A. Ibrahim, A. M. Amer, and I. B. Otazu. 2014. "Rare aggressive natural killer cell leukemia presented with bone marrow fibrosis - a diagnostic challenge." *Springerplus* 3:390. doi: 10.1186/2193-1801-3-390.

[144] Ankita, G., and D. Shashi. 2016. "Pulmonary Lymphomatoid Granulomatosis- a Case Report with Review of Literature." *Indian J Surg Oncol* 7:484-87. doi: 10.1007/s13193-016-0525-1.

[145] Oprea, C., C. Cainap, R. Azoulay, E. Assaf, E. Jabbour, S. Koscielny, S. Lapusan, D. Vanel, J. Bosq, and V. Ribrag. 2005. "Primary diffuse large B-cell non-Hodgkin lymphoma of the paranasal sinuses: a report of 14 cases." *Br J Haematol* 131:468-71. doi: 10.1111/j.1365-2141.2005.05787.x.

[146] Lee, W. J., H. J. Kang, C. H. Won, S. E. Chang, J. H. Choi, and M. W. Lee. 2016. "Cutaneous Extranodal Natural Killer/T-Cell Lymphomas Histopathologically Mimicking Benign Inflammatory Disease." *Am J Dermatopathol*. doi: 10.1097/DAD.0000000000000620.

[147] Ko, Y. H., E. Y. Cho, J. E. Kim, S. S. Lee, J. R. Huh, H. K. Chang, W. I. Yang, C. W. Kim, S. W. Kim, and H. J. Ree. 2004. "NK and NK-like T-cell lymphoma in extranasal sites: a comparative clinicopathological study according to site and EBV status." *Histopathology* 44:480-9. doi: 10.1111/j.1365-2559.2004.01867.x.

[148] Quintanilla-Martinez, L., P. M. Jansen, M. C. Kinney, S. H. Swerdlow, and R. Willemze. 2013. "Non-mycosis fungoides cutaneous T-cell lymphomas: report of the 2011 Society for Hematopathology/European Association for Haematopathology workshop." *Am J Clin Pathol* 139:491-514. doi: 10.1309/AJCP83AOQTMLOJTM.

[149] Toro, J. R., M. Beaty, L. Sorbara, M. L. Turner, J. White, D. W. Kingma, M. Raffeld, and E. S. Jaffe. 2000. "gamma delta T-cell lymphoma of the skin: a clinical, microscopic, and molecular study." *Arch Dermatol* 136:1024-32.

[150] Willemze, R., and C. J. Meijer. 2006. "Classification of cutaneous T-cell lymphoma: from Alibert to WHO-EORTC." *J Cutan Pathol* 33 Suppl 1:18-26. doi: 10.1111/j.0303-6987.2006.00494.x.

[151] Jaffe, E. S., A. Nicolae, and S. Pittaluga. 2013. "Peripheral T-cell and NK-cell lymphomas in the WHO classification: pearls and pitfalls." *Mod Pathol* 26 Suppl 1:S71-87. doi: 10.1038/modpathol.2012.181.

[152] Iqbal, J., D. D. Weisenburger, A. Chowdhury, M. Y. Tsai, G. Srivastava, T. C. Greiner, C. Kucuk, K. Deffenbacher, J. Vose, L. Smith, W. Y. Au, S. Nakamura, M. Seto, J. Delabie, F. Berger, F. Loong, Y. H. Ko, I. Sng, X. Liu, T. P. Loughran, J. Armitage, W. C. Chan, and T. cell Lymphoma Project International Peripheral. 2011. "Natural killer cell lymphoma shares strikingly similar molecular features with a group of non-hepatosplenic gammadelta T-cell lymphoma and is highly

sensitive to a novel aurora kinase A inhibitor in vitro." *Leukemia* 25:348-58. doi: 10.1038/leu.2010.255.

[153] Kimura, H., Y. Ito, S. Kawabe, K. Gotoh, Y. Takahashi, S. Kojima, T. Naoe, S. Esaki, A. Kikuta, A. Sawada, K. Kawa, K. Ohshima, and S. Nakamura. 2012. "EBV-associated T/NK-cell lymphoproliferative diseases in nonimmunocompromised hosts: prospective analysis of 108 cases." *Blood* 119:673-86. doi: 10.1182/blood-2011-10-381921.

[154] Asada, H. 2007. "Hypersensitivity to mosquito bites: a unique pathogenic mechanism linking Epstein-Barr virus infection, allergy and oncogenesis." *J Dermatol Sci* 45:153-60. doi: 10.1016/j.jdermsci.2006.11.002.

[155] Takeuchi, K., M. Yokoyama, S. Ishizawa, Y. Terui, K. Nomura, K. Marutsuka, M. Nunomura, N. Fukushima, T. Yagyuu, H. Nakamine, F. Akiyama, K. Hoshi, K. Matsue, K. Hatake, and K. Oshimi. 2010. "Lymphomatoid gastropathy: a distinct clinicopathologic entity of self-limited pseudomalignant NK-cell proliferation." *Blood* 116:5631-7. doi: 10.1182/blood-2010-06-290650.

[156] Mansoor, A., S. Pittaluga, P. L. Beck, W. H. Wilson, J. A. Ferry, and E. S. Jaffe. 2011. "NK-cell enteropathy: a benign NK-cell lymphoproliferative disease mimicking intestinal lymphoma: clinicopathologic features and follow-up in a unique case series." *Blood* 117:1447-52. doi: 10.1182/blood-2010-08-302737.

[157] Wong, K. F., Y. M. Zhang, and J. K. Chan. 1999. "Cytogenetic abnormalities in natural killer cell lymphoma/leukaemia--is there a consistent pattern?" *Leuk Lymphoma* 34:241-50. doi: 10.3109/10428199909050949.

[158] Siu, L. L., J. K. Chan, and Y. L. Kwong. 2002. "Natural killer cell malignancies: clinicopathologic and molecular features." *Histol Histopathol* 17:539-54.

[159] Tien, H. F., I. J. Su, J. L. Tang, M. C. Liu, F. Y. Lee, Y. C. Chen, and S. M. Chuang. 1997. "Clonal chromosomal abnormalities as direct evidence for clonality in nasal T/natural killer cell lymphomas." *Br J Haematol* 97:621-5.

[160] Ko, Y. H., K. E. Choi, J. H. Han, J. M. Kim, and H. J. Ree. 2001. "Comparative genomic hybridization study of nasal-type NK/T-cell lymphoma." *Cytometry* 46:85-91.

[161] Nakashima, Y., H. Tagawa, R. Suzuki, S. Karnan, K. Karube, K. Ohshima, K. Muta, H. Nawata, Y. Morishima, S. Nakamura, and M. Seto. 2005. "Genome-wide array-based comparative genomic hybridization of natural killer cell lymphoma/leukemia: different genomic alteration patterns of aggressive NK-cell leukemia and extranodal Nk/T-cell lymphoma, nasal type." *Genes Chromosomes Cancer* 44:247-55. doi: 10.1002/gcc.20245.

[162] Sun, H. S., I. J. Su, Y. C. Lin, J. S. Chen, and S. Y. Fang. 2003. "A 2.6 Mb interval on chromosome 6q25.2-q25.3 is commonly deleted in human nasal natural killer/T-cell lymphoma." *Br J Haematol* 122:590-9.

[163] Iqbal, J., C. Kucuk, R. J. Deleeuw, G. Srivastava, W. Tam, H. Geng, D. Klinkebiel, J. K. Christman, K. Patel, K. Cao, L. Shen, K. Dybkaer, I. F. Tsui, H. Ali, N. Shimizu, W. Y. Au, W. L. Lam, and W. C. Chan. 2009. "Genomic analyses reveal global functional alterations that promote tumor growth and novel tumor suppressor genes in natural killer-cell malignancies." *Leukemia* 23:1139-51. doi: 10.1038/leu.2009.3.

[164] Huang, Y., A. de Reynies, L. de Leval, B. Ghazi, N. Martin-Garcia, M. Travert, J. Bosq, J. Briere, B. Petit, E. Thomas, P. Coppo, T. Marafioti, J. F. Emile, M. H. Delfau-Larue, C. Schmitt, and P. Gaulard. 2010. "Gene expression profiling identifies emerging oncogenic pathways operating in extranodal NK/T-cell lymphoma, nasal type." *Blood* 115:1226-37. doi: 10.1182/blood-2009-05-221275.

[165] Shapiro-Shelef, M., K. I. Lin, L. J. McHeyzer-Williams, J. Liao, M. G. McHeyzer-Williams, and K. Calame. 2003. "Blimp-1 is required for the formation of immunoglobulin secreting plasma cells and pre-plasma memory B cells." *Immunity* 19:607-20.

[166] Martins, G. A., L. Cimmino, M. Shapiro-Shelef, M. Szabolcs, A. Herron, E. Magnusdottir, and K. Calame. 2006. "Transcriptional repressor Blimp-1 regulates T cell homeostasis and function." *Nat Immunol* 7:457-65. doi: 10.1038/ni1320.

[167] Codogno, P., and A. J. Meijer. 2006. "Atg5: more than an autophagy factor." *Nat Cell Biol* 8:1045-7. doi: 10.1038/ncb1006-1045.

[168] Yousefi, S., R. Perozzo, I. Schmid, A. Ziemiecki, T. Schaffner, L. Scapozza, T. Brunner, and H. U. Simon. 2006. "Calpain-mediated cleavage of Atg5 switches autophagy to apoptosis." *Nat Cell Biol* 8:1124-32. doi: 10.1038/ncb1482.

[169] Ray, M. E., G. Wistow, Y. A. Su, P. S. Meltzer, and J. M. Trent. 1997. "AIM1, a novel non-lens member of the betagamma-crystallin superfamily, is associated with the control of tumorigenicity in human malignant melanoma." *Proc Natl Acad Sci U S A* 94:3229-34.

[170] Kucuk, C., X. Hu, J. Iqbal, P. Gaulard, D. Klinkebiel, A. Cornish, B. J. Dave, and W. C. Chan. 2013. "HACE1 is a tumor suppressor gene candidate in natural killer cell neoplasms." *Am J Pathol* 182:49-55. doi: 10.1016/j.ajpath.2012.09.012.

[171] Rotin, D., and S. Kumar. 2009. "Physiological functions of the HECT family of ubiquitin ligases." *Nat Rev Mol Cell Biol* 10:398-409. doi: 10.1038/nrm2690.

[172] Zhang, L., M. S. Anglesio, M. O'Sullivan, F. Zhang, G. Yang, R. Sarao, P. N. Mai, S. Cronin, H. Hara, N. Melnyk, L. Li, T. Wada, P. P. Liu, J. Farrar, R. J. Arceci, P. H. Sorensen, and J. M. Penninger. 2007. "The E3 ligase HACE1 is a critical chromosome 6q21 tumor suppressor involved in multiple cancers." *Nat Med* 13:1060-9. doi: 10.1038/nm1621.

[173] Karube, K., M. Nakagawa, S. Tsuzuki, I. Takeuchi, K. Honma, Y. Nakashima, N. Shimizu, Y. H. Ko, Y. Morishima, K. Ohshima, S. Nakamura, and M. Seto. 2011. "Identification of FOXO3 and PRDM1 as tumor-suppressor gene candidates in

NK-cell neoplasms by genomic and functional analyses." *Blood* 118:3195-204. doi: 10.1182/blood-2011-04-346890.

[174] Chen, Y. W., T. Guo, L. Shen, K. Y. Wong, Q. Tao, W. W. Choi, R. K. Au-Yeung, Y. P. Chan, M. L. Wong, J. C. Tang, W. P. Liu, G. D. Li, N. Shimizu, F. Loong, E. Tse, Y. L. Kwong, and G. Srivastava. 2015. "Receptor-type tyrosine-protein phosphatase kappa directly targets STAT3 activation for tumor suppression in nasal NK/T-cell lymphoma." *Blood* 125:1589-600. doi: 10.1182/blood-2014-07-588970.

[175] Li, T., T. Hongyo, M. Syaifudin, T. Nomura, Z. Dong, N. Shingu, S. Kojya, S. Nakatsuka, and K. Aozasa. 2000. "Mutations of the p53 gene in nasal NK/T-cell lymphoma." *Lab Invest* 80:493-9.

[176] Quintanilla-Martinez, L., J. L. Franklin, I. Guerrero, L. Krenacs, K. N. Naresh, C. Rama-Rao, K. Bhatia, M. Raffeld, and I. T. Magrath. 1999. "Histological and immunophenotypic profile of nasal NK/T cell lymphomas from Peru: high prevalence of p53 overexpression." *Hum Pathol* 30:849-55.

[177] Hongyo, T., Y. Hoshida, S. Nakatsuka, M. Syaifudin, S. Kojya, W. I. Yang, Y. H. Min, H. Chan, C. H. Kim, Y. Harabuchi, T. Himi, M. Inuyama, K. Aozasa, and T. Nomura. 2005. "p53, K-ras, c-kit and beta-catenin gene mutations in sinonasal NK/T-cell lymphoma in Korea and Japan." *Oncol Rep* 13:265-71.

[178] Hoshida, Y., T. Hongyo, X. Jia, Y. He, K. Hasui, Z. Dong, W. J. Luo, M. F. Ham, T. Nomura, and K. Aozasa. 2003. "Analysis of p53, K-ras, c-kit, and beta-catenin gene mutations in sinonasal NK/T cell lymphoma in northeast district of China." *Cancer Sci* 94:297-301.

[179] Nakatsuka, S., T. Hongyo, M. Syaifudin, T. Nomura, N. Shingu, and K. Aozasa. 2002. "Mutations of p53, c-kit, K-ras, and beta-catenin gene in non-Hodgkin's lymphoma of adrenal gland." *Jpn J Cancer Res* 93:267-74.

[180] Katayama, H., K. Sasai, H. Kawai, Z. M. Yuan, J. Bondaruk, F. Suzuki, S. Fujii, R. B. Arlinghaus, B. A. Czerniak, and S. Sen. 2004. "Phosphorylation by aurora kinase A induces Mdm2-mediated destabilization and inhibition of p53." *Nat Genet* 36:55-62. doi: 10.1038/ng1279.

[181] Hongyo, T., T. Li, M. Syaifudin, R. Baskar, H. Ikeda, Y. Kanakura, K. Aozasa, and T. Nomura. 2000. "Specific c-kit mutations in sinonasal natural killer/T-cell lymphoma in China and Japan." *Cancer Res* 60:2345-7.

[182] Kurniawan, A. N., T. Hongyo, E. S. Hardjolukito, M. F. Ham, T. Takakuwa, R. Kodariah, Y. Hoshida, T. Nomura, and K. Aozasa. 2006. "Gene mutation analysis of sinonasal lymphomas in Indonesia." *Oncol Rep* 15:1257-63.

[183] Quintanilla-Martinez, L., M. Kremer, G. Keller, M. Nathrath, A. Gamboa-Dominguez, A. Meneses, L. Luna-Contreras, A. Cabras, H. Hoefler, A. Mohar, and F. Fend. 2001. "p53 Mutations in nasal natural killer/T-cell lymphoma from

Mexico: association with large cell morphology and advanced disease." *Am J Pathol* 159:2095-105. doi: 10.1016/S0002-9440(10)63061-1.

[184] Takakuwa, T., T. Li, H. Kanno, S. Nakatsuka, and K. Aozasa. 1999. "No evidence of replication error phenotype in nasal nK/T cell lymphoma." *Int J Cancer* 84:623.

[185] Jiang, L., Z. H. Gu, Z. X. Yan, X. Zhao, Y. Y. Xie, Z. G. Zhang, C. M. Pan, Y. Hu, C. P. Cai, Y. Dong, J. Y. Huang, L. Wang, Y. Shen, G. Meng, J. F. Zhou, J. D. Hu, J. F. Wang, Y. H. Liu, L. H. Yang, F. Zhang, J. M. Wang, Z. Wang, Z. G. Peng, F. Y. Chen, Z. M. Sun, H. Ding, J. M. Shi, J. Hou, J. S. Yan, J. Y. Shi, L. Xu, Y. Li, J. Lu, Z. Zheng, W. Xue, W. L. Zhao, Z. Chen, and S. J. Chen. 2015. "Exome sequencing identifies somatic mutations of DDX3X in natural killer/T-cell lymphoma." *Nat Genet* 47:1061-6. doi: 10.1038/ng.3358.

[186] Lee, S., H. Y. Park, S. Y. Kang, S. J. Kim, J. Hwang, S. Lee, S. H. Kwak, K. S. Park, H. Y. Yoo, W. S. Kim, J. I. Kim, and Y. H. Ko. 2015. "Genetic alterations of JAK/STAT cascade and histone modification in extranodal NK/T-cell lymphoma nasal type." *Oncotarget* 6:17764-76. doi: 10.18632/oncotarget.3776.

[187] Kucuk, C., B. Jiang, X. Hu, W. Zhang, J. K. Chan, W. Xiao, N. Lack, C. Alkan, J. C. Williams, K. N. Avery, P. Kavak, A. Scuto, E. Sen, P. Gaulard, L. Staudt, J. Iqbal, W. Zhang, A. Cornish, Q. Gong, Q. Yang, H. Sun, F. d'Amore, S. Leppa, W. Liu, K. Fu, L. de Leval, T. McKeithan, and W. C. Chan. 2015. "Activating mutations of STAT5B and STAT3 in lymphomas derived from gammadelta-T or NK cells." *Nat Commun* 6:6025. doi: 10.1038/ncomms7025.

[188] Choi, S., J. H. Go, E. K. Kim, H. Lee, W. M. Lee, C. S. Cho, and K. Han. 2016. "Mutational Analysis of Extranodal NK/T-Cell Lymphoma Using Targeted Sequencing with a Comprehensive Cancer Panel." *Genomics Inform* 14:78-84. doi: 10.5808/GI.2016.14.3.78.

[189] Dobashi, A., N. Tsuyama, R. Asaka, Y. Togashi, K. Ueda, S. Sakata, S. Baba, K. Sakamoto, K. Hatake, and K. Takeuchi. 2016. "Frequent BCOR aberrations in extranodal NK/T-Cell lymphoma, nasal type." *Genes Chromosomes Cancer* 55:460-71. doi: 10.1002/gcc.22348.

[190] Shen, L., A. C. Liang, L. Lu, W. Y. Au, Y. L. Kwong, R. H. Liang, and G. Srivastava. 2002. "Frequent deletion of Fas gene sequences encoding death and transmembrane domains in nasal natural killer/T-cell lymphoma." *Am J Pathol* 161:2123-31. doi: 10.1016/S0002-9440(10)64490-2.

[191] Takakuwa, T., Z. Dong, S. Nakatsuka, S. Kojya, Y. Harabuchi, W. I. Yang, S. Nagata, and K. Aozasa. 2002. "Frequent mutations of Fas gene in nasal NK/T cell lymphoma." *Oncogene* 21:4702-5. doi: 10.1038/sj.onc.1205571.

[192] Aozasa, K., T. Takakuwa, T. Hongyo, and W. I. Yang. 2008. "Nasal NK/T-cell lymphoma: epidemiology and pathogenesis." *Int J Hematol* 87:110-7. doi: 10.1007/s12185-008-0021-7.

[193] Chiang, A. K., Q. Tao, G. Srivastava, and F. C. Ho. 1996. "Nasal NK- and T-cell lymphomas share the same type of Epstein-Barr virus latency as nasopharyngeal carcinoma and Hodgkin's disease." *Int J Cancer* 68:285-90. doi: 10.1002/(SICI)1097-0215(19961104)68:3<285::AID-IJC3>3.0.CO;2-Y.

[194] Rickinson, A. B., and D. J. Moss. 1997. "Human cytotoxic T lymphocyte responses to Epstein-Barr virus infection." *Annu Rev Immunol* 15:405-31. doi: 10.1146/annurev.immunol.15.1.405.

[195] Rickinson, A. B., R. J. Murray, J. Brooks, H. Griffin, D. J. Moss, and M. G. Masucci. 1992. "T cell recognition of Epstein-Barr virus associated lymphomas." *Cancer Surv* 13:53-80.

[196] Khanna, R., S. R. Burrows, J. Nicholls, and L. M. Poulsen. 1998. "Identification of cytotoxic T cell epitopes within Epstein-Barr virus (EBV) oncogene latent membrane protein 1 (LMP1): evidence for HLA A2 supertype-restricted immune recognition of EBV-infected cells by LMP1-specific cytotoxic T lymphocytes." *Eur J Immunol* 28:451-8. doi: 10.1002/(SICI)1521-4141(199802)28:02<451::AID-IMMU451>3.0.CO;2-U.

[197] Shen, L., A. K. Chiang, W. P. Liu, G. D. Li, R. H. Liang, and G. Srivastava. 2001. "Expression of HLA class I, beta(2)-microglobulin, TAP1 and IL-10 in Epstein-Barr virus-associated nasal NK/T-cell lymphoma: Implications for tumor immune escape mechanism." *Int J Cancer* 92:692-6.

[198] Teruya-Feldstein, J., E. S. Jaffe, P. R. Burd, H. Kanegane, D. W. Kingma, W. H. Wilson, D. L. Longo, and G. Tosato. 1997. "The role of Mig, the monokine induced by interferon-gamma, and IP-10, the interferon-gamma-inducible protein-10, in tissue necrosis and vascular damage associated with Epstein-Barr virus-positive lymphoproliferative disease." *Blood* 90:4099-105.

[199] Au, W. Y., A. Pang, C. Choy, C. S. Chim, and Y. L. Kwong. 2004. "Quantification of circulating Epstein-Barr virus (EBV) DNA in the diagnosis and monitoring of natural killer cell and EBV-positive lymphomas in immunocompetent patients." *Blood* 104:243-9. doi: 10.1182/blood-2003-12-4197.

[200] Robbins, K. T., L. M. Fuller, M. Vlasak, B. Osborne, B. S. Jing, W. S. Velasquez, and J. A. Sullivan. 1985. "Primary lymphomas of the nasal cavity and paranasal sinuses." *Cancer* 56:814-9.

[201] Logsdon, M. D., C. S. Ha, V. S. Kavadi, F. Cabanillas, M. A. Hess, and J. D. Cox. 1997. "Lymphoma of the nasal cavity and paranasal sinuses: improved outcome and altered prognostic factors with combined modality therapy." *Cancer* 80:477-88.

[202] Li, Y. X., P. A. Coucke, J. Y. Li, D. Z. Gu, X. F. Liu, L. Q. Zhou, R. O. Mirimanoff, Z. H. Yu, and Y. R. Huang. 1998. "Primary non-Hodgkin's lymphoma of the nasal cavity: prognostic significance of paranasal extension and the role of radiotherapy and chemotherapy." *Cancer* 83:449-56.

[203] Kim, W. S., S. Y. Song, Y. C. Ahn, Y. H. Ko, C. H. Baek, D. Y. Kim, S. S. Yoon, H. G. Lee, W. K. Kang, H. J. Lee, C. H. Park, and K. Park. 2001. "CHOP followed by involved field radiation: is it optimal for localized nasal natural killer/T-cell lymphoma?" *Ann Oncol* 12:349-52.

[204] Chim, C. S., S. Y. Ma, W. Y. Au, C. Choy, A. K. Lie, R. Liang, C. C. Yau, and Y. L. Kwong. 2004. "Primary nasal natural killer cell lymphoma: long-term treatment outcome and relationship with the International Prognostic Index." *Blood* 103:216-21. doi: 10.1182/blood-2003-05-1401.

[205] Aviles, A., N. R. Diaz, N. Neri, S. Cleto, and A. Talavera. 2000. "Angiocentric nasal T/natural killer cell lymphoma: a single centre study of prognostic factors in 108 patients." *Clin Lab Haematol* 22:215-20.

[206] Lee, J., C. Suh, Y. H. Park, Y. H. Ko, S. M. Bang, J. H. Lee, D. H. Lee, J. Huh, S. Y. Oh, H. C. Kwon, H. J. Kim, S. I. Lee, J. H. Kim, J. Park, S. J. Oh, K. Kim, C. Jung, K. Park, and W. S. Kim. 2006. "Extranodal natural killer T-cell lymphoma, nasal-type: a prognostic model from a retrospective multicenter study." *J Clin Oncol* 24:612-8. doi: 10.1200/JCO.2005.04.1384.

[207] Suzuki, R., J. Suzumiya, M. Yamaguchi, S. Nakamura, J. Kameoka, H. Kojima, M. Abe, T. Kinoshita, T. Yoshino, K. Iwatsuki, Y. Kagami, T. Tsuzuki, M. Kurokawa, K. Ito, K. Kawa, K. Oshimi, and N. K-cell Tumor Study Group. 2010. "Prognostic factors for mature natural killer (NK) cell neoplasms: aggressive NK cell leukemia and extranodal NK cell lymphoma, nasal type." *Ann Oncol* 21:1032-40. doi: 10.1093/annonc/mdp418.

[208] Cai, Q., X. Luo, G. Zhang, H. Huang, H. Huang, T. Lin, W. Jiang, Z. Xia, and K. H. Young. 2014. "New prognostic model for extranodal natural killer/T cell lymphoma, nasal type." *Ann Hematol* 93:1541-9. doi: 10.1007/s00277-014-2089-x.

[209] Jo, J. C., D. H. Yoon, S. Kim, B. J. Lee, Y. J. Jang, C. S. Park, J. Huh, S. W. Lee, J. S. Ryu, and C. Suh. 2012. "Clinical features and prognostic model for extranasal NK/T-cell lymphoma." *Eur J Haematol* 89:103-10. doi: 10.1111/j.1600-0609.2012.01796.x.

[210] Vasquez, J., M. Serrano, L. Lopez, C. Pacheco, and S. Quintana. 2016. "Predictors of survival of natural killer/T-cell lymphoma, nasal type, in a non-Asian population: a single cancer centre experience." *Ecancermedicalscience* 10:688. doi: 10.3332/ecancer.2016.688.

[211] Lee, J., Y. H. Park, W. S. Kim, S. S. Lee, B. Y. Ryoo, S. H. Yang, K. W. Park, J. H. Kang, J. O. Park, S. H. Lee, K. Kim, C. W. Jung, Y. S. Park, Y. H. Im, W. K. Kang, M. H. Lee, Y. H. Ko, Y. C. Ahn, and K. Park. 2005. "Extranodal nasal type NK/T-cell lymphoma: elucidating clinical prognostic factors for risk-based stratification of therapy." *Eur J Cancer* 41:1402-8. doi: 10.1016/j.ejca.2005.03.010.

[212] Kim, S. J., D. H. Yoon, A. Jaccard, W. J. Chng, S. T. Lim, H. Hong, Y. Park, K. M. Chang, Y. Maeda, F. Ishida, D. Y. Shin, J. S. Kim, S. H. Jeong, D. H. Yang, J. C. Jo, G. W. Lee, C. W. Choi, W. S. Lee, T. Y. Chen, K. Kim, S. H. Jung, T. Murayama, Y. Oki, R. Advani, F. d'Amore, N. Schmitz, C. Suh, R. Suzuki, Y. L. Kwong, T. Y. Lin, and W. S. Kim. 2016. "A prognostic index for natural killer cell lymphoma after non-anthracycline-based treatment: a multicentre, retrospective analysis." *Lancet Oncol* 17:389-400. doi: 10.1016/S1470-2045(15)00533-1.

[213] Kim, S. J., B. S. Kim, C. W. Choi, J. Choi, I. Kim, Y. H. Lee, and J. S. Kim. 2007. "Ki-67 expression is predictive of prognosis in patients with stage I/II extranodal NK/T-cell lymphoma, nasal type." *Ann Oncol* 18:1382-7. doi:10.1093/annonc/mdm183.

[214] Jiang, L., P. Li, H. Wang, J. Liu, X. Zhang, H. Qiu, and B. Zhang. 2014. "Prognostic significance of Ki-67 antigen expression in extranodal natural killer/T-cell lymphoma, nasal type." *Med Oncol* 31:218. doi: 10.1007/s12032-014-0218-y.

[215] Lei, K. I., L. Y. Chan, W. Y. Chan, P. J. Johnson, and Y. M. Lo. 2002. "Diagnostic and prognostic implications of circulating cell-free Epstein-Barr virus DNA in natural killer/T-cell lymphoma." *Clin Cancer Res* 8:29-34.

[216] Ito, Y., H. Kimura, Y. Maeda, C. Hashimoto, F. Ishida, K. Izutsu, N. Fukushima, Y. Isobe, J. Takizawa, Y. Hasegawa, H. Kobayashi, S. Okamura, H. Kobayashi, M. Yamaguchi, J. Suzumiya, R. Hyo, S. Nakamura, K. Kawa, K. Oshimi, and R. Suzuki. 2012. "Pretreatment EBV-DNA copy number is predictive of response and toxicities to SMILE chemotherapy for extranodal NK/T-cell lymphoma, nasal type." *Clin Cancer Res* 18:4183-90. doi: 10.1158/1078-0432.CCR-12-1064.

[217] Wang, Z. Y., Q. F. Liu, H. Wang, J. Jin, W. H. Wang, S. L. Wang, Y. W. Song, Y. P. Liu, H. Fang, H. Ren, R. Y. Wu, B. Chen, X. M. Zhang, N. N. Lu, L. Q. Zhou, and Y. X. Li. 2012. "Clinical implications of plasma Epstein-Barr virus DNA in early-stage extranodal nasal-type NK/T-cell lymphoma patients receiving primary radiotherapy." *Blood* 120:2003-10. doi: 10.1182/blood-2012-06-435024.

[218] Suzuki, R., M. Yamaguchi, K. Izutsu, G. Yamamoto, K. Takada, Y. Harabuchi, Y. Isobe, H. Gomyo, T. Koike, M. Okamoto, R. Hyo, J. Suzumiya, S. Nakamura, K. Kawa, K. Oshimi, and N. K-cell Tumor Study Group. 2011. "Prospective measurement of Epstein-Barr virus-DNA in plasma and peripheral blood mononuclear cells of extranodal NK/T-cell lymphoma, nasal type." *Blood* 118:6018-22. doi: 10.1182/blood-2011-05-354142.

[219] Lin, C. W., Y. H. Chen, Y. C. Chuang, T. Y. Liu, and S. M. Hsu. 2003. "CD94 transcripts imply a better prognosis in nasal-type extranodal NK/T-cell lymphoma." *Blood* 102:2623-31. doi: 10.1182/blood-2003-01-0295.

[220] Bossard, C., K. Belhadj, F. Reyes, N. Martin-Garcia, F. Berger, J. A. Kummer, J. Briere, A. C. Baglin, S. Cheze, J. Bosq, V. Ribrag, C. Gisselbrecht, N. Mounier, and P. Gaulard. 2007. "Expression of the granzyme B inhibitor PI9 predicts

outcome in nasal NK/T-cell lymphoma: results of a Western series of 48 patients treated with first-line polychemotherapy within the Groupe d'Etude des Lymphomes de l'Adulte (GELA) trials." *Blood* 109:2183-9. doi: 10.1182/blood-2006-07-033142.

[221] Kwong, Y. L., A. W. Pang, A. Y. Leung, C. S. Chim, and E. Tse. 2014. "Quantification of circulating Epstein-Barr virus DNA in NK/T-cell lymphoma treated with the SMILE protocol: diagnostic and prognostic significance." *Leukemia* 28:865-70. doi: 10.1038/leu.2013.212.

In: Benign and Malignant Disorders …
Editors: Ling Zhang and Lubomir Sokol

ISBN: 978-1-53612-999-1
© 2018 Nova Science Publishers, Inc.

Chapter 10

CLINICAL INTERVENTION AND NOVEL THERAPEUTIC STRATEGIES FOR EXTRANODAL NK/T CELL LYMPHOMA, NASAL TYPE

George Yang, Daniel Grass, Kamran Ahmed and Sungjune Kim
H. L. Moffitt Cancer Center and Research Institute, Tampa, FL, US

ABSTRACT

Extranodal NK/T cell lymphoma, nasal type (ENKTL) represents an aggressive non-Hodgkin lymphoma primarily endemic to East Asian and Latin American populations. Treatment of this disease requires thorough understanding of its pathogenesis related to the Epstein-Barr virus. This chapter will describe relevant clinicopathologic features, differential diagnosis, workup, prognostic tools and current evidence for the treatment and management of ENKTL. Of particular importance when evaluating ENKTL is risk stratification through a variety of prognostic models – patients in different risk echelons are subsequently treated with radiotherapy or chemotherapy alone, chemoradiation, systemic therapy or bone marrow transplantation. Despite recent advances in therapy, ENKTL remains a challenging clinical entity, and future therapeutic methods being explored include targeted molecular therapy and immunotherapy.

1. INTRODUCTION

Non-Hodgkin lymphoma (NHL) is comprised of a diverse array of malignancies caused by aberrations in the B-, T- or natural killer (NK) cell lineages. NHLs are primarily of a nodal origin, though some rarer subsets originate at extranodal sites [1]. These extranodal lymphomas make up approximately one third of NHL cases in the

United States of America (USA) and have increased in incidence more than nodal lymphomas over the last several decades [2].

Peripheral T-cell lymphomas (PTCLs) are a heterogeneous group of mature, postthymic malignancies originating from T or NK cell lineage. Within this designation is extranodal NK/T-cell lymphoma, nasal type (ENKTL-NT). This rare form of aggressive NHL with 5-year overall survival rate of 40% to 50% [3]. ENKTL-NT is most prevalent in East Asia and Latin America and is strongly associated with Epstein-Barr virus (EBV)-related pathogenesis [4]. It typically affects the upper aerodigestive tract, such as the nasal cavity or nasopharynx, and frequently extends locoregionally into the surrounding anatomic regions such as orbits, paranasal sinuses and adjacent lymph nodes. In some instances ENKTL-NT may develop in the skin, gastrointestinal tract, testis or lungs. Even more rarely, it may also present as only nodal presentation, or extranodal manifestation companying with disseminated lymphadenopathy, leukemic phase, or bone marrow involvement [5].

ENKTL-NT is a NHL caused by genetic insults in the NK or T-cell lineages and uniform Epstein-Bar Virus (EBV)-infection or reactivation. ENKTL-NT was previously termed angiocentric T-cell lymphoma due to its proclivity for angio-invasion/destruction [6] and it is the most common cause of the syndrome termed "lethal midline granuloma." Other names previously given to this disease include: polymorphic reticulosis, midline malignant reticulosis, idiopathic midline destructive disease and lymphomatoid granulomatosis [7]. These lymphoma cells are typically $CD2^+$, $CD56^{+bright}$, cytoplasmic $CD3\varepsilon^+$, $CD16^{+/-}$, have germline T-cell receptor (TCR) configuration and express cytotoxic granule-associated proteins, such as TIA, perforin, granzyme B and T-cell restricted intracellular antigen 1 (TIA-1) [8, 9]. A recent study suggests that stratification based on TCR subtype may not accurately identify distinct NK or T-cell groups, suggesting that further molecular characterization is needed for risk analysis [10]. Regardless, further molecular characterization can aid in separating ENKTL-NT from other disorders of NK or T-cells, which can be difficult to distinguish using conventional cytomorphology and immunohistochemistry approaches.

ENKTL-NT is most common in Far East Asia (e.g., China, Korea and Japan) and in Latin America (e.g., Mexico, South and Central America). In these areas the incidence of disease among T cell lymphomas can be over 10% [11-14]. It is rarely identified in the USA, Europe, Africa, South Asia and the Middle East. A recent analysis in the USA identified that the incidence, although very rare, is the highest in the Asian Pacific Islander and Hispanic populations and is rising [15]. This increasing incidence may be due to immigration into the USA [16] or alternatively preliminary evidence suggests lifestyle practices or environmental exposures to pesticides/chemical solvents may be a contributing factor [17]. The median age at diagnosis is 52 years, though some rare cases may occur in children [18]. ENKTL-NT predominantly affects men with a male to female ratio of 2:1.

2. MOLECULAR CHARACTERIZATION OF ENKTL-NT

The etiology and molecular pathogenesis of ENKTL-NT has not been fully elucidated, but is thought to partially originate from an EBV infection of NK or T-cells. ENKTL-NT is uniformly EBV$^+$, where monoclonal episomal EBV DNA and EBV latent membrane protein-1 (LMP-1) are detectable [4]; for this reason EBV testing is an inclusive diagnostic criterion. In fact, circulating EBV DNA titer can be employed as a marker to gauge tumor burden and response to treatment [19].

In depth molecular characterization has identified that chromosome 6q21 is frequently deleted with the corresponding residing putative tumor suppressor genes, *FOX03, PRDM1* and *HACE1* [20-23]. The loss of *PRDM1* function may result from CpG island promoter hypermethylation [24] or microRNA (miR)-223 aberrant expression [25]. Next generation sequencing analyses have also identified mutations in other tumor suppressor genes, including *TP53, KMT2D* and *ARID1A* [26]. Similar to other malignancies, a combination of genetic aberrations likely contributes to ENKTL-NT pathobiology.

A recent study has identified that approximately 80% of ENKTL-NT tumor specimens express programmed cell death ligand-1 (PD-L1), a target for multiple immunotherapies [27]. This elevated PD-L1 expression may be due to chronic EBV infection, which portends a better prognosis [28].

3. CLINICAL FEATURES

ENKTL-NT tumors are characterized as locally destructive and necrotizing midfacial lesions that frequently invade cartilage, bone and soft tissues adjacent to the nasal cavity. Presenting symptoms are dependent on the location and extent of the disease. Frequently, patients may complain of a sensation of nasal obstruction associated with a remitting sinus-like infection that is unresponsive to supportive care or antibiotic treatment. If confined only to the nasal cavity, patients may present with perpetual rhinorrhea or epistaxis. Additionally, sinus pressure, headaches, visual changes, halitosis, tenderness along the hard palate or facial swelling may be observed. Constitutional 'B-symptoms' may also be evident, which are most common when the tumor has extends beyond the nasal cavity. Lymph nodes involvement is associated with advanced disease, but rarely is observed as the primary disease site. Approximately 10% of patients may have bone marrow involvement [29].

On physical exam, extensive friable and granular tissue may be seen along the anterior nasal cavity walls in conjunction with perforation of the nasal septum [7].

Oronasal fistulas may occur due to concomitant mucosal ulceration and palatal necrosis [30].

Proper diagnosis requires referral to ear-nose-throat (ENT) and medical oncology specialists with expertise in lymphoma, as this is a unique entity compared to other NHLs. Appropriate work-up includes a thorough physical exam, panendoscopy with biopsy of suspicious sites, standard laboratory studies, EBV DNA titers, bilateral superior iliac crest bone marrow biopsies and imaging with positron emission tomography with computed tomography (PET-CT) imaging [31].

4. Differential Diagnosis

The differential diagnosis of extranodal NK/T cell lymphoma includes other T and NK cell malignancies as well as other EBV-associated lymphoproliferative disorders, we have discussed a list of diseases that could mimic extranodal NK/T cell lymphoma such as carcinoma (e.g., nasopharyngeal carcinoma, metastatic neuroendocrine neoplasm), chronic active viral infection, or reactive or inflammatory situations (e.g., Herpes simplex or EBV infection, benign inflammatory dermatosis, reactive lymphoid hyperplasia, Wegener granulomatosis, mosquito bite hypersensitivity, hydroa vaccinifome like lymphoma), a list of T-cell lymphomas (primary cutaneous $\gamma\delta$ T-cell lymphoma, primary cutaneous CD8 positive aggressive epidermotropic cytotoxic T-cell lymphoma, mycosis fungoides, subcutaneous panniculitis-like T-cell Lymphoma, primary cutaneous CD56-positive peripheral T-cell lymphoma, monomorphic epitheliotropic intestinal T-cell lymphoma in gastrointestinal tract, and NK-cell enteropathy (Lymphomatoid Gastropathy) and a rare entity namely blastic plasmacytoid dendritic cell neoplasm, in addition to aggressive or indolent NK cell neoplasms (aggressive NK cell leukemia)

Several other EBV-associated lymphoid neoplasms also need to be differentiated from extranodal NK cell lymphoma.

ENKTL-NT can rarely involve bone marrow and peripheral blood. This manifestation is similar to an aggressive NK cell leukemia. Aggressive NK cell leukemia cells frequently expresses CD16, in contrast to extranodal NK/T cell lymphoma which is predominantly CD16 negative. Clonal, episomal EBV involvement is common in both malignancies.

Lymphomatoid granulomatosis is an EBV-associated lymphoma that appears at extranodal sites, however malignant cells are of B-cell origin and express B cell markers such as CD20 or PAX5. This is in contrast to ENKTL-NT, which is of NK or T cell origin [32].

EBV-positive mucocutaneous ulcers (EMCU) are isolated circumscribed ulcerated lesions that occur most commonly in elderly individuals in cases of immunosuppression. These lesions most commonly occur in the oropharynx but can also be observed in the skin and GI tract and consist of a polymorphous inflammatory infiltrate mixed with scattered EBV-infected B cells. In addition, there are cells in EMCU resembling Hodgkin/Reed-Sternberg cells both morphologically and immunophenotypically, which is rarely found in ENKTL-NT. Moreover, EBV-positive mucocutaneous ulcers show benign course and excellent response to therapy [33, 34].

EBV-positive diffuse large B cell lymphoma, NOS is a variant of DLBCL that presents at extranodal sites and can exhibit angiodestruction, angioinvasion, and tissue necrosis. Nasal presentation is rare and the tumor cells express B cell markers (CD20, CD79a) with clonal immunoglobulin gene rearrangements and CD30 expression in a majority of cases [35, 36].

EBV-positive plasmacytoma is a plasma cell neoplasm that may present in a similar clinical and morphologic fashion. However, these neoplasms are characterized by diffuse proliferation of predominantly mature appearing plasma cells (CD138+, MUM1+) with a brisk reactive, CD8+, TIA-1+ and cytotoxic T-cell infiltrate in the background. These patients have considerably more favorable outcome compared to ENKL-NT [37].

In contrast to EBV-positive plasmacytoma is EBV positive plasmablastic lymphoma occurring in the nasal cavity. The latter is an aggressive non-Hodgkin's lymphoma which arises frequently primarily HIV infected patients. As a clinical entity it is challenging to treat with high rates of relapse and death [38].

Taken together, a sole identification of episomal clonal EBV is insufficient for diagnosis of ENKTL-NT. Of importance, other lymphomas of B- or plasma cell origin could also be EBV positive, which should be excluded besides the aforementioned reactive or neoplastic disorders.

5. PROGNOSTIC PARAMETERS

5.1. International Prognostic Index

ENKTL-NT is a relatively recently recognized distinct entity in the WHO classification of lymphoid neoplasms. The International Prognostic Index (IPI) was initially developed for aggressive B-cell lymphomas and used as a predictive system for peripheral T- cell lymphomas. However, it has varied correlations when used for ENTKL-NT (See Table 1). The reported limited usefulness of the International Prognostic Index stems primarily from the categorization of most ENKTL-NT as "favorable" prognosis subgroup, with only 0-7% of ENTKL-NT categorized as high-risk, despite the relatively poor clinical outcome (Kim et al., Blood 2005) [39]. Despite this limitation many studies continue to utilize IPI with mixed results.

Table 1. International Prognostic Index

International Prognostic Index
Risk factors - assign 1 point if present
Age >60 years
Stage III or IV disease
Performance status 2-4
Extranodal involvement >1 site
Elevated serum LDH

Risk categories	
0 or 1	Low
2	Low-intermediate
3	High-intermediate
4 or 5	High-intermediate

5.2. The Nature of Tumor Cells

In general, the prognostic features of ENKTL-NT include features unique to the disease state as well as oncologic features. Tumor invasiveness, defined as bony invasion or destruction, or direct tumor invasion of the skin was an independently significant prognostic factor for unfavorable disease free survival (DFS) and overall survival as well as low probability of complete remission (CR) in nasal stage IE/IIE. Other groups have noted shortened overall survival in patients with extranasal disease compared to nasal presentations [40]. Factors that have been well studied in other disease sites such as age, performance status, stage, and involved lymph node status are useful in ENKTL-NT as well [41].

5.3. Anatomic Location

Lee et al. proposed two subtypes, upper aerodigestive tract NK/T cell lymphoma (UNKTL) and extra-upper aerodigestive tract NK/T-cell (EUNKTL), which have been identified as having significantly different survival rates. UNKTL includes all lymphomas involving the nasal cavity, nasopharynx, and upper aerodigestive tract. EUNKTL was defined as all sites not including those for UNKTL. Patients with EUNKTL in their study had more advanced stage at diagnosis, higher LDH, higher IPI, poorer performance status and worse response to anthracycline-based chemotherapy. Survival rates were significantly different; 20% for EUNKTL compared to 54% with UNKTL (p = 0.0068) [40].

5.4. EBV DNA Level

EBV is closely associated with ENTKL-NT, with distinct expression of the markers related to EBV status. EBV has been shown in >90% of tumor tissue, with plasma EBV DNA detected in >80% of patients. Multiple studies have demonstrated that high EBV-DNA load is associated with advanced stage, B-symptoms, elevated LDH levels and worse clinical response. Plasma EBV-DNA levels prior to initiation of treatment as well as serial analysis of levels following chemotherapy suggested that patients with low-pretreatment EBV-DNA load tended to respond more favorably compared to patients with high pretreatment level [42]. In this study by Wang et al. (Blood 2012), patients with early stage ENKTL receiving primary radiotherapy with EBV-DNA levels >500 copies/mL had lower estimated progression free survival (PFS) (52 vs. 79 percent) and overall survival (OS) (66% vs. 97%) at three years compared to those with EBV-DNA levels ≤500 copies/mL. In addition, patients with undetectable EBV-DNA levels following treatment compared to those with detectable levels had significantly higher PFS (78 vs 51%) and OS (92 vs 70 percent) at three years [42]. Thus, EBV-DNA levels have been proposed as not only a prognostic factor but also as a stratification tool prior to and following therapy to identify appropriate patients who would benefit from early systemic therapy. High Ki-67 index has been associated with worse OS and DFS compared to low Ki-67 index, and was more frequently elevated in patients with B symptoms and bulky disease. With regards to bone marrow involvement, EBV-encoded RNA-1 *in situ* hybridization (EBER-1 ISH) in bone marrow specimens was evaluated with clinical stage I/II disease. Of the 91 patients evaluated, 17 (18.7%) exhibited positivity for EBER-1 ISH, and these patients had significantly poorer overall survival compared to those with negative EBER-1 ISH. These findings suggest that EBER-1 ISH should be evaluated in patients with localized disease as an additional stratification tool [43].

5.5. Select Protein Expression

The role of select protein expressions has been explored as a potential prognostic feature for ENTKL-NT. Bossard et al. analyzed a cohort of patients receiving chemotherapy for expression of active caspase-3 (aC3), granzyme B protease inhibitor 9 (PI9) and Bcl-2 proteins. This study showed that the absence of PI9 and low apoptotic index were associated with poor outcome, suggesting that loss of PI9 expression may represent a prognostic feature for poor clinical outcome [44]. Other factors such as increased cyclooxygenase-2 expression have been shown to correlate with poor treatment response, high systemic recurrence and overall unfavorable prognosis. Shim et al. reported that fewer COX-2 positive patients achieved complete response in contrast to

COX-2 negative patients, with 54% 2-year systemic recurrence free survival in COX-2 positive patients compared to 100% in COX-2 negative patients, as well as decreased 5-year overall survival (32 vs. 70%) [45].

5.6. Imaging Findings

The use of (18)F-fluorodeoxyglucose (18F-FDG/PET) has an established important role in accurate staging and response assessment of several distinct types of aggressive lymphomas, however until relatively recently its role in ENKTL was unclear. Jiang et al. conducted a prospective trial of treatment naïve ENKTL with pre and post-treatment 18F-FDG/PET imaging and stratification based on maximum standard uptake value (SUVMax). Their results showed a significant difference in post-therapy with18F-FDG/PET decreased SUVMax as a significant predictor of PFS and overall survival [46].

6. RISK STRATIFICATION

In an effort to clarify the prognostic features of ENKTL, several groups have performed retrospective reviews to investigate prognostic models of ENKTL. A new model, the NK/T cell lymphoma prognostic index (NKPI) was proposed. The Korean Prognostic Index model was based on four adverse factors: "B" symptoms (constitutional symptoms of fevers, night sweats, and weight loss), increased serum lactate dehydrogenase (LDH), stage ≥ III, and regional lymph node involvement. Patients with higher numbers of adverse factors (0, 1, 2, 3-4) were shown to have correspondingly lower survival rates (81, 63, 34, 7%, respectively). This new model demonstrated a stratification of patients into four risk groups, which better identified high risk patients compared to the IPI [47].

A prognostic model proposed by Dai et al. included the use of beta-2 microglobulin to lymphocyte ratio index (betaLRI) and lactate dehydrogenase to lymphocyte ratio index (LLRI) as potential models for ENKTL. This retrospective review of pre-treatment betaLRI and LLRI noted improved stratification of stage IE/IIE ENKTL compared to the IPI and Korean Prognostic Index [48].

In the era of non-anthracyoline based chemotherapies, Kim etal proposed the prognostic index of natural killer lymphoma (PINK) with inclusion of Epstein-Barr virus DNA titer (PINK-E) based on a retrospective analysis of 527 patients;. This stratification utilized four risk factors: age, stage, non-nasal type, and distant lymph node involvement in conjunction with blood EBV DNA levels to differentiate three risk levels. Low risk (no or one risk factor), intermediate (two risk factors) and high risk (≥3 risk factors) were significantly associated with overall and progression-free survival. These findings were confirmed in a validation cohort and may prove valuable for future risk stratification [49].

7. TREATMENT FOR EXTRANODAL NK/T CELL LYMPHOMA

Treatment for extranodal NK/T cell lymphoma, nasal type (ENTKL-NT) is guided by initial stage, nasal or extranasal involvement and performance status. Early stage ENTKL-NT comprises the majority (70-90%) of cases. Current National Comprehensive Cancer Network (NCCN) guidelines are currently equivocal regarding the optimal therapy for early stage disease with regards to radiation alone, sequential chemotherapy and RT, or concurrent chemoradiotherapy. Due to the rarity of the disease, treatment recommendations have been derived from retrospective studies and a few phase I/II studies.

7.1. Radiation Therapy Alone for Early Stage Disease

Radiation therapy is an important initial component for early stage ENTKL-NT to help achieve complete response (CR). Several studies have shown the benefit of radiotherapy either alone or as part of chemoradiotherapy (CRT) as compared to chemotherapy alone for early stage disease. Primary radiation therapy alone for early stage patients appears to have reasonable results in a well selected patient population based on risk factor stratification. Patients with multiple risk factors of age ≥60 years, ECOG ≥ 2, regional lymph node involvement, local tumor invasion, elevated LDH, high Ki-67 proliferation index and EBV DNA ≥6.1 x 10^7 copies/mL indicate high risk disease and are not suitable for radiotherapy alone. Li et al. [50] demonstrated that appropriately risk-stratified patients with stage I ENTKL-NT treated with primary RT achieved complete response rate of 95.4% with comparable 5-year overall survival, PFS and local control compared to historical data. A substantial number of patients treated with radiation therapy alone did develop systemic extranodal dissemination (17%), whereas only 5% of patients had local relapse or lymph node relapse supporting a role for systemic therapy. Other retrospective studies have shown a significant difference between combination therapy (chemoradiation) and radiation alone [51]. However, the large scale multi-institutional retrospective study of 1273 patients from China has demonstrated that the low risk patients based on 5 independent prognostic factors (stage, age, performance status, lactate dehydrogenase, primary tumor invasion) did not benefit from the addition of chemotherapy suggesting that in a carefully selected low risk patients RT alone should be preferred choice [52].

Table 2. Selected studies on treatment of extranodal NK/T cell lymphoma, nasal type

Study - Year	Disease/Stage	Number	Treatment	ORR	CR	OS	PFS
Cheung et al - 2002	Newly diagnosed, stage I/II	18	RT alone (50 Gy)	78%	78%	5 y: 30%	5 y: 31%
Li et al - 2006	Newly diagnosed, stage I/II	31	RT alone (50 Gy)	100%	97%	5 y: 66%	5 y: 61%
Kim et al - 2001	Newly diagnosed, stage I/II	17	CHOP + RT (45 Gy)	58%	58%	3 y: 59%	-
Yamaguchi et al - 2009	Newly diagnosed, stage I/II	27	Concurrent RT (50 Gy) + 2/3 DeVIC	81%	77%	2 y: 78%	2 y: 67%
Kim et al - 2009	Newly diagnosed, stage I/II	30	Concurrent RT (40 Gy) + cisplatin + VIPD	83%	80%	3 y: 86%	3 y: 85%
Jiang et al - 2012	Newly diagnosed, stage I/II	26	LVP + sandwiched RT (56 Gy)	89%	81%	2 y: 89%	2 y: 81%
Wang et al - 2013	Newly diagnosed, stage I/II	27	GELOX + sandwiched RT (56 Gy)	96%	74%	2 y: 86%	2 y: 86%
Yamaguchi et al - 2011	Newly diagnosed, stage IV or relapsed/refractory	38	SMILE	79%	45%	1 y: 55%	1 y: 53%
Kwong et al - 2012	Newly diagnosed, any stage or relapsed/refractory	87	SMILE ± sandwiched RT (50 Gy)	81%	66%	5 y: 50%	4 y: 64%
Jaccard et al - 2011	Relaped/Refractory	19	AspaMetDex	78%	61%	2 y: 40%	2 y: 40%

Dose of radiation and delineation of treatment field are important considerations, with most studies accepting ≥50 Gy as more likely to achieve favorable response [53, 54]. The role of higher doses of radiation has been investigated as well, with RT doses greater than 54 Gy or more were shown to improve both overall survival and disease free survival compared to doses <54 Gy [55]. Treatment field design for RT include involved field (IF), extended field (EF), and nodal irradiation. The extended field should include all macroscopic lesions noted on endoscopy, paranasal sinus, palate, and nasopharynx.

The use of modern techniques such as intensity-modulated radiotherapy (IMRT) has been reported with improved dosimetric and normal tissue constraints and some reports of improved overall survival, progression-free survival in retrospective studies [56]. IMRT provides a lower mean parotid dose, which theoretically can decrease the risk of parotid gland dysfunction as a late toxicity [57] for tumors involving the head and neck region. Prophylactic cervical nodal irradiation (PCNI) appears to have no benefit for patients with IE ENTKL-NT – this was evaluated in a retrospective review of 35 patients receiving prophylactic cervical lymph node irradiation with no benefit for PFS or OS when compared to a similar cohort of patients who did not receive PCNI as part of chemoradiation. This lack of benefit was present regardless of primary tumor site or degree of local tumor invasion [58].

7.2. Chemotherapy for Localized Disease

7.2A. Anthracycline-Based Chemotherapy

Historically, anthracycline-based chemotherapy regimens were utilized as part of chemoradiation due to success in other aggressive lymphomas [59] such as CHOP based regimens (cyclophosphamide, doxorubicin, vincristine, prednisolone) [60]. This regimen combined with involved field radiation to 45 Gy for early stage ENTKL-NT led to suboptimal complete response rates and correspondingly low overall survival of 58% and 59% respectively. Multiple attempts to increase the efficacy of CHOP based regimens by manipulating drug dosages and cycle numbers or modification of the agents have been largely unsuccessful [61]. The lack of response to anthracycline-based chemotherapy is thought to be related to the intrinsic property of the malignant cells. NK-cells, and therefore NK/T cell lymphomas express high P-glycoprotein [62]. This results in minimal residual disease (MDR) and has necessitated the development of non-MDR dependent chemotherapy regimens to overcome this obstacle.

Table 3. Chemotherapy regimens

Regimen	Protocol
AspaMetDex	*E. coli* L-asparaginase: 6000 U/m² IM: days 2, 4, 6, and 8
	Methotrexate: 3000 mg/m² IV: day 1
	Dexmethasone: 40 mg PO: days 1-4
2/3 DeVIC	Dexamethasone: 40 mg IV: days 1-3
	Etoposide: 67 mg/m² IV, days 1-3
	Ifosfamide: 1000 mg/m² IV, days 1-3
	Carboplatin: 200 mg/m² IV, day 1
VIPD	Etoposide: 100 mg/m² IV: days 1-3
	Ifosfamide: 1200 mg/m² IV, days 1-3
	Cisplatin: 33 mg/m² IV: days 1-3
	Dexamethasone: 40 mg IV or PO: days 1-3
LVP	*E. coli* L-asparaginase: 6000 U/m² IV, days 1-5
	Vincristine: 1.4 mg/m² IV: day 1
	Prednisolone: 100 mg PO: days 1-5
GELOX	Gemcitabine: 1000 mg/m² IV: days 1 and 8
	E. coli L-asparaginase: 6000 U/m² IM: days 1-7
	Oxaliplatin: 130 mg/m² IV: day 1
SMILE	Dexamethasone: 40 mg IV or PO: days 2-4
	Methotrexate: 2000 mg/m² IV: day 1
	Ifosfamide: 1500 mg/m² IV: days 2-4
	E. coli L-asparaginase: 6000 U/m² IM: Even days 8-20
	Etoposide: 100 mg/m² IV: days 2-4

7.2B. L-Asparaginase-Based Chemotherapy for Localized Disease

L-asparaginase is a chemotherapy agent, which was found to be effective in multiple hematologic malignancies. It is an enzyme that interacts with asparagine and removes the amine group, releasing aspartate and ammonia. This mechanism of action exploits the fact that hematologic cells are unable to synthesize asparagine, and must rely on the presence of the amino acid in the blood for normal function. Thus, the enzyme cuts the supply of asparagine in the bloodstream and induces cell death. L-asparaginase was previously employed as a single agent in relapsed/refractory NK/T cell lymphomas. Subsequently, this agent has been increasingly incorporated into chemotherapy regimens with sandwiched radiotherapy.

A phase II study of stage I/II patients were treated with LVP (L-asparaginase, vincristine, prednisolone) for 6 courses with radiation therapy occurring after 2 courses of CT [63]. ORR was 92% and CR was achieved in 42% after 2 cycles. At completion of

RT and CT, ORR was 89% with 81% of CR. Two-year OS and PFS were 88.5% and 80.6%, respectively with median follow-up of 27 months. Only 2.7% patients were noted to have grade 3 leukopenia and 23.1% of patients had grade 3 radiation-related mucositis.

In addition to the LVP/RT regimen there was a prospective study investigating GELOX (gemcitabine, L-asparaginase and oxaliplatin). Twenty seven patients with stage I/II disease achieved ORR of 93% and CR of 56% after 2 cycles, and after completion of sandwich radiation therapy of 56 Gy and 2-4 cycles of GELOX the ORR was 96% with a CR of 74%. Two-year OS and PFS were both 86% with median follow-up of 27 months. This regimen was comparatively more intense with 33.3% of patients experiencing grade 3-4 leukopenia and 15% of patients having grade 3 radiation related mucositis. Local and systemic failure rates were 15% and 11% [64].

The SMILE regimen (dexamethasone, methotrexate, ifosfamide, L-asparaginase, and etoposide) is the most intense protocol for early stage disease. A prospective study of 29 patients with newly diagnosed stage I/II disease showed an ORR of 86% and CR in 69% after 2-3 cycles of chemotherapy. At the completion of radiation therapy with 50 Gy and remainder of SMILE treatment cycles (6 total) ORR increased to 89.7% with no change in CR rates. Remission was maintained in 90% of patients who achieved CR during follow-up. This combination of chemotherapy is by far more toxic with grade 3-4 neutropenia occurring in 61% of patients despite routine administration of G-CSF, as well as 7% treatment related mortality [65].

Modifications of the SMILE regimen have been attempted, as described in a phase II study of 28 patients with stage I/II disease, treated with concurrent MIDLE (methotrexate, ifosfamide, dexamethasone, L-asparaginase, and etoposide) and radiation with 36-44 Gy with increased dose of methotrexate compared to the SMILE regimen. This resulted in final CR rates of 82.1% and ORR of 85.7%. The study achieved 3 year PFS and OS of 74.1% and 81.5%, respectively with a median follow-up of 46 months [66].

7.2C. Localized Extra-Nasal Disease

There is very limited evidence supporting management of localized non-nasal NK/T cell lymphoma. A small retrospective review of 13 patients with localized non-nasal disease treated with CHOP-based chemotherapy and sandwiched radiation or surgery resulted in ORR of 69% and CR of 54%. Three-year OS was 50%. The scant amount of data for localized non-nasal lymphoma suggests that systemic therapy with radiotherapy should be utilized when applicable, but with relatively limited results when compared to nasal disease.

7.2D. Chemoradiation for Early Stage Disease

There is substantial retrospective data support for the role of radiation therapy in ENTKL-NT, and several prospective studies have suggested that concurrent chemoradiation (CRT) is an effective strategy in the treatment of localized ENTKL-NT. In Japanese phase I/II study (JCOG0211), patients with high risk stage I/II nasal disease were treated with concurrent radiation (50 Gy) and 3 courses of dexamethasone, etoposide, ifosfamide, and carboplatin (DeVIC). They demonstrated 5-year PFS and OS rates of 67% and 73% respectively, with a few grade 3-4 late toxicities [64]. A similar Korean phase II study evaluated patients undergoing concurrent CRT with cisplatin and radiation therapy (RT) (40-52.8 Gy) followed by three cycles of etoposide, ifosfamide, cisplatin, and dexamethasone (VIPD) in 30 patients with stage I/II nasal ENTKL-NT. Complete response rate was 73% after initial chemoradiation which increased to 80% after VIPD chemotherapy. Three-year PFS and OS were 85% and 86%, respectively [67]. These studies support the use of concurrent chemoradiation in patients with stage I/II disease.

Chemotherapy and RT has been delivered sequentially or concurrently. Data regarding timing of radiation therapy indicates that upfront radiation therapy has improved outcomes when compared to chemotherapy followed by RT [55]. A retrospective analysis of 105 Japanese patients receiving RT alone, CRT showed complete response rates for patients receiving initial RT was superior to those receiving initial chemotherapy (83% vs 20%) (?) The more recent large multi-institutional retrospective analysis of 1273 Chinese patients also confirmed that RT used before chemotherapy given a significant 5-year overall survival advantage (72.2% vs. 58.3%, p = 0.004) [52].

7.3. Systemic Treatment

7.3A. Advanced Stage and Relapsed/Refractory NK/T Cell Lymphoma

Advanced stage and refractory and relapsed disease has significantly worse response to therapy compared to initial and localized disease. Treatment regimens for refractory, relapsed and advanced stage ENTKL-NT include L-asparaginase based chemotherapy with radiation therapy. A series of 45 patients with relapsed and refractory nasal type ENTKL-NT were treated with L-asparaginase based salvage regimen for a median of three cycles followed by primary involved field radiation with a median dose of 50 Gy and with 85% of patients receiving ≥50 Gy. CR rate was 55.6% and overall 3- and 5-year overall survival of 82.2% and 66.9%, respectively. This study demonstrated that L-asparaginase chemotherapy with RT was effective for refractory and relapsed nasal ENTKL-NT [63]. The combination of L-asparaginase with other chemotherapy agents has been evaluated as well. L-asparaginase, methotrexate and dexamethasone (AspaMetDex) was evaluated in a small study of 19 patients with ENTKL-NT treated with 3 cycles of chemotherapy and consolidative radiation therapy afterwards. Complete response and overall response rates after the three cycles of chemotherapy were 61% and

78%, respectively, with median PFS and overall survival of 1 year. The absence of serum EBV-DNA and anti-asparaginase antibodies was statistically significantly associated with better outcome [68].

A recent phase II study from the NK-cell Tumor Study Group evaluated SMILE protocol (dexamethasone, methotrexate, ifosfamide, L-asparaginase and etoposide) in the setting of newly diagnosed stage IV, relapsed, and refractory ENTKL-NT. Twenty-eight of the 38 patients (74%) completed the planned treatment with overall response rate and complete response rates of 79% and 45%. They noted no difference between treatment naïve patients compared to those with relapsed/refractory disease. One year PFS and overall survival were 53% and 55% respectively. Radiation therapy was not utilized in this study. As with the SMILE regimen for localized disease almost all the patients developed grade 4 myelosuppression and 61% of patients had infectious complications [69]. Interestingly, a separate analysis noted that EBV-DNA copy number was correlative and predictive the response with the SMILE regimen, with incidence of grade 4 non-hematologic toxicity being significantly higher in patients with >10^4 copies/mL of plasma EBV-DNA - 86% vs. 26% (p = 0.002) or >10^5 copies/mL of whole blood (EBV-DNA – 100% vs. 29% (p = 0.007) [70].

The Asia Lymphoma Study Group also evaluated the SMILE regimen in a similar patient cohort in 87 newly diagnosed, relapsed/refractory patients. Overall response rate was 81% and complete response of 66% - both newly diagnosed and relapsed/refractory had similar results. The 4 year disease free survival was 64% and 5 year overall survival was 50%. These results suggest that compared to historical data the SMILE regimen is an acceptable option for this patient group [65]. These studies indicate that newly diagnosed advanced stage and relapsed/refractory NK/T cell lymphoma should be treated with L-asparaginase based and non-MDR susceptible chemotherapy.

7.3B. Stem Cell Transplantation for ENTKL-NT

The role of high dose chemotherapy (HDT) with hematopoietic stem cell transplantation has been evaluated in multiple small retrospective series. Stem cell transplantation includes both autologous and allogeneic sources. High dose therapy with autologous stem cell transplantation (HDT-ASCT) was investigated in the study with 18 patients by Au et al. In the update of the original study there was a trend towards better overall survival in patients who received ASCT at complete remission 1 (CR1) compared to historically matched controls, with no disease relapse beyond 6 months [71]. More recently reported larger retrospective studies have evaluated patients who underwent HDT-ASCT with similar results. A 47 patient analysis showed that in patients with CR and subsequent HDT-ASCT the 5-year disease specific survival rates were significantly higher in the transplanted group compared to historical non-transplanted controls (87% vs. 68%, p = 0.027). These patients were risk stratified according to NK/T-cell prognostic index. There was no statistical significant difference between disease-specific survival

(DSS) rates between transplanted patients and control groups for low risk patients (87% vs 69%, p = 0.534). However, there was a substantial DSS benefit for high risk patients when compared to the historical control (100% vs 51.2%, p = 0.05[72]. Allogenic stem cell transplant has also been analyzed in the management of ENTKL-NT in case reports and small retrospective series. A study of 22 chemosensitive and chemorefractory patients underwent allogenic HSCT, with 2 year PFS and overall survival rates (OS) of 32% and 40% [73]. Overall the quality of evidence for patients undergoing either allogenic or autologous HSCT is very limited and restricts the ability to make definitive recommendations.

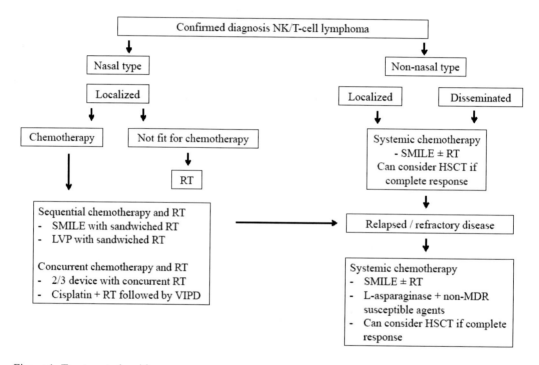

Figure 1. Treatment algorithm.

8. FUTURE THERAPEUTIC DIRECTIONS

The challenges of developing treatment regimens for rare diseases have been a persistent problem in ENTKL-NT. The relative rarity of the disease makes designing large prospective randomized trials extremely challenging, and the breadth of time that spans much of the retrospective data in the literature confounds analysis and interpretation as well. The disease that was considered a lethal condition in past, has significantly improved clinical outcome, due to the development of novel chemotherapy regimens, and more sophisticated modern radiation techniques.

Table 4. Hematopoietic stem cell transplantation, selected trials

Study/Year	Disease/Stage	Number	Allogenic (n)	Autogenic (n)	DSS	PFS	OS
Au et al, 2003	I-IV	18	-	18	-		Improved OS in CR1 compared to historic control
Lee et al, 2008	Low to high risk	47	-	47	Low risk 5 y: 87% High risk 5y: 100%	-	
Suzuki et al, 2006	I-IV	22	6	16	-	-	2 y: 54.5%
Suzuki et al, 2011	I-IV	134	74	60	-		2 y: 69% (allo) vs 41% (auto)
Murashige et al 2005	Chemosensitive /refractory	22	22	0	-	2 y: 34%	2 y: 40%

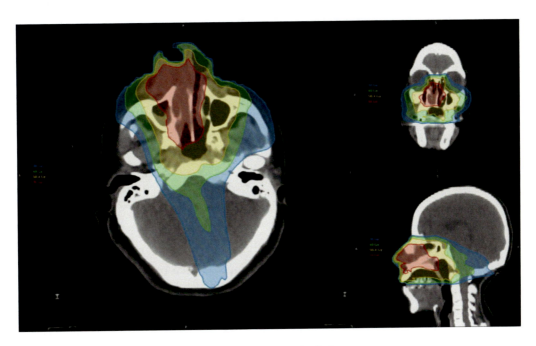

Figure 2. Radiation treatment planning: axial, coronal, sagittal views.

Targeted therapy: Various surface markers have been investigated in ENTKL-NT. CD38 is a type II glycosylated protein with a transmembrane domain near the N-terminus, and is a pleiotropic glycoprotein. A retrospective study of 94 patients found that the majority of the NKL cases were CD38 positive, with strong expression being significantly correlated with poor outcomes. This is notable as daratumumab is an investigational anti-cancer agent targeting CD38 which has been utilized in other hematologic malignancies [74]. The *STAT3* and STAT-5b mutations have been evaluated *in vitro*, with these mutations being associated with increased phosphorylated protein and growth advantage in NK/T cell lines – these findings suggest that the JAK-STAT pathway may represent a potential therapeutic target [75]. Positive expression of CD30 antigen detected in about 50% of patients with ENTKL-NT could be attractive target for brentuximab vedotin [76].

Immunotherapy: it has been utilized in number of other malignancies however has to date not played a significant role in the treatment of ENTKL-NT. The expression of programmed cell death 1 (PD1) and programmed cell death ligand 1 (PDL-1) in ENTKL-NT was evaluated with notable rates of PD-L1 expression [27]. This may represent an opportunity for immune therapy agents such as nivolumab, pembrolizumab and other checkpoint inhibitors as well. The adoptive immunotherapy has been utilized in the setting of EBV latent membrane protein (LMP)-1 and LMP-2a-specific cytotoxic T lymphocytes, stimulated with LMP1/2a RNA-transferred dendritic cells. Cho et al. demonstrated in 10 patients 100% OS and 90% in patients who received the treatment following response to standard therapy. This small trial demonstrated potential post-remission therapeutic approach of a novel immune based therapy [77].

While modern chemotherapy regimens and radiation techniques have improved survival and response rates significantly over the past two decades, there is substantial room for improvement to find less toxic and more effective regimens. These future treatment modalities will likely include immunotherapy approaches including chimeric-antigen-receptor (CAR) T cell therapy.

CONCLUSION

Extranodal NK/T lymphoma, nasal type is a rare condition that has increasingly more effective chemotherapy and radiation therapy regimens, which offer a better outcome for a majority of patients with early stage disease. Future challenges include development of less toxic therapies for early stage disease and more effective therapeutic approaches for patients with advance stage disease. The better understanding of pathobiology of this disease will ultimately result in discovery of novel targets for modern therapeutic approaches. A global collaboration of clinical investigators is necessary to test novel therapies in large prospective clinical studies.

REFERENCES

[1] Swerdlow SH, Campo E, Pileri SA, et al. The 2016 revision of the World Health Organization classification of lymphoid neoplasms. *Blood.* 2016;127(20):2375-2390.

[2] Wu XC, Andrews P, Chen VW, Groves FD. Incidence of extranodal non-Hodgkin lymphomas among whites, blacks, and Asians/Pacific Islanders in the United

States: anatomic site and histology differences. *Cancer Epidemiol.* 2009;33(5):337-346.

[3] Suzuki R. Pathogenesis and treatment of extranodal natural killer/T-cell lymphoma. *Semin Hematol.* 2014;51(1):42-51.

[4] Kanavaros P, Lescs MC, Briere J, et al. Nasal T-cell lymphoma: a clinicopathologic entity associated with peculiar phenotype and with Epstein-Barr virus. *Blood.* 1993;81(10):2688-2695.

[5] Tse E, Kwong YL. How I treat NK/T-cell lymphomas. *Blood.* 2013;121(25):4997-5005.

[6] Liang X, Greffe B, Garrington T, Graham DK. Precursor natural killer cell leukemia. *Pediatr Blood Cancer.* 2008;50(4):876-878.

[7] Gourin CG, Johnson JT, Selvaggi K. Nasal T-cell lymphoma: case report and review of diagnostic features. *Ear Nose Throat J.* 2001;80(7):458-460.

[8] Lima M. Extranodal NK/T cell lymphoma and aggressive NK cell leukaemia: evidence for their origin on CD56+bright CD16-/+dim NK cells. *Pathology.* 2015;47(6):503-514.

[9] Pongpruttipan T, Sukpanichnant S, Assanasen T, et al. Extranodal NK/T-cell lymphoma, nasal type, includes cases of natural killer cell and alphabeta, gammadelta, and alphabeta/gammadelta T-cell origin: a comprehensive clinicopathologic and phenotypic study. *Am J Surg Pathol.* 2012;36(4):481-499.

[10] Hong M, Lee T, Young Kang S, Kim SJ, Kim W, Ko YH. Nasal-type NK/T-cell lymphomas are more frequently T rather than NK lineage based on T-cell receptor gene, RNA, and protein studies: lineage does not predict clinical behavior. *Mod Pathol.* 2016;29(5):430-443.

[11] Vose J, Armitage J, Weisenburger D, International TCLP. International peripheral T-cell and natural killer/T-cell lymphoma study: pathology findings and clinical outcomes. *J Clin Oncol.* 2008;26(25):4124-4130.

[12] William BM, Armitage JO. International analysis of the frequency and outcomes of NK/T-cell lymphomas. *Best Pract Res Clin Haematol.* 2013;26(1):23-32.

[13] Chihara D, Ito H, Matsuda T, et al. Differences in incidence and trends of haematological malignancies in Japan and the United States. *Br J Haematol.* 2014;164(4):536-545.

[14] Sun J, Yang Q, Lu Z, et al. Distribution of lymphoid neoplasms in China: analysis of 4,638 cases according to the World Health Organization classification. *Am J Clin Pathol.* 2012;138(3):429-434.

[15] Haverkos BM, Pan Z, Gru AA, et al. Extranodal NK/T Cell Lymphoma, Nasal Type (ENKTL-NT): An Update on Epidemiology, Clinical Presentation, and Natural History in North American and European Cases. *Curr Hematol Malig Rep.* 2016.

[16] Au WY, Gascoyne RD, Klasa RD, et al. Incidence and spectrum of non-Hodgkin lymphoma in Chinese migrants to British Columbia. *Br J Haematol.* 2005;128(6):792-796.

[17] Xu JX, Hoshida Y, Yang WI, et al. Life-style and environmental factors in the development of nasal NK/T-cell lymphoma: a case-control study in East Asia. *Int J Cancer.* 2007;120(2):406-410.

[18] Au WY, Weisenburger DD, Intragumtornchai T, et al. Clinical differences between nasal and extranasal natural killer/T-cell lymphoma: a study of 136 cases from the International Peripheral T-Cell Lymphoma Project. *Blood.* 2009;113(17):3931-3937.

[19] Kwong YL, Pang AW, Leung AY, Chim CS, Tse E. Quantification of circulating Epstein-Barr virus DNA in NK/T-cell lymphoma treated with the SMILE protocol: diagnostic and prognostic significance. *Leukemia.* 2014;28(4):865-870.

[20] Siu LL, Wong KF, Chan JK, Kwong YL. Comparative genomic hybridization analysis of natural killer cell lymphoma/leukemia. Recognition of consistent patterns of genetic alterations. *Am J Pathol.* 1999;155(5):1419-1425.

[21] Siu LL, Chan V, Chan JK, Wong KF, Liang R, Kwong YL. Consistent patterns of allelic loss in natural killer cell lymphoma. *Am J Pathol.* 2000;157(6):1803-1809.

[22] Nakashima Y, Tagawa H, Suzuki R, et al. Genome-wide array-based comparative genomic hybridization of natural killer cell lymphoma/leukemia: different genomic alteration patterns of aggressive NK-cell leukemia and extranodal Nk/T-cell lymphoma, nasal type. *Genes Chromosomes Cancer.* 2005;44(3):247-255.

[23] Yoon J, Ko YH. Deletion mapping of the long arm of chromosome 6 in peripheral T and NK cell lymphomas. *Leuk Lymphoma.* 2003;44(12):2077-2082.

[24] Kucuk C, Iqbal J, Hu X, et al. PRDM1 is a tumor suppressor gene in natural killer cell malignancies. *Proc Natl Acad Sci U S A.* 2011;108(50):20119-20124.

[25] Liang L, Nong L, Zhang S, et al. The downregulation of PRDM1/Blimp-1 is associated with aberrant expression of miR-223 in extranodal NK/T-cell lymphoma, nasal type. *J Exp Clin Cancer Res.* 2014;33:7.

[26] Choi S, Go JH, Kim EK, et al. Mutational Analysis of Extranodal NK/T-Cell Lymphoma Using Targeted Sequencing with a Comprehensive Cancer Panel. *Genomics Inform.* 2016;14(3):78-84.

[27] Jo JC, Kim M, Choi Y, et al. Expression of programmed cell death 1 and programmed cell death ligand 1 in extranodal NK/T-cell lymphoma, nasal type. *Ann Hematol.* 2016.

[28] Kim WY, Jung HY, Nam SJ, et al. Expression of programmed cell death ligand 1 (PD-L1) in advanced stage EBV-associated extranodal NK/T cell lymphoma is associated with better prognosis. *Virchows Arch.* 2016;469(5):581-590.

[29] Au WY, Ma SY, Chim CS, et al. Clinicopathologic features and treatment outcome of mature T-cell and natural killer-cell lymphomas diagnosed according to the

World Health Organization classification scheme: a single center experience of 10 years. *Ann Oncol.* 2005;16(2):206-214.

[30] Cleary KR, Batsakis JG. Sinonasal lymphomas. *Ann Otol Rhinol Laryngol.* 1994;103(11):911-914.

[31] Horwitz SM, Zelenetz AD, Gordon LI, et al. NCCN Guidelines Insights: Non-Hodgkin's Lymphomas, Version 3.2016. *J Natl Compr Canc Netw.* 2016;14(9):1067-1079.

[32] Song JY, Pittaluga S, Dunleavy K, et al. Lymphomatoid granulomatosis--a single institute experience: pathologic findings and clinical correlations. *Am J Surg Pathol.* 2015;39(2):141-156.

[33] Nelson AA, Harrington AM, Kroft S, Dahar MA, Hamadani M, Dhakal B. Presentation and management of post-allogeneic transplantation EBV-positive mucocutaneous ulcer. *Bone Marrow Transplant.* 2016;51(2):300-302.

[34] Roberts TK, Chen X, Liao JJ. Diagnostic and therapeutic challenges of EBV-positive mucocutaneous ulcer: a case report and systematic review of the literature. *Exp Hematol Oncol.* 2015;5:13.

[35] Beltran BE, Morales D, Quinones P, Medeiros LJ, Miranda RN, Castillo JJ. EBV-positive diffuse large b-cell lymphoma in young immunocompetent individuals. *Clin Lymphoma Myeloma Leuk.* 2011;11(6):512-516.

[36] Hong JY, Yoon DH, Suh C, et al. EBV-positive diffuse large B-cell lymphoma in young adults: is this a distinct disease entity? *Ann Oncol.* 2015;26(3):548-555.

[37] Loghavi S, Khoury JD, Medeiros LJ. Epstein-Barr virus-positive plasmacytoma in immunocompetent patients. *Histopathology.* 2015;67(2):225-234.

[38] Castillo JJ, Reagan JL. Plasmablastic lymphoma: a systematic review. *TheScientificWorldJournal.* 2011;11:687-696.

[39] Kim TM, Park YH, Lee SY, et al. Local tumor invasiveness is more predictive of survival than International Prognostic Index in stage I(E)/II(E) extranodal NK/T-cell lymphoma, nasal type. *Blood.* 2005;106(12):3785-3790.

[40] Lee J, Park YH, Kim WS, et al. Extranodal nasal type NK/T-cell lymphoma: elucidating clinical prognostic factors for risk-based stratification of therapy. *Eur J Cancer.* 2005;41(10):1402-1408.

[41] Li YX, Fang H, Liu QF, et al. Clinical features and treatment outcome of nasal-type NK/T-cell lymphoma of Waldeyer ring. *Blood.* 2008;112(8):3057-3064.

[42] Wang ZY, Liu QF, Wang H, et al. Clinical implications of plasma Epstein-Barr virus DNA in early-stage extranodal nasal-type NK/T-cell lymphoma patients receiving primary radiotherapy. *Blood.* 2012;120(10):2003-2010.

[43] Lee J, Suh C, Huh J, et al. Effect of positive bone marrow EBV in situ hybridization in staging and survival of localized extranodal natural killer/T-cell lymphoma, nasal-type. *Clin Cancer Res.* 2007;13(11):3250-3254.

[44] Bossard C, Belhadj K, Reyes F, et al. Expression of the granzyme B inhibitor PI9 predicts outcome in nasal NK/T-cell lymphoma: results of a Western series of 48 patients treated with first-line polychemotherapy within the Groupe d'Etude des Lymphomes de l'Adulte (GELA) trials. *Blood.* 2007;109(5):2183-2189.

[45] Shim SJ, Yang WI, Shin E, et al. Clinical significance of cyclooxygenase-2 expression in extranodal natural killer (NK)/T-cell lymphoma, nasal type. *Int J Radiat Oncol Biol Phys.* 2007;67(1):31-38.

[46] Jiang C, Zhang X, Jiang M, et al. Assessment of the prognostic capacity of pretreatment, interim, and post-therapy (18)F-FDG PET/CT in extranodal natural killer/T-cell lymphoma, nasal type. *Ann Nucl Med.* 2015;29(5):442-451.

[47] Lee J, Suh C, Park YH, et al. Extranodal natural killer T-cell lymphoma, nasal-type: a prognostic model from a retrospective multicenter study. *J Clin Oncol.* 2006;24(4):612-618.

[48] Dai W, Jia B, Yang J, et al. Development of new prognostic model based on pretreatment betaLRI and LLRI for stage IE/IIE upper aerodigestive tract ENKTL, nasal type. *Oncotarget.* 2017;8(21):34787-34795.

[49] Kim SJ, Yoon DH, Jaccard A, et al. A prognostic index for natural killer cell lymphoma after non-anthracycline-based treatment: a multicentre, retrospective analysis. *Lancet Oncol.* 2016;17(3):389-400.

[50] Li YX, Wang H, Jin J, et al. Radiotherapy alone with curative intent in patients with stage I extranodal nasal-type NK/T-cell lymphoma. *Int J Radiat Oncol Biol Phys.* 2012;82(5):1809-1815.

[51] Dong LH, Zhang LJ, Wang WJ, et al. Sequential DICE combined with l-asparaginase chemotherapy followed by involved field radiation in newly diagnosed, stage IE to IIE, nasal and extranodal NK/T-cell lymphoma. *Leuk Lymphoma.* 2016;57(7):1600-1606.

[52] Yang Y, Zhu Y, Cao JZ, et al. Risk-adapted therapy for early-stage extranodal nasal-type NK/T-cell lymphoma: analysis from a multicenter study. *Blood.* 2015;126(12):1424-1432; quiz 1517.

[53] Isobe K, Uno T, Tamaru J, et al. Extranodal natural killer/T-cell lymphoma, nasal type: the significance of radiotherapeutic parameters. *Cancer.* 2006;106(3):609-615.

[54] Yahalom J, Illidge T, Specht L, et al. Modern radiation therapy for extranodal lymphomas: field and dose guidelines from the International Lymphoma Radiation Oncology Group. *International journal of radiation oncology, biology, physics.* 2015;92(1):11-31.

[55] Huang MJ, Jiang Y, Liu WP, et al. Early or up-front radiotherapy improved survival of localized extranodal NK/T-cell lymphoma, nasal-type in the upper aerodigestive tract. *Int J Radiat Oncol Biol Phys.* 2008;70(1):166-174.

[56] Wang H, Li YX, Wang WH, et al. Mild toxicity and favorable prognosis of high-dose and extended involved-field intensity-modulated radiotherapy for patients with early-stage nasal NK/T-cell lymphoma. *Int J Radiat Oncol Biol Phys.* 2012;82(3):1115-1121.

[57] Shen Q, Ma X, Hu W, Chen L, Huang J, Guo Y. Intensity-modulated radiotherapy versus three-dimensional conformal radiotherapy for stage I-II natural killer/T-cell lymphoma nasal type: dosimetric and clinical results. *Radiat Oncol.* 2013;8:152.

[58] Wang L, Xia ZJ, Lu Y, Zhang YJ. Prophylactic cervical lymph node irradiation provides no benefit for patients of stage IE extranodal natural killer/T cell lymphoma, nasal type. *Med Oncol.* 2015;32(1):320.

[59] Suzuki R. Treatment of advanced extranodal NK/T cell lymphoma, nasal-type and aggressive NK-cell leukemia. *Int J Hematol.* 2010;92(5):697-701.

[60] Kim WS, Song SY, Ahn YC, et al. CHOP followed by involved field radiation: is it optimal for localized nasal natural killer/T-cell lymphoma? *Ann Oncol.* 2001;12(3):349-352.

[61] Kim SJ, Kim WS. Treatment of localized extranodal NK/T cell lymphoma, nasal type. *Int J Hematol.* 2010;92(5):690-696.

[62] Wang B, Li XQ, Ma X, Hong X, Lu H, Guo Y. Immunohistochemical expression and clinical significance of P-glycoprotein in previously untreated extranodal NK/T-cell lymphoma, nasal type. *Am J Hematol.* 2008;83(10):795-799.

[63] Yong W, Zheng W, Zhang Y, et al. L-asparaginase-based regimen in the treatment of refractory midline nasal/nasal-type T/NK-cell lymphoma. *Int J Hematol.* 2003;78(2):163-167.

[64] Yamaguchi M, Tobinai K, Oguchi M, et al. Concurrent chemoradiotherapy for localized nasal natural killer/T-cell lymphoma: an updated analysis of the Japan clinical oncology group study JCOG0211. *J Clin Oncol.* 2012;30(32):4044-4046.

[65] Kwong YL, Kim WS, Lim ST, et al. SMILE for natural killer/T-cell lymphoma: analysis of safety and efficacy from the Asia Lymphoma Study Group. *Blood.* 2012;120(15):2973-2980.

[66] Yoon DH, Kim SJ, Jeong SH, et al. Phase II trial of concurrent chemoradiotherapy with L-asparaginase and MIDLE chemotherapy for newly diagnosed stage I/II extranodal NK/T-cell lymphoma, nasal type (CISL-1008). *Oncotarget.* 2016.

[67] Kim SJ, Kim K, Kim BS, et al. Phase II trial of concurrent radiation and weekly cisplatin followed by VIPD chemotherapy in newly diagnosed, stage IE to IIE, nasal, extranodal NK/T-Cell Lymphoma: Consortium for Improving Survival of Lymphoma study. *J Clin Oncol.* 2009;27(35):6027-6032.

[68] Jaccard A, Gachard N, Marin B, et al. Efficacy of L-asparaginase with methotrexate and dexamethasone (AspaMetDex regimen) in patients with refractory or relapsing extranodal NK/T-cell lymphoma, a phase 2 study. *Blood.* 2011;117(6):1834-1839.

[69] Yamaguchi M, Suzuki R, Kwong YL, et al. Phase I study of dexamethasone, methotrexate, ifosfamide, L-asparaginase, and etoposide (SMILE) chemotherapy for advanced-stage, relapsed or refractory extranodal natural killer (NK)/T-cell lymphoma and leukemia. *Cancer Sci.* 2008;99(5):1016-1020.

[70] Ito Y, Kimura H, Maeda Y, et al. Pretreatment EBV-DNA copy number is predictive of response and toxicities to SMILE chemotherapy for extranodal NK/T-cell lymphoma, nasal type. *Clin Cancer Res.* 2012;18(15):4183-4190.

[71] Au WY, Lie AK, Liang R, et al. Autologous stem cell transplantation for nasal NK/T-cell lymphoma: a progress report on its value. *Ann Oncol.* 2003;14(11):1673-1676.

[72] Lee J, Au WY, Park MJ, et al. Autologous hematopoietic stem cell transplantation in extranodal natural killer/T cell lymphoma: a multinational, multicenter, matched controlled study. *Biol Blood Marrow Transplant.* 2008;14(12):1356-1364.

[73] Murashige N, Kami M, Kishi Y, et al. Allogeneic haematopoietic stem cell transplantation as a promising treatment for natural killer-cell neoplasms. *Br J Haematol.* 2005;130(4):561-567.

[74] Wang L, Wang H, Li PF, et al. CD38 expression predicts poor prognosis and might be a potential therapy target in extranodal NK/T cell lymphoma, nasal type. *Ann Hematol.* 2015;94(8):1381-1388.

[75] Lee S, Park HY, Kang SY, et al. Genetic alterations of JAK/STAT cascade and histone modification in extranodal NK/T-cell lymphoma nasal type. *Oncotarget.* 2015;6(19):17764-17776.

[76] Feng Y, Rao H, Lei Y, et al. CD30 expression in extranodal natural killer/T-cell lymphoma, nasal type among 622 cases of mature T-cell and natural killer-cell lymphoma at a single institution in South China. *Chin J Cancer.* 2017;36(1):43.

[77] Cho SG, Kim N, Sohn HJ, et al. Long-term Outcome of Extranodal NK/T Cell Lymphoma Patients Treated With Postremission Therapy Using EBV LMP1 and LMP2a-specific CTLs. *Mol Ther.* 2015;23(8):1401-1409.

In: Benign and Malignant Disorders …
Editors: Ling Zhang and Lubomir Sokol

ISBN: 978-1-53612-999-1
© 2018 Nova Science Publishers, Inc.

Chapter 11

AGGRESSIVE NATURAL KILLER (NK) CELL LEUKEMIA

Xiaohui Zhang, MD, PhD
Department of Hematopathology and Laboratory Medicine
H. Lee Moffitt Cancer Center and Research Institute, Tampa, FL, US

ABSTRACT

Aggressive natural killer cell leukemia is an extremely rare disease characterized by the abnormal proliferation of neoplastic cells originating from Natural Killer (NK) cells, with a fulminant clinical course and dismal prognosis. The disease is strongly associated with the reactivation of the Epstein-Barr virus (EBV) and often presents with coagulopathy, hemophagocytic lymphohistocytosis (HLH) and multi-organ failure. Aggressive NK cell leukemia cells exhibit a unique immunophenotype: CD2+/cytoplasmic CD3+/CD56+/TCR-. There are no specific cytogenetic abnormalities identified, although array based comparative genomic hybridization showed frequent loss of chromsome 7q, 17p and gain of chromosome 1q, which could be useful to differentiate it from extranodal NK/T-cell lymphoma. The exact pathogenesis of aggressive NK cell leukemia is illusive despite the recent introduction of whole genomic sequencing and other advanced molecular technologies. Recent studies showed that *PRDM1* and *FOXO3* are two tumor suppressor genes that play critical roles in NK cell neoplasms. The presence of the *STAT5B* mutation and *HACE1* hypermethylation at CpG-177 is found in EBV-positive aggressive natural killer cell leukemia, while *STAT3* (Y640F) and *PTPN2* (G224V) mutations have been reported in EBV-negative aggressive natural killer cell leukemia. However, the role of the above listed genes in the development of aggressive NK cell leukemia is unclear. The chapter aims to review the natural history of aggressive NK cell leukemia, emphasizing the diagnosis and differential diagnosis of this entity.

1. INTRODUCTION

Aggressive natural killer (NK) cell leukemia is a very rare, systemic neoplastic proliferation of NK cells with an extremely aggressive clinical course. It is most often associated with the Epstein-Barr virus (EBV), but rarely can be EBV negative [1, 2]. It was initially recognized in the mid-1980s and thought to be an aggressive large granular lymphocyte (LGL) leukemia of non-T cell type, since morphologically the proliferating cells resembled large granular lymphocytes but expressed a natural killer cell phenotype (surface CD3(-), CD4(-), CD8(-), CD16(+), CD56(+), and TCR αβ and TCR γδ(-))[3-5]. Subsequently, many of the case reports or case series reported the association with EBV [6-8].The term "aggressive NK-cell leukemia/lymphoma" was first adopted in 1990 to describe this aggressive NK-cell-derived malignancy with peripheral blood and systemic involvement [9]. The terminology of "leukemia/lymphoma" has been used to reflect the systemic nature and extensive multi-organ involvement of this disease. Aggressive natural killer (NK) cell leukemia was separated from LGL leukemia and was recognized in the World Health Organization (WHO) classification of tumors of hematopoietic and lymphoid tissues (2001 and 2008 editions) as a distinct entity of mature NK cell neoplasm characterized by the primary involvement of peripheral blood and bone marrow with a fulminant clinical course [10].

2. EPIDEMIOLOGY AND ETIOLOGY

Aggressive NK cell leukemia is more prevalent in Asians than in Caucasians, with the majority of cases reported from East Asia including China and Japan [11, 12]. It typically occurs in adolescents or young adults, but can develop in older patients (median age, 30-40 years) [10, 13, 14]. Men and women are equally affected.

There is a strong association between aggressive NK cell leukemia and EBV, although cases with negative EBV have been reported, particularly those arising from chronic lymphoproliferative disorder of NK cells [15]. The exact pathogenetic role of EBV and the definite etiology of aggressive NK cell leukemia remain unclear. The disease can occur *de novo* or develop from pre-existing systemic EBV related T/NK cell lymphoproliferative disorders, such as chronic active EBV infection, nasal NK/T cell lymphoma, and mosquito bite allergy [16-18].

3. CLINICAL FEATURES

Patients with aggressive NK cell leukemia typically present with fevers, generalized lymphadenopathy, hepatosplenomegaly, and the presence of atypical lymphocytes with large azurophilic cytoplasmic granules in the peripheral blood, and bone marrow [11, 19-21]. The number of circulating neoplastic cells in peripheral blood can be variable, ranging from low or even absent, to high. Those who present with absent or low circulating neoplastic cells often present with generalized lymphadenopathy [22, 23]. Bone marrow involvement can be diffuse or patchy. While any organ can be involved, skin involvement is uncommon, and can manifest as a non-specific skin rash.

Patients usually have cytopenias (anemia, neutropenia, and thrombocytopenia), and markedly elevated serum lactate dehydrogenase levels and Fas Ligand (FasL) [24, 25]. Secondary complications include disseminated intravascular coagulopathy (DIC), hemophagocytic lymphohistocytosis (HLH) or multi-organ failure [2, 9, 11, 26, 27]. Concurrent HLH is present in up to 60% of the patients [28], occurring at the time diagnosis or later on during the disease course.

4. DIAGNOSIS

4.1. Morphological Findings

The diagnosis of aggressive NK cell leukemia is usually based on peripheral blood examination and bone marrow aspiration. Aggressive NK cell leukemia cells in the peripheral blood can have variable cytology, ranging from normal-appearing large granular lymphocytes to atypical and immature large granular lymphocytes [10, 13, 29]. When resembling normal looking large granular lymphocytes, the neoplastic cells usually have moderate to abundant slightly basophilic cytoplasm with coarse azurophilic granules and a round nucleus with condensed or slightly immature chromatin and inconspicuous nucleoli (Figure 1).When the neoplastic cells show atypical features, they can show variable cell sizes and shapes, enlarged and irregular nuclei with irregular nuclear contours and often times immature chromatin and distinct nucleoli (Figure 2). The numbers of circulating aggressive NK cell leukemia cells in peripheral blood range from less than 5% to more than 80% of lymphocytes.

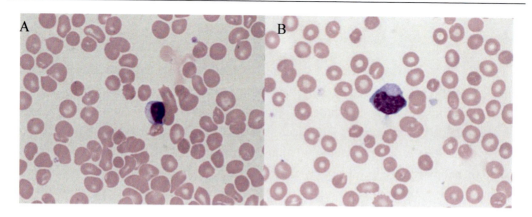

Figure 1. Aggressive NK cell leukemia cells resembling reactive large granular lymphocytes. The cells show moderate to abundant slightly basophilic cytoplasm with coarse azurophilic granules and nucleus with condensed or slightly immature chromatin (A and B, Wright-Giemsa stain, 1000x).

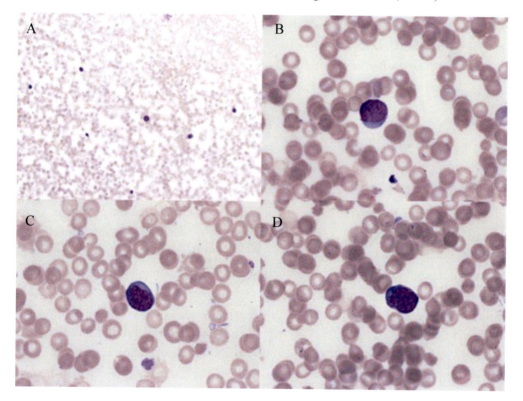

Figure 2. Aggressive NK cell leukemia cells with atypical features. The cells show variable sizes and shapes (A, Wright-Giemsa stain, 200x), and they can have enlarged, irregular nuclei with irregular nuclear contours and sometimes immature chromatin and distinct nucleoli. Few cytoplasmic azurophilic granules can also be seen (B-D, Wright-Giemsa stain, 1000x).

Bone marrow involvement varies from diffuse interstitial to subtle and focal or patchy [11] (Figure 3, and Figure 4). The infiltrating neoplastic cells are monomorphous cells with moderate amounts of pale or amphophilic cytoplasm, and round or irregular nuclei. Hemophagocytoses may be seen, which can be a morphologic hint to the diagnosis of complicating HLH, although definitive diagnosis of HLH requires clinical and laboratory correlation [30]. Apoptotic bodies, necrosis, angioinvasion and angiodestruction may be seen [13, 20, 22]. Bone marrow stromal damage and dyserythropoiesis are also common findings [24].

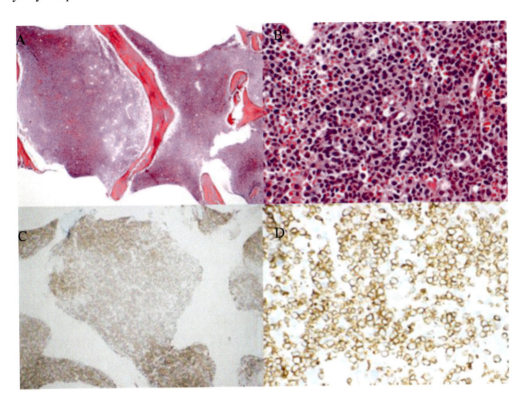

Figure 3. Diffuse bone marrow involvement by aggressive NK cell leukemia. The bone marrow is diffusely infiltrated by aggressive NK cell leukemia cells (A, H&E stain, 40x; B, H&E stain, 400x). The neoplastic cells are stained with CD3 in cytoplasmic staining pattern (C, immunohistochemical stain, 40x; D, immunohistochemical stain, 400x).

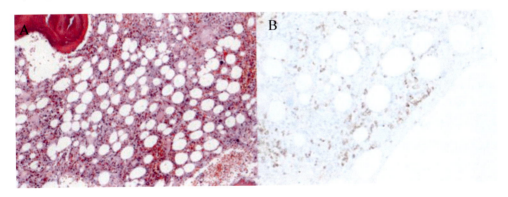

Figure 4. Patchy involvement by aggressive NK cell leukemia in bone marrow. In this case, the bone marrow is infiltrated by aggressive NK cell leukemia cells in a focal and patchy pattern, which is better highlighted by immunostains for CD3, CD56 and other markers (A, H&E stain, 100x; B, CD3 immunohistochemical stain, 200x).

Besides peripheral blood and bone marrow, the diagnosis can also be established by tissue biopsy, such as biopsy from the liver or the spleen [31]. The normal structure of the involved organ is disrupted by the neoplastic cells, which are monomorphic or pleomorphic cells infiltrating into the parenchyma, such as portal areas and sinusoids in liver, and cords and sinuses of red pulp in spleen [31]. Lymph node biopsy can show diffuse effacement by neoplastic cells infiltrating in paracortical and sinus areas. Skin involvement shows atypical dermal lymphoid infiltrate with a perivascular and interstitial pattern [1, 32]. Necrosis and angioinvasion can often be seen.

4.2. Immunophenotyping

Immunophenotyping is the key to the diagnosis of aggressive NK cell leukemia. The neoplastic NK cells exhibit a CD56 bright+/CD16 dim+ and CD57- immunophenotype with markedly increased Ki-67 proliferation index [33]. Flow cytometry is both sensitive and specific for the early diagnosis of aggressive NK cell leukemia. By immunohistochemistry or flow cytometric analysis, the neoplastic cells are CD2+, surface CD3(-), cytoplasmic CD3ε+, CD56+ and cytotoxic markers positive. The immunophenotype is identical to that of extranodal NK/T-cell lymphoma, except that CD16 expression is seen in 50~75% of the cases [11]. CD57 is usually negative. CD3, CD4, CD5, TCRαβ and TCRγδ are consistently absent. CD7 is frequently absent (Figure 5, Figure 6 and Figure 7). Expression of CD8 is observed in a subset (approximately 30%) of the cases [34]. In addition, NK cell receptors, also known as killer-cell immunoglobulin-like receptors (KIRs), such as CD158a/h, CD158b, and CD158e are lost or show low level expression [33, 35].

Aggressive NK cell leukemia has a strong association with EBV infection or reactivation. EBV is positive in the majority of cases (more than 90% of cases) [10, 13]. However, rare cases of EBV-negative aggressive NK cell leukemia have been reported [1, 2, 11, 36, 37]. EBV-negative aggressive NK cell leukemia patients appear to be older than EBV-positive cases, with a median age of 63 years. The morphologic and immunophenotypic features, clinical presentation and course are similar to EBV-positive aggressive NK cell leukemia, although few reports did describe a slightly longer overall survival with a range from 11 months to 4 years when comparing with EBV-positive aggressive NK cell leukemia [37, 38]. Of note, blastoid cytology with fine chromatin and coarse azuropilic cytoplasmic granules has been described.

Similar to other NK cell neoplasms, aggressive NK cell leukemia cases do not show clonal T cell receptor gene rearrangement. When clonal T cell receptor gene rearrangement is present, clinicians and pathologists should interpret it with caution as the clonality could be a false positive or represent reactive T-cells in the background.

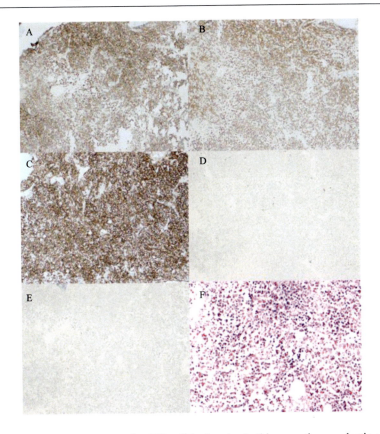

Figure 5. Immunophenotype of aggressive NK cell leukemia. In this case, the neoplastic cells are positive for cytoplasmic CD2 (A, immunohistochemical stain, 100x), cytoplasmic CD3 (B, immunohistochemical stain, 100x), CD56 (C, immunohistochemical stain, 100x), and EBER (F, in situ hybridization, 200x), and negative for CD5 and CD7 (D and E. immunohistochemical stain, 100x).

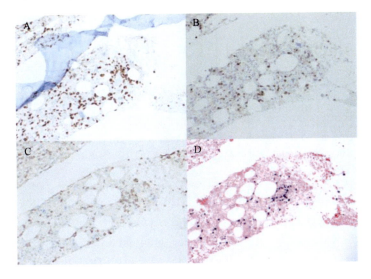

Figure 6. Immunophenotypes of aggressive NK cell leukemia. The neoplastic cells are positive for cytoplasmic CD3 (A, immunohistochemical stain, 200x), CD56 (C, immunohistochemical stain, 200x), and EBER (D, in situ hybridization, 200x), and negative for CD5 (B. immunohistochemical stain, 200x).

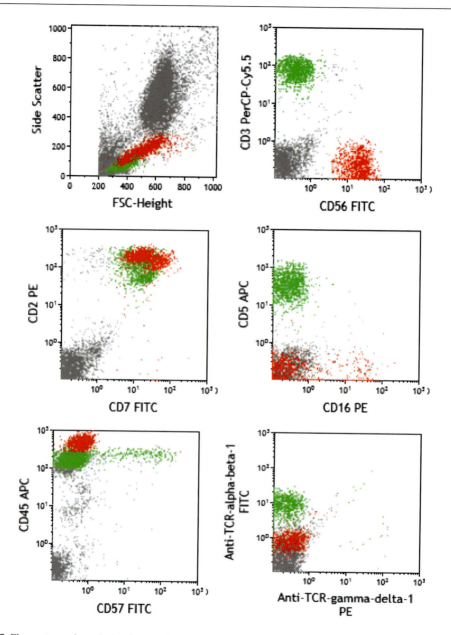

Figure 7. Flow cytometric analysis of aggressive NK cell leukemia cells. The neoplastic NK cells (red dots) are positive for CD45 (bright), CD2, CD7, CD56 and negative for surface CD3, CD5, CD16, CD57, TCRαβ and TCR γδ. T cells are colored green.

In summary, the diagnosis of aggressive NK cell leukemia requires the integration of clinical presentation, cytology and immunophenotype. Key features include aggressive clinical course, typical or atypical large granular lymphocyte cytology, and immunophenotype of NK cells (cytoplasmic CD3, CD56), EBV positivity (in majority of the cases), lack of myeloid or B cell antigens, and germline configuration of T cell receptor genes.

5. GENETIC, MOLECULAR FEATURES AND PATHOGENESIS

While there are no cytogenetic abnormalities specific to aggressive NK cell leukemia, several clonal cytogenetic abnormalities have been reported. These cytogenetic changes can be used as evidence of clonal proliferation of the neoplastic cells in aggressive NK cell leukemia. The most common ones involve chromosomes 6q and 11q, including 6q21-23 deletion and 11q deletion [39]. Deletion of 6q may result in the loss of several tumor suppressor genes e.g., *PRDM1, ATG5, AIM1, and HACE1*. Reports have shown that NK cell lymphoma/leukemia, including extranodal NK/T cell lymphoma and aggressive NK cell leukemia, can show clonal cytogenetic abnormalities in two-thirds of the cases [39]. The cytogenetic changes in extranodal NK/T cell lymphoma and aggressive NK cell leukemia include loss of 3p, 6q, 11q, and 12q [39, 40]. One array-based comparative genomic hybridization (CGH) study on 10 aggressive NK-cell leukemia cases and 17 extranodal NK/T-cell [NK/T] lymphomas, nasal type, reported that there were differences in the genomic alteration pattern. In the former, loss of 7p and 17p13.1 and gain of 1q were more frequent than in the latter, suggesting that the loss of 7p and 17p13.1 may be associated with leukemogenesis of aggressive NK-cell leukemia [41].

Molecular features and molecular pathogenesis of aggressive NK cell leukemia are largely unknown. It has been suggested that EBV plays an important role in disease progression, but not in oncogenesis of aggressive NK cell leukemia [23]. In aggressive NK cell leukemia cases, there is a clonal episomal form of EBV, but the neoplastic cells do not express EBV-associated latent membrane protein (LMP-1) or EBV nuclear antigen-2 (EBNA-2) proteins, thus suggesting that these EBV-related proteins are not involved in malignant transformation of NK cells [23]. The *STAT5B* mutation (N642H) and *HACE1* hypermethylation at CpG-177 island have been reported in EBV-positive aggressive NK cell leukemia [32], while *STAT3* mutation (Y640F) and *PTPN2* (G224V) have been reported in EBV-negative aggressive NK cell leukemia [1]. It was proposed that a combination of *PTPN2* inactivation and *STAT3* mutation might result in uncontrolled activation of the JAK/STAT pathway [1].

FOXO3 and *PRDM1* are tumor suppressor genes recently identified to be involved in the pathogenesis of NK cell neoplasms including extranodal NK cell lymphoma and aggressive NK cell leukemia [42]. These two genes are located in chromosome 6q21-23 region, which is frequently deleted [39]. *PRDM1*(PR domain zinc finger protein 1) is a repressive transcription factor involved in terminal differentiation of immunoblasts and plasma cells. *FOXO3* is a transcription factor belonging to FoxO family that regulates multiple cellular processes. Mutational deletion of *FOXO3* has been identified in B-cell lymphoproliferative disorders and acute lymphoblastic leukemia [43]. In an *in vitro* study, induced expression of *FOXO3* results in its nuclear translocation and decreased AKT expression, further inhibiting proliferation in NK cell lines. Induced expression of

PRDM1 could suppress cell proliferation not only in NK cell lines but also in other cell lines [44]. Therefore, *FOXO3* function is more NK-cell lineage specific, suggesting that its loss may play more important roles in the pathogenesis.

HACE1 is another tumor suppressor gene located in 6q21 and encodes E3 ubiquitin ligase. Its role in NK cell neoplasms is controversial. Deletion of HACE1 was detected in NK cell lines and biopsy specimens of aggressive NK cell neoplasms, leading to its mRNA down regulation [45]. However, a study by Sako and colleagues showed decreased HACE1 mRNA induced by hypermethylation of CpG-177 island did not alter its protein production and function of NK cells, suggesting that HACE1 was not a key regulator in NK cell lymphoma/leukemia [46].

6. DIFFERENTIAL DIAGNOSIS

6.1. Chronic Lymphoproliferative Disorder of NK Cells and T-Cell Large Granular Lymphocytic Leukemia (T-LGL)

Both chronic lymphoproliferative disorder of NK cells (CLPD-NK) and T-LGLL share similar cytological features with a subset of aggressive NK cell leukemia cases. The cases of CLPD-NK typically have a persistent increase in circulating mature NK cells in the peripheral blood (>6 months, ≥2000/μL by WHO 2008 criteria, or >80% of total lymphocytes [47]). Patients have a higher median age than aggressive EBV positive NK cell leukemia patients (60 years of age vs 30-40 years of age), and have an indolent clinical course. The majority of the patients are asymptomatic, but can infrequently present with cytopenias. Lymphadenopathy, hepatomegaly, splenomegaly and cutaneous lesions are rare [48]. CLPD-NK cells are typically surface CD3 negative, cytoplasmic CD3ε positive, brightly CD16 positive and CD57 positive (majority of cases). A subset of cases have diminished or absent expression of CD56 [20, 49, 50]. Aberrantly lost expression of CD2, CD7, CD57, or co-expression of CD5 and CD8 can be present [49, 51]. Abnormal expression of KIR antigens, such as uniform expression of a single KIR, or absence of all KIR antigens, can be seen in CLPD-NK cell cases [50-52]. Chronic lymphoproliferative disorder of NK cells is negative for EBV infection.

In summary, CLPD-NK and aggressive NK cell leukemia differ from the following aspects: CLPD-NK occurs in older patients, and show dramatically different clinical course from aggressive NK cell leukemia. Cytologically, the large granular lymphocytes lack cytological atypia. Phenotypically chronic lymphoproliferative disorder of NK cells frequently express CD16 and CD57, whereas in aggressive NK cell leukemia the cells express bright CD56, dim or negative CD16 (vast majority of the cases) and lack CD57 expression [35]. In contrast to aggressive NK cell leukemia, CLPD-NK is not associated with the EBV infection. However, despite these differences it can be challenging to distinguish CLPD-NK from early stage EBV negative aggressive NK cell leukemia which only shows subtle bone marrow infiltrate [53]. Of note, it has been reported that the more aggressive form of NK cell lymphoma/leukemia can arise from indolent chronic lymphoproliferative disorder of NK cells [15, 54], which requires careful investigation before rendering a final diagnosis.

T-LGLL cells typically show large granular lymphocyte cytology with no atypia or immature appearance, except for rare aggressive forms. Phenotypically the cells are surface CD3 positive, CD8 positive, CD57 positive, CD16 positive and T-cell receptor αβ positive cytotoxic cells [55]. T cell receptor genes are usually clonally rearranged.

6.2. Extranodal T/NK Cell Lymphoma, Nasal Type

Extranodal T/NK cell lymphoma, nasal type, shows morphologic and immunophenotypic overlap with aggressive NK cell leukemia. Similar to aggressive NK cell leukemia, extranodal T/NK cell lymphoma is more prevalent in Asians, is associated with an EBV infection, and is a highly aggressive disease. However, extranodal T/NK cell lymphoma typically presents with localized extranodal involvement. Presence of large areas of geographic necrosis is a helpful morphologic feature usually not seen in aggressive NK cell leukemia. When extranodal NK/T-cell lymphoma shows multiorgan involvement, the two diseases can show overlap features and it may be difficult to distinguish [56]. Although it has been suggested that aggressive NK cell leukemia may represent the leukemic counterpart of extranodal NK/T-cell lymphoma, the current consensus based on the differences identified on array based CGH is that the two represent distinct entities.

6.3. Systemic EBV-Positive T-Cell Lymphoma of Childhood and Young Adults

Systemic EBV-positive T-cell lymphoma of childhood and young adults is a fulminant disease characterized by a clonal proliferation of EBV infected T cells [57]. Similar to aggressive NK cell leukemia, it is prevalent in Asia and can present with concurrent HLH. It occurs shortly after an acute EBV infection and presents with fevers, hepatosplenomegaly and pancytopenia. The disease progresses rapidly and eventually causes death. However, it occurs most often in children and young adults. In contrast to aggressive NK cell leukemia, the involved cells are T cells, and immunophenotypically the cells are CD2 positive, surface CD3 positive, TIA-1 positive, granzyme B positive and CD56 negative. T cell receptor genes show clonal rearrangement [58].

The expression patterns of the useful immunophenotypic markers in the aforementioned entities are summarized in Table 1[19].

Table 1. The different expression patterns of immunophenotypic markers in aggressive NK cell leukemia and other T/NK cell lymphomas/leukemias

Diseases	Surface CD3	Cytoplasmic CD3	CD56	CD16	CD2	CD5	CD7	CD4	CD8	CD57	EBV	TCR
ANKL	-	+	+	-	+	-	+	-	+/-	-	+#	-
ENKTL	-	+	+	-	+/-	-	+	-	+/-	-	+	-
CLPD-NK	-	+	-	+	+	-	+	-	-	+	-	-
T-LGL	+	+	-/+	+/-	+	dim+	+	-	+	+	-	+
SEBVTL	+	+	-	ND	+	ND	ND	+/-	+/-	ND	+	+

*Abbreviations: ANKL: aggressive NK cell leukemia; ENKTL: extranodal NK/T cell lymphoma; CLPD-NK: chronic lymphoproliferative disorder of NK cells; SEBVTL: Systemic EBV-positive T-cell lymphoma of childhood and young adults; ND: not determined.
Majority of cases. A small subset of cases can be negative [1].

7. TREATMENT AND PROGNOSIS

A standard treatment protocol has not been established for aggressive NK cell leukemia. The response to conventional chemotherapy is poor, and the complete remission rate is below 20% [59]. Systemic chemotherapy followed by an allogeneic stem cell transplant is the only approach which can lead to longer survival.

The prognosis of aggressive NK cell leukemia is very poor, with a median survival of 2 months [11, 13]. Refractoriness to chemotherapy is common. The disease is usually complicated by coagulopathy, HLH, and multi-organ failure. A detailed discussion on therapeutic strategies and clinical outcomes will be followed in a separate chapter.

REFERENCES

[1] Nicolae, A., et al., EBV-negative Aggressive NK-cell Leukemia/Lymphoma: Clinical, Pathologic, and Genetic Features. *Am. J. Surg. Pathol.*, 2017. 41(1): p. 67-74.

[2] Zhang, Q., et al., Six cases of aggressive natural killer-cell leukemia in a Chinese population. *Int. J. Clin. Exp. Pathol.*, 2014. 7(6): p. 3423-31.

[3] Sheridan, W., et al., Leukemia of non-T lineage natural killer cells. *Blood*, 1988. 72(5): p. 1701-7.

[4] Fernandez, L.A., et al., Aggressive natural killer cell leukemia in an adult with establishment of an NK cell line. *Blood*, 1986. 67(4): p. 925-30.

[5] Koizumi, S., et al., Malignant clonal expansion of large granular lymphocytes with a Leu-11+, Leu-7- surface phenotype: in vitro responsiveness of malignant cells to recombinant human interleukin 2. *Blood*, 1986. 68(5): p. 1065-73.

[6] Kawa-Ha, K., et al., CD3-negative lymphoproliferative disease of granular lymphocytes containing Epstein-Barr viral DNA. *J. Clin. Invest.*, 1989. 84(1): p. 51-5.

[7] Hart, D. N., et al., Epstein-Barr viral DNA in acute large granular lymphocyte (natural killer) leukemic cells. *Blood*, 1992. 79(8): p. 2116-23.

[8] Gelb, A.B., et al., Epstein-Barr virus-associated natural killer-large granular lymphocyte leukemia. *Hum. Pathol.*, 1994. 25(9): p. 953-60.

[9] Imamura, N., et al., Aggressive natural killer cell leukaemia/lymphoma: report of four cases and review of the literature. Possible existence of a new clinical entity originating from the third lineage of lymphoid cells. *Br. J. Haematol.*, 1990. 75(1): p. 49-59.

[10] Chan, J. K. C., et al., Aggressive NK-cell leukemia, in World Health Organization classification of tumours of haematopoietic and lymphoid tissues, S.H. Swerdlow, et al., Editors. 2008, *International Agency for Research on Cancer*: Lyon, France. p. 276-277.

[11] Bhandari, A., et al., Increased expression of matrix metalloproteinase-2 in nasal polyps. *Acta Otolaryngol.*, 2004. 124(10): p. 1165-70.

[12] Ruskova, A., Thula, R. and Chan, G. Aggressive Natural Killer-Cell Leukemia: report of five cases and review of the literature. *Leuk. Lymphoma*, 2004. 45(12): p. 2427-38.

[13] Ko, Y. H., Chan, J. K. C. and Quintanilla-Martinez, L. Virally-associated T-cell and NK-cell neoplasms, in *Hematopathology*, E.S. Jaffe, et al., Editors. 2016, Elsevier: Philadelphia, PA. p. 565-598.

[14] Greer, J. P. and Mosse, C. A. Natural killer-cell neoplasms. *Curr. Hematol. Malig. Rep.*, 2009. 4(4): p. 245-52.

[15] Ohno, Y., et al., Acute transformation of chronic large granular lymphocyte leukemia associated with additional chromosome abnormality. *Cancer*, 1989. 64(1): p. 63-7.

[16] Ishihara, S., et al., Hypersensitivity to mosquito bites conceals clonal lymphoproliferation of Epstein-Barr viral DNA-positive natural killer cells. *Jpn. J. Cancer Res.*, 1997. 88(1): p. 82-7.

[17] Kimura, H., et al., EBV-associated T/NK-cell lymphoproliferative diseases in nonimmunocompromised hosts: prospective analysis of 108 cases. *Blood*, 2012. 119(3): p. 673-86.

[18] Soler, J., et al., Aggressive natural killer cell leukaemia/lymphoma in two patients with lethal midline granuloma. *Br. J. Haematol.*, 1994. 86(3): p. 659-62.

[19] Nava, V. E. and Jaffe, E. S. The pathology of NK-cell lymphomas and leukemias. *Adv. Anat. Pathol.*, 2005. 12(1): p. 27-34.

[20] Chan, J. K., et al., Nonnasal lymphoma expressing the natural killer cell marker CD56: a clinicopathologic study of 49 cases of an uncommon aggressive neoplasm. *Blood*, 1997. 89(12): p. 4501-13.

[21] Song, S. Y., et al., Aggressive natural killer cell leukemia: clinical features and treatment outcome. *Haematologica*, 2002. 87(12): p. 1343-5.

[22] Mori, N., et al., Lymphomatous features of aggressive NK cell leukaemia/lymphoma with massive necrosis, haemophagocytosis and EB virus infection. *Histopathology*, 2000. 37(4): p. 363-71.

[23] Akashi, K. and S. Mizuno, Epstein-Barr virus-infected natural killer cell leukemia. *Leuk. Lymphoma*, 2000. 40(1-2): p. 57-66.

[24] Ryder, J., et al., Aggressive natural killer cell leukemia: report of a Chinese series and review of the literature. *Int. J. Hematol.*, 2007. 85(1): p. 18-25.

[25] Makishima, H., et al., Chemokine system and tissue infiltration in aggressive NK-cell leukemia. *Leuk. Res.*, 2007. 31(9): p. 1237-45.

[26] Kwong, Y. L., et al., Large granular lymphocyte leukemia. A study of nine cases in a Chinese population. *Am. J. Clin. Pathol.*, 1995. 103(1): p. 76-81.

[27] Okuda, T., et al., Hemophagocytic syndrome associated with aggressive natural killer cell leukemia. *Am. J. Hematol.*, 1991. 38(4): p. 321-3.

[28] Li, C., et al., Abnormal immunophenotype provides a key diagnostic marker: a report of 29 cases of de novo aggressive natural killer cell leukemia. *Transl. Res.*, 2014. 163(6): p. 565-77.

[29] Lima, M., Aggressive mature natural killer cell neoplasms: from epidemiology to diagnosis. *Orphanet. J. Rare Dis.*, 2013. 8: p. 95.

[30] Morimoto, A., Y. Nakazawa, and E. Ishii, Hemophagocytic lymphohistiocytosis: Pathogenesis, diagnosis, and management. *Pediatr. Int.*, 2016. 58(9): p. 817-25.

[31] Gao, L. M., et al., Aggressive natural killer-cell leukemia with jaundice and spontaneous splenic rupture: a case report and review of the literature. *Diagn. Pathol.*, 2013. 8: p. 43.

[32] Gao, L. M., et al., Clinicopathologic Characterization of Aggressive Natural Killer Cell Leukemia Involving Different Tissue Sites. *Am. J. Surg. Pathol.*, 2016. 40(6): p. 836-46.

[33] Li, Y., et al., Flow Cytometric Immunophenotyping Is Sensitive for the Early Diagnosis of De Novo Aggressive Natural Killer Cell Leukemia (ANKL): A Multicenter Retrospective Analysis. *PLoS One*, 2016. 11(8): p. e0158827.

[34] Suzuki, K., et al., Clinicopathological states of Epstein-Barr virus-associated T/NK-cell lymphoproliferative disorders (severe chronic active EBV infection) of children and young adults. *Int. J. Oncol.*, 2004. 24(5): p. 1165-74.

[35] Lima, M., et al., Aggressive mature natural killer cell neoplasms: report on a series of 12 European patients with emphasis on flow cytometry based immunophenotype and DNA content of neoplastic natural killer cells. *Leuk. Lymphoma*, 2015. 56(1): p. 103-12.

[36] Matano, S., et al., Monomorphic agranular natural killer cell lymphoma/leukemia with no Epstein-Barr virus association. *Acta Haematol.*, 1999. 101(4): p. 206-8.

[37] Park, J. A., et al., Favorable outcome in a child with EBV-negative aggressive NK cell leukemia. *Int. J. Hematol.*, 2013. 97(5): p. 673-6.

[38] Ko, Y. H., et al., Aggressive natural killer cell leukemia: is Epstein-Barr virus negativity an indicator of a favorable prognosis? *Acta Haematol.*, 2008. 120(4): p. 199-206.

[39] Wong, K. F., Zhang, Y. M. and Chan, J. K. Cytogenetic abnormalities in natural killer cell lymphoma/leukaemia--is there a consistent pattern? *Leuk. Lymphoma*, 1999. 34(3-4): p. 241-50.

[40] Siu, L. L., Chan, J. K. and Kwong, Y. L. Natural killer cell malignancies: clinicopathologic and molecular features. *Histol. Histopathol.*, 2002. 17(2): p. 539-54.

[41] Nakashima, Y., et al., Genome-wide array-based comparative genomic hybridization of natural killer cell lymphoma/leukemia: different genomic alteration patterns of aggressive NK-cell leukemia and extranodal Nk/T-cell lymphoma, nasal type. *Genes Chromosomes Cancer*, 2005. 44(3): p. 247-55.

[42] Karube, K., et al., Identification of FOXO3 and PRDM1 as tumor-suppressor gene candidates in NK-cell neoplasms by genomic and functional analyses. *Blood*, 2011. 118(12): p. 3195-204.

[43] Thelander, E. F., et al., Characterization of 6q deletions in mature B cell lymphomas and childhood acute lymphoblastic leukemia. *Leuk. Lymphoma*, 2008. 49(3): p. 477-87.

[44] Karube, K., et al., Lineage-specific growth inhibition of NK cell lines by FOXO3 in association with Akt activation status. *Exp. Hematol.*, 2012. 40(12): p. 1005-1015 e6.

[45] Kucuk, C., et al., HACE1 is a tumor suppressor gene candidate in natural killer cell neoplasms. *Am. J. Pathol.*, 2013. 182(1): p. 49-55.

[46] Sako, N., et al., HACE1, a potential tumor suppressor gene on 6q21, is not involved in extranodal natural killer/T-cell lymphoma pathophysiology. *Am. J. Pathol.*, 2014. 184(11): p. 2899-907.

[47] Morice II, W. G., T-cell and NK-cell large granular lymphocyte proliferations, in *Hematopathology*, Jaffe, E. S. et al., Editors. 2016, Elsevier: Philadelphia, PA. p. 599-607.

[48] Lima, M., et al., Clinicobiological, immunophenotypic, and molecular characteristics of monoclonal CD56-/+dim chronic natural killer cell large granular lymphocytosis. *Am. J. Pathol.*, 2004. 165(4): p. 1117-27.

[49] Morice, W. G., The immunophenotypic attributes of NK cells and NK-cell lineage lymphoproliferative disorders. *Am. J. Clin. Pathol.*, 2007. 127(6): p. 881-6.

[50] Morice, W. G., et al., Chronic lymphoproliferative disorder of natural killer cells: a distinct entity with subtypes correlating with normal natural killer cell subsets. *Leukemia*, 2010. 24(4): p. 881-4.

[51] Morice, W. G., et al., Demonstration of aberrant T-cell and natural killer-cell antigen expression in all cases of granular lymphocytic leukaemia. *Br. J. Haematol.*, 2003. 120(6): p. 1026-36.

[52] Zambello, R., et al., Expression and function of KIR and natural cytotoxicity receptors in NK-type lymphoproliferative diseases of granular lymphocytes. *Blood*, 2003. 102(5): p. 1797-805.

[53] Shi, M., et al., A case of lymphoproliferative disorder of NK-cells: aggressive immunophenotype but indolent behavior. *Clin. Case Rep.*, 2015. 3(9): p. 740-3.

[54] Huang, Q., et al., An aggressive extranodal NK-cell lymphoma arising from indolent NK-cell lymphoproliferative disorder. *Am. J. Surg. Pathol.*, 2005. 29(11): p. 1540-3.

[55] Watters, R. J., Liu, X. and Loughran, T. P. Jr., T-cell and natural killer-cell large granular lymphocyte leukemia neoplasias. *Leuk. Lymphoma*, 2011. 52(12): p. 2217-25.

[56] Chan, J. K., Natural killer cell neoplasms. *Anat. Pathol.*, 1998. 3: p. 77-145.

[57] Swerdlow, S. H., et al., The 2016 revision of the World Health Organization classification of lymphoid neoplasms. *Blood*, 2016. 127(20): p. 2375-90.

[58] Pillai, V., et al., Mature T- and NK-cell non-Hodgkin lymphoma in children and young adolescents. *Br. J. Haematol.*, 2016. 173(4): p. 573-81.

[59] Suzuki, R., Treatment of advanced extranodal NK/T cell lymphoma, nasal-type and aggressive NK-cell leukemia. *Int. J. Hematol.*, 2010. 92(5): p. 697-701.

In: Benign and Malignant Disorders …
Editors: Ling Zhang and Lubomir Sokol

ISBN: 978-1-53612-999-1
© 2018 Nova Science Publishers, Inc.

Chapter 12

CLINICAL MANIFESTATION AND MANAGEMENT OF AGGRESSIVE NATURAL KILLER CELL LEUKEMIA

Emilie Wang, MD[1], Ling Zhang, MD[2] and Lubomir Sokol, MD PhD[3]

[1]Department of Internal Medicine, University of South Florida, Tampa, FL, US

[2]Department of Pathology-hematopathology, H Lee Moffitt Cancer Center, Tampa, FL, US

[3]Division of Hematology-Oncology, H Lee Moffitt Cancer Center, Tampa, FL, US

ABSTRACT

Aggressive natural killer cell leukemia (ANKL) is an Epstein - Barr virus (EBV) associated lymphoid neoplasm which is rarely encountered in Western countries. This disease is associated with a very aggressive clinical course and has poor clinical outcome with survival as short as a few weeks. Clinically, this disease manifests as an acute illness with B symptoms, circulating neoplastic natural killer (NK) cells, cytopenias, organomegaly, coagulopathy, and hemophagocytic lymphohistiocytosis (HLH) often resulting in multiorgan failure. ANKL is usually refractory to conventional chemotherapy therapies. Given its rarity, there are not any standard treatment regimens established. The SMILE protocol including dexamethasone, methotrexate, ifosfamide, L-asparaginase, and etoposide is the most commonly adopted for initial therapy. The pediatric acute lymphoblastic leukemia protocols followed by allogeneic hematopoietic stem cell transplant (allo-HSCT) were attempted and benefited to a subgroup of patients. Novel therapies including pembrolizumab (anti-PD1) or brentuximab vedotin have been tested in a limited number of patients. Improved understanding of the pathobiology of this disease and early diagnosis are critical to improve clinical outcomes of patients with this disease in the future.

Keywords: aggressive natural killer cell leukemia, T cell lymphoma, large granular lymphocytic leukemia

1. INTRODUCTION

Aggressive natural killer cell leukemia (ANKL) is a rare and aggressive lymphoid neoplasm associated with the Epstein - Barr virus [1] and accounts for less than 0.1% of all lymphoid neoplasms [2]. Unlike the indolent chronic lymphoproliferative disorder of NK cells (CLPD-NK), patients with ANKL frequently present with fulminant organ failure due to disseminated intravascular coagulation (DIC), hemophagocytic lymphohistiocytosis (HLH), or direct infiltration with malignant cells leading to death within a few weeks [3]. ANKL has been shown to be generally refractory to most common chemotherapy regimens. However, induction therapy with an intensive acute lymphoblastic leukemia (ALL)-like regimen followed by allogeneic stem cell transplantation has shown better outcomes in a limited number of cases [4, 5].

2. CLINICAL PRESENTATION

ANKL can be further subdivided into EBV positive and EBV negative. In both conditions, ANKL presents as an acute illness with B symptoms, organomegaly, cytopenias, and lymphadenopathy. Most patients present with complaints such as fever, fatigue, easy bruising, and abdominal pain. While anemia and thrombocytopenia are observed in the majority of patients, severe neutropenia is less common. Laboratory workup reveals elevated liver enzymes and lactate dehydrogenase (LDH) levels. Imaging studies show hepatosplenomegaly and occasionally lymphadenopathy. Peripheral blood smears and bone marrow biopsies reveal the presence of normal appearing or atypical large granular lymphocytes [6-10].

The course of ANKL is often complicated with fulminant liver failure, disseminated intravascular coagulopathy, central nervous system (CNS) involvement, and sepsis [11]. Hemorrhagic complications are thought to be associated with either low plasma level of coagulation factors from severe hepatic failure or more likely from consumptive coagulopathy such as DIC due to destructive angioinvasive and necrotic nature of the disease in patients with ANKL [7, 11, 12]. Several case reports have documented the presence of hemorrhagic shock a few days after chemotherapy was initiated due to treatment-induced apoptosis of blood vessels infiltrated with leukemia cells [11]. This vascular destructive behavior may also explain the multiorgan failure which is a commonly observed complication.

2.1. Hemophagocytic Lymphohistiocytosis

ANKL is frequently associated with HLH, a condition which is also frequently triggered by an EBV infection. Since the vast majority of patients with ANKL are EBV positive, it is not uncertain whether EBV or leukemic cells alone trigger this condition. HLH work-up should be included as a part of the initial evaluation. The diagnosis of HLH is based on the HLH 2004 trial, which includes laboratory evaluation of ferritin, soluble CD25, triglycerides and NK cell activity in addition to a bone marrow biopsy and aspiration or involved tissue biopsy. Some patients may initially be misdiagnosed with HLH alone and treated for this condition prior to a final diagnosis of ANKL [13]. Out of six cases of ANKL reported by Nanjing Drum Tower Hospital in China, four patients developed HLH [13]. In addition to the typical presentation of fever, organomegaly, cytopenias, and lymphadenopathy, some patients' clinical course was complicated with acute renal failure and cavitary effusions.

2.2. Coagulopathy

DIC is another frequent complication of ANKL. Coagulation studies including testing for prothrombin time, activated partial thromboplastin time, fibrin degradation products, D-dimer, and peripheral blood schistocytes should also be included in the initial work-up. Due to the fulminant course of this complication, a prompt correction of coagulation abnormalities with fresh frozen plasma, cryoprecipitates, and platelet transfusions with frequent coagulation test monitoring are very important aspects in the management of this aggressive disease.

2.3. Central Nervous System Involvement

Central nervous system (CNS) involvement is not uncommon, especially in patients with relapsed or refractory disease. However, the reports of patients with CNS ANKL are limited [14-16]. In low level of CNS involvement, EBV DNA viral load can be a very helpful diagnostic test. CNS symptoms can be due to HLH in some patients with negative cerebrospinal fluid cytology or flow cytometry.

2.4. Extraocular Muscle Involvement

Case reports have documented ANKL extraocular muscle (EOM) involvement, as a rare feature of the disease [13, 17]. Of note, only 8% of myeloid leukemias and 12% of lymphoid leukemias have orbital involvement with intraocular involvement, far more common than extraocular infiltration. The mechanisms of EOM infiltration by leukemia including ANKL are not well understood. Kincaid and Green reported that EOM was identified in only 1.3% of leukemia patients per autopsy [18]. Most frequently orbital involvement is thought to be due to its proximity to the bone marrow density located in the greater wing of the sphenoid and zygoma. However, another theory suggested that leukemic cell infiltration via the ophthalmic artery might seed the EOM [19].

Because of varied clinical presentations of ANKL, a rapid and early diagnosis of EOM involvement might be difficult. Unfortunately, for most patients, ANKL is a catastrophic disease that almost always leads death in a short period of time.

3. DIAGNOSTIC TESTS

The diagnostic workup of this disease is described more extensively in Chapter 11. Briefly, diagnostic tests such as complete blood count and differential, comprehensive metabolic panel, EBV viral load, computer axial tomography imaging of the chest, abdomen and pelvis, bone marrow biopsy, or biopsy of the involved tissue with hemopathology review and immunotyping are essential (Table 1). The priority is to examine circulating atypical lymphoid cells and submit the specimen for flow cytometry study using appropriate parameters including CD2, surface CD3, cytoplasmic CD3, CD5, CD7, CD8, TCR-αβ and -γδ, CD25, CD30, CD20, CD16, CD56, and CD57 in order to differentiate ANKL and other T/NK cell lymphoproliferative disorders. Typical immunophenotype of ANKL cells is an absence of surface CD3 antigen and positive for CD2, cytoplasmic CD3ε and strongly positive for CD56 expression [6, 10, 20]. A combination of fine needle aspiration (FNA) and core biopsy of the spleen or liver with immunohistochemistry, flow cytometry, and fluorescence in situ hybridization (FISH) for common translocations may be optimal for diagnosis. Hematopathology review of all histopathology slides prepared from the paraffin blocks is also extremely important, and rebiopsy is often required if the biopsy sample is non-diagnostic. Cytoplasmic CD3ε, CD56, cytotoxic markers (e.g., TIA, grazyme B and perforin) immunohistochemical (IHC) staining and, of importance, EBER-ISH (in situ hybridization) for detection of EBV infection should be included in the diagnostic panel [10, 21, 22].

Table 1. Diagnosis and work up of ANKL per NCCN guidelines

Diagnosis	*Essential Tests* -Hematopathology review with at least one paraffin block representative of tumor. -Excisional or incisional biopsy preferred -For tumors not easily accessible, consider FNA and core biopsy with: 　-Immunohistochemistry 　-Flow cytometry 　-PCR for T-cell receptor gene rearrangements 　-FISH for common translocations -cCD3ε, CD56, EBER-ISH included in an IHC panel
Workup	*Essential Evaluations* -History and physical exam including symptoms and performance status -Lab Tests 　-CBC/Differential 　-CMP 　-LDH 　-Uric acid 　-EBV viral load -Bone marrow biopsy -CT abdomen/pelvis with contrast

CBC: complete blood count, CMP: comprehensive metabolic panel, LDH: lactate dehydrogenase, ISH: In situ hybridization, IHC: immunohistochemical stain.

4. TREATMENT OF ANKL

A variety of chemotherapy regimens have been utilized in ANKL. However, no standard treatment approach has been established. Since ANKL cells express P-glycoprotein, a transmembrane efflux pump encoded by the multidrug resistance 1 gene, conventional chemotherapy regimens such as CHOP (cyclophosphamide, doxorubicin, vincristine, and prednisone) are not effective in most cases [23]. Agents such as methotrexate and L-asparaginase, not affected by P-glycoprotein, have been more successful in treatment [24, 25]. After achieving remission with initial induction chemotherapy, consolidation with allogeneic hematopoietic cell transplantation should be considered as demonstrated in selected patients with ANKL [26, 27]. The outcome of transplant depends on the disease response prior to transplant. Generally, patients in complete remission do significantly better than patients with partial response.

Suzuki et al., reported that 3 out of 13 patients achieved complete remission with an anthracycline based regimen compared to 0 out of 8 patients who did not receive an anthracycline [28]. Interestingly, anthracyclines such as doxorubicin may not be the best option as P-glycoproteins found on NK cells have a molecular weight between 70 to 80 kDa compared to the classic 170 kDa P-glycoprotein. The smaller weight of NK P-glycoproteins does not allow transport of anthracycline into the cancer cells [29]. More investigation must be conducted to evaluate the efficacy of distinct anthracycline containing regimens in ANKL.

Another chemotherapy agent that has been studied is L-asparaginase [30, 31]. Jung et al., compared the response of dexamethasone, methotrexate, ifosfamide, L-asparaginase, and etoposide (SMILE) against etoposide, ifosfamide, dexamethasone, and L-asparaginase (VIDL). Out of the 13 patients who underwent therapy with SMILE as the first line chemotherapy, 5 had complete or partial response. Five patients received VIDL, two of which had complete response. Additionally, the overall response rate of all patients enrolled in the trial was 33% while the median progression free survival and median overall survival (OS) was 3.9 and 7.0 months respectively [32]. Despite its promising potential, L-asparaginase may be difficult to administer for those patients with hepatic failure.

Due to the rarity of ANKL, very few prospective studies have been conducted and recommendations for treatment with SMILE regimen are derived from observations of cases with extranodal NK/T cell lymphoma, nasal type (ENKL) [2]. Despite genetic differences, ANKL and advanced-stage ENKL share many similarities including responsiveness to chemotherapy and prognosis [33]. Yamaguchi and colleagues have conducted both a phase I and phase II study assessing the efficacy of SMILE in ENKL patients (Table 2). While the results of the phase II study were encouraging with an overall response rate (ORR) of 79% (90% CI, 65% to 89%), the majority of patients were observed to have grade 4 neutropenia (92%) [30]. Given the poor bone marrow function in patients with ANKL, elderly patients (more than 65 years of age) with organ impairment frequently do not tolerate the high intensity SMILE regimen. Therefore, the committee of NK-cell Tumor Study Group recommends to start therapy with L-asparaginase and steroids and then with dose reduced chemotherapy such as SMILE (Figure 1).

Pembrolizumab, an anti-programmed death 1 (PD1) antibody, has recently been shown as a potential salvage therapy in patients with relapsed/refractory ANKL who were previously treated with L-asparaginase based regimens. In a small case series of 7 patients with NK/T-cell lymphoma who failed a median of 2 regimens, including those with L-asparaginase and allogenic stem cell transplant, all patients responded, based on clinical, radiologic, morphologic, and molecular (circulating EBV DNA) criteria. Five patients achieved complete remission (CR) and remained in CR after a median follow up of 6 months. These patients received a median of 7 cycles of pembrolizumab [34].

Another treatment option with promising results is the combination of brentuximab vedotin with bendamustine. Several mature subtypes of T and B cell lymphomas express CD30 antigen, the therapeutic target of the anti-CD30 antibody-drug-conjugate brentuximab vedotin. A case report described a 17-year-old female diagnosed with abdominal NK/T-cell lymphoma that was initially treated with an L-asparaginase based regimen (gemcitabine, cisplastin, ifosfamide, etoposide, and dexamethasone). Despite initial response, the patient unfortunately relapsed and subsequently underwent salvage therapy with brentuximab vedotin and bendamustine. After 3 cycles of treatment, the patient achieved CR and subsequently underwent allogeneic transplant and remained disease free 5 months post-transplant [35].

Given the relatively young age of ANKL patients, consolidation therapy with HSCT should be explored after complete remission is achieved. A study conducted by the NK Tumor Study Group evaluated the overall survival of 40 transplanted patients with NK neoplasm, which included NK precursor acute leukemia (n=4), blastic NK cell lymphoma (n=11), aggressive NK cell leukemia (n=3), and nasal-type extranodal NK-cell lymphoma (n=22). Twenty-five patients received autologous transplant and fifteen received an allograft. Of these, one patient with ANKL underwent autologous transplant and two ANKL patients underwent allogenic transplant. The patient who underwent autologous ANKL survived 16 months after transplant, while the allogenic transplant candidates passed away an average of 6 months post transplant. Out of the 40 patients with NK neoplasms, the overall 4-year survival was 39% for all transplanted patients with a median follow up of 50 months compared to 21% of individuals who did not have transplant. The 4-year overall survival was 68% for those who were in complete remission prior to transplant, significantly better compared to those who achieved remission but did not undergo transplant [26].

The largest report of transplant outcomes in ANKL was recently published using the International Blood and Marrow Transplant Research database [36]. This study included twenty-one patients with ANKL from nineteen sites, of whom fourteen were in CR at the time of alloHSCT. Although ANKL is more prevalent among Asians, the majority of patients in this study were Caucasians (71%). The majority of patients were treated with L-asparaginase containing regimen prior to transplant. Two year progression free survival (PFS) and OS were 20% and 24%, respectively with medium follow up of 25 months. Additionally, nonrelapse mortality at 2 years was 21% with reported relapse/progression of 59% [36]. Patients who achieved CR prior to transplant had a significantly improved PFS compared to those who had active disease at time of transplant (30% vs. 0%, $p = 0.001$) [36]. This study highlights the important role of alloHSCT in achieving a durable response in patients with ANKL in CR prior to transplant.

Supportive care strategies are an essential component of treatment approaches for these patients. Due to the high incidence of DIC as described earlier in this chapter, transfusions with coagulation factors such as fresh frozen plasma, fibrinogen, and platelets as critically important to prevent hemorrhagic complications [11]. Administration of steroids prior and following chemotherapy may improve hepatic function. While there is limited data regarding the optimal therapeutic strategy for these patients, recent developments in immunotherapy such as pembrolizumab are promising.

Table 2. Summary of clinical trials in ANKL

Study	Dx	N	Therapy	ORR	CR	PFS	OS	Reference
L-asparaginase based regimen (VIDL, SMILE)	ANKL	21	VIDL (24%); SMILE 1st line (62%), 2nd line (14%)	VIDL: 40% SMILE: 38% Overall: 33%	NA	3.9 mo	7.0 mo	[32]
Phase I SMILE	ENKL	6	SMILE	67%	50%	NA	NA	[31]
Phase II SMILE	ENKL	38	SMILE	79%	45%	NA	55%	[30]
HSCT (allo/auto) vs nontransplant	NK neoplasms	228	HSCT	NA	NA	NA	4 yr survival: HSCT 39% No HSCT 21%	[26]
Allogenic HSCT	ANKL	21	AlloHSCT	NA	NA	20%	24%	[36]
Pembrolizumab	ENKL	7	Pembrolizumab salvage therapy after failed L-asparaginase regimen	NA	71%	NA	NA	[34]
Brentuximab vedotin/ Bendamustine	ENKL	1	Brentuximab vedotin/Bendamustine salvage therapy after L-asparaginase based regimen	NA	100%	NA	NA	[35]

Dx: diagnosis, ORR: objective response rate, CR: complete remission, PFS: progression free survival, OS: overall survival.

5. PROGNOSIS OF ANKL

The prognosis of advanced stage ANKL is overall very poor despite the use of multiagent chemotherapy. Currently, the median survival ranges between 2 and 6 months [28]. Unfortunately, some patients expire from hemorrhagic complications several days after treatment initiation [11]. Others have had shown a long-term remission after chemotherapy and hematopoietic cell transplantation [26, 36].

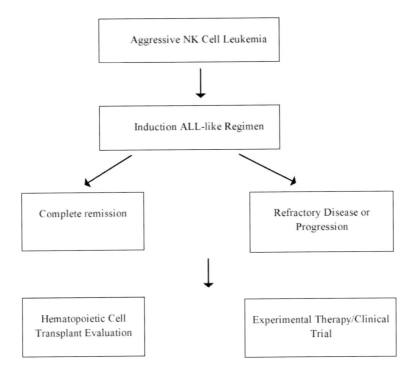

Figure 1. Therapeutic algorithm of ANKL.

Since EBV negative cases of ANKL are rare, there is limited data on overall prognosis in this population. Some reports have suggested that EBV negative ANKL has a less aggressive course compared to the EBV positive disease with survival rates ranging from 11 months to 4 years [37, 38]. However, more recently there have been case reports that disputed this claim [28, 39]. In a recent report of seven EBV negative ANKL patients by Nicolae and colleagues, the median survival was 8 weeks which is comparable with the reported median survival in the EBV positive counterparts [39]. The longer survival rates of EBV negative ANKL are thought to be due to the lack of up regulation of multidrug resistance genes associated with EBV which leads to improved response to chemotherapy and overall survival [40, 41].

CONCLUSION

ANKL is an aggressive, frequently EBV-associated, lymphoid malignancy with fulminant clinical course,. Despite advances in chemotherapy, immunotherapy and hematopoietic stem cell transplant, this disease is incurable in the majority of patients. An improved understanding of the pathobiology of this disease along with early diagnosis and therapeutic interventions are necessary to significantly change clinical outcomes of patients with this aggressive disease.

REFERENCES

[1] Hart, D. N., Baker, B. W., Inglis, M. J., et al. Epstein-Barr viral DNA in acute large granular lymphocyte (natural killer) leukemic cells. *Blood.* 1992;79(8):2116-2123.

[2] Suzuki, R. Treatment of advanced extranodal NK/T cell lymphoma, nasal-type and aggressive NK-cell leukemia. *Int. J. Hematol.* 2010;92(5):697-701.

[3] Han, A. R., Lee, H. R., Park, B. B., et al. Lymphoma-associated hemophagocytic syndrome: clinical features and treatment outcome. *Ann. Hematol.* 2007;86(7):493-498.

[4] Ebihara, Y., Manabe, A., Tanaka, R., et al. Successful treatment of natural killer (NK) cell leukemia following a long-standing chronic active Epstein-Barr virus (CAEBV) infection with allogeneic bone marrow transplantation. *Bone Marrow Transplant.* 2003;31(12):1169-1171.

[5] Okamura, T., Kishimoto, T., Inoue, M., et al. Unrelated bone marrow transplantation for Epstein-Barr virus-associated T/NK-cell lymphoproliferative disease. *Bone Marrow Transplant.* 2003;31(2):105-111.

[6] Ruskova, A., Thula, R., Chan, G. Aggressive Natural Killer-Cell Leukemia: report of five cases and review of the literature. *Leuk. Lymphoma.* 2004;45(12):2427-2438.

[7] Kwong, Y. L., Wong, K. F., Chan, L. C., et al. Large granular lymphocyte leukemia. A study of nine cases in a Chinese population. *Am. J. Clin. Pathol.* 1995;103(1):76-81.

[8] Imamura, N., Kusunoki, Y., Kawa-Ha, K., et al. Aggressive natural killer cell leukaemia/lymphoma: report of four cases and review of the literature. Possible existence of a new clinical entity originating from the third lineage of lymphoid cells. *Br. J. Haematol.* 1990;75(1):49-59.

[9] Chan, J. K. Natural killer cell neoplasms. *Anat. Pathol.* 1998;3:77-145.

[10] Chan JKC, Jaffe ES, Ra;floaer E, Lp YO. Aggressive NK cell leukemia. In: press W, ed. *WHO classification of tumours of Haematopoietic and lymphoid tissues*. Lyon, France: IARC:276.

[11] Okuno, Y., Tatetsu, H., Nosaka, K., Mitsuya, H. Three cases of aggressive natural killer cell leukemia with a lethal hemorrhagic complication. *J. Clin. Exp. Hematop.* 2012;52(2):101-106.

[12] Quintanilla-Martinez, L., Jaffe, E. S. Commentary: aggressive NK cell lymphomas: insights into the spectrum of NK cell derived malignancies. *Histopathology.* 2000;37(4):372-374.

[13] Zhang, Q., Jing, W., Ouyang, J., Zeng, H., George, S. K., Liu, Z. Six cases of aggressive natural killer-cell leukemia in a Chinese population. *International journal of clinical and experimental pathology.* 2014;7(6):3423-3431.

[14] Ichikawa, S., Fukuhara, N., Yamamoto, J., et al. Successful allogeneic hematopoietic stem cell transplantation for aggressive NK cell leukemia. *Intern. Med.* 2010;49(17):1907-1910.

[15] Nichols, G. E., Normansell, D. E., Williams, M. E. Lymphoproliferative disorder of granular lymphocytes: nine cases including one with features of CD56 (NKH1)-positive aggressive natural killer cell lymphoma. *Mod. Pathol.* 1994;7(8):819-824.

[16] Wong, K. F., Chan, J. K., Ma, S. K., Lai, K. Y. Aggressive pleomorphic CD2+, CD3-, CD56+ lymphoma with t(5;9)(q31;q34) abnormality. *Cancer Genet. Cytogenet.* 1995;82(1):73-75.

[17] Kiratli, H., Balci, K. E., Himmetoglu, C., Uner, A. Isolated extraocular muscle involvement as the ophthalmic manifestation of leukaemia. *Clin. Exp. Ophthalmol.* 2009; 37(6):609-613.

[18] Kincaid, M. C., Green, W. R. Ocular and orbital involvement in leukemia. *Surv. Ophthalmol.* 1983;27(4):211-232.

[19] Aydin, A., Cakir, A., Ersanli, D. Isolated extraocular muscle involvement as the ophthalmic manifestation of leukaemia: an alternative explanation. *Clin. Exp. Ophthalmol.* 2010;38(6):651.

[20] Sokol, L., Loughran, T. P., Jr. Large granular lymphocyte leukemia. *Oncologist.* 2006;11(3):263-273.

[21] *National Comprehensive Cancer Network.* T-Cell Lymphomas. https://www.nccn.org/professionals/physician_gls/pdf/t-cell.pdf. Accessed August 17, 2017.

[22] Morice, W. G., Kurtin, P. J., Leibson, P. J., Tefferi, A., Hanson, C. A. Demonstration of aberrant T-cell and natural killer-cell antigen expression in all cases of granular lymphocytic leukaemia. *Br. J. Haematol.* 2003;120(6):1026-1036.

[23] Egashira, M., Kawamata, N., Sugimoto, K., Kaneko, T., Oshimi, K. P-glycoprotein expression on normal and abnormally expanded natural killer cells and inhibition of P-glycoprotein function by cyclosporin A and its analogue, PSC833. *Blood.* 1999;93(2):599-606.

[24] Ishida, F., Ko, Y. H., Kim, W. S., et al. Aggressive natural killer cell leukemia: therapeutic potential of L-asparaginase and allogeneic hematopoietic stem cell transplantation. *Cancer Sci.* 2012;103(6):1079-1083.

[25] Tse, E., Kwong, Y. L. How, I. treat NK/T-cell lymphomas. *Blood.* 2013;121(25):4997-5005.

[26] Suzuki, R., Suzumiya, J., Nakamura, S., et al. Hematopoietic stem cell transplantation for natural killer-cell lineage neoplasms. *Bone Marrow Transplant.* 2006;37(4):425-431.

[27] Ito, T., Makishima, H., Nakazawa, H., et al. Promising approach for aggressive NK cell leukaemia with allogeneic haematopoietic cell transplantation. *Eur. J. Haematol.* 2008;81(2):107-111.

[28] Suzuki, R., Suzumiya, J., Nakamura, S., et al. Aggressive natural killer-cell leukemia revisited: large granular lymphocyte leukemia of cytotoxic NK cells. *Leukemia.* 2004;18(4):763-770.

[29] Trambas, C., Wang, Z., Cianfriglia, M., Woods, G. Evidence that natural killer cells express mini P-glycoproteins but not classic 170 kDa P-glycoprotein. *Br. J. Haematol.* 2001;114(1):177-184.

[30] Yamaguchi, M., Kwong, Y. L., Kim, W. S., et al. Phase II study of SMILE chemotherapy for newly diagnosed stage IV, relapsed, or refractory extranodal natural killer (NK)/T-cell lymphoma, nasal type: the NK-Cell Tumor Study Group study. *J. Clin. Oncol.* 2011;29(33):4410-4416.

[31] Yamaguchi, M., Suzuki, R., Kwong, Y. L., et al. Phase I study of dexamethasone, methotrexate, ifosfamide, L-asparaginase, and etoposide (SMILE) chemotherapy for advanced-stage, relapsed or refractory extranodal natural killer (NK)/T-cell lymphoma and leukemia. *Cancer Sci.* 2008;99(5):1016-1020.

[32] Jung, K. S., Cho, S. H., Kim, S. J., Ko, Y. H., Kang, E. S., Kim, W. S. L-asparaginase-based regimens followed by allogeneic hematopoietic stem cell transplantation improve outcomes in aggressive natural killer cell leukemia. *J. Hematol. Oncol.* 2016;9:41.

[33] Nakashima, Y., Tagawa, H., Suzuki, R., et al. Genome-wide array-based comparative genomic hybridization of natural killer cell lymphoma/leukemia: different genomic alteration patterns of aggressive NK-cell leukemia and extranodal Nk/T-cell lymphoma, nasal type. *Genes, chromosomes & cancer.* 2005;44(3):247-255.

[34] Kwong, Y. L., Chan, T. S. Y., Tan, D., et al. PD1 blockade with pembrolizumab is highly effective in relapsed or refractory NK/T-cell lymphoma failing l-asparaginase. *Blood.* 2017;129(17):2437-2442.

[35] Poon, L. M., Kwong, Y. L. Complete remission of refractory disseminated NK/T cell lymphoma with brentuximab vedotin and bendamustine. *Ann. Hematol.* 2016;95(5):847-849.

[36] Hamadani, M., Kanate, A. S., DiGilio, A., et al. Allogeneic Hematopoietic Cell Transplantation for Aggressive NK Cell Leukemia. A Center for International Blood and Marrow Transplant Research Analysis. *Biol Blood Marrow Transplant.* 2017;23(5):853-856.

[37] Matano, S., Nakamura, S., Nakamura, S., et al. Monomorphic agranular natural killer cell lymphoma/leukemia with no Epstein-Barr virus association. *Acta Haematol.* 1999;101(4):206-208.

[38] Osuji, N., Matutes, E., Morilla, A., Del Giudice, I., Wotherspoon, A., Catovsky, D. Prolonged treatment response in aggressive natural killer cell leukemia. *Leuk. Lymphoma.* 2005;46(5):757-763.

[39] Nicolae, A., Ganapathi, K. A., Pham, T. H., et al. EBV-negative Aggressive NK-cell Leukemia/Lymphoma: Clinical, Pathologic, and Genetic Features. *Am. J. Surg. Pathol.* 2017;41(1):67-74.

[40] Kim, J. H., Kim, W. S., Park, C. SNARK, a novel downstream molecule of EBV latent membrane protein 1, is associated with resistance to cancer cell death. *Leuk. Lymphoma.* 2008;49(7):1392-1398.

[41] Ko, Y. H,. Park, S., Kim, K., Kim, S. J., Kim, W. S. Aggressive natural killer cell leukemia: is Epstein-Barr virus negativity an indicator of a favorable prognosis? *Acta Haematol.* 2008;120(4):199-206.

In: Benign and Malignant Disorders …
Editors: Ling Zhang and Lubomir Sokol

ISBN: 978-1-53612-999-1
© 2018 Nova Science Publishers, Inc.

Chapter 13

NATURAL KILLER CELL DYSFUNCTION IN PRIMARY AND ACQUIRED HEMOPHAGOCYTIC LYMPHOHISTIOCYTOSIS

*Seongseok Yun[1] and Ling Zhang[2],**
[1]Department of Hematology and Oncology and
[2]Department of Hematopathology and Laboratory Medicine,
H. Lee Moffitt Cancer Center and Research Institutue, Tampa, FL, US

ABSTRACT

Hemophagocytic lymphohistiocytosis (HLH) is a rare but life threatening disease that affects individuals of different age and ethnic background and clinically characterized by profound cytopenias, fever, hepatosplenomegly, and hemophagocytosis in bone marrow and other tissues, occuring either as a familial disorder or in association with a variety of conditions including infection, malignancy, autoimmunity, immune deficiency or compromised status or metabolic disease. Dysregulations of cytotoxic T-cells and natural killer (NK) cells were shown to play a pirvotal role in familial HLH development, which is mainly attributed to several gene mutations (PRF1 (Perforin 1/Pore forming protein-1), UNC13D (Protein unc-13 Homolog D), Munc18-2 (mammalian uncoordinated 18-2), Rab27a (Ras-related protein Rab27a), *STX11* (Syntaxin 11), SH2D1A (SH2 domain containing 1A), or BIRC4 (Baculoviral IAP repeat containing protein 4)) that are related to NK and T-cell granule-mediated cytotoxic function. Nevertheless, the exact pathogenesis of NK-cells in acquired HLH has been poorly understood. The book chapter will summarize clinicopathologic characteristics of HLH with a focus on the genetic alterations in familial HLH that are related to NK cell defects as well as the potential mechanisms of NK cell dysfunctions in acquired HLH.

---

* Corresponding Author address Email:Ling.Zhang@moffitt.org.

Keywords: hemophagocytic lymphohistiocytosis (HLH), NK-cell

1. INTRODUCTION

Hemophagocytic lymphohistiocytosis (HLH) is a rare disorder characterized by clinical findings such as fever, splenomegaly, profound cytopenia, and hemophagocytosis in the bone marrow, lymph node, spleen or extranodal lymphoid tissues. Because of its first description as histiocytic medullary reticulosis in 1939, HLH was thought to be from neoplastic proliferation of histiocytes [1]. Potential familial linkage of HLH was first described by Farquhar JW and Claireaux AF in 1952 [2]. A case of simultaneous development of HLH in both father and son reported in 1965 suggested that HLH could be associated with infectious etiology [3]. Since then, HLH was shown to be associated with a variety of pathologic conditions including autoimmune diseases, immune deficient or compromised status, malignancies, infections, genetic defect, and NK-cell dysfunction, leading to macrophage activation, hypercytokinemia, and eventually multiple organ failure. Based on potentially differences in pathogenesis, clinically, HLH is subcategorized into primary HLH and acquired HLH. For genetic HLH, it can further subgrouped into two: familial HLH (FHLH) and immune deficiencies. The latter mainly encompasses Griscelli syndrome, Chediak-Higashi syndrome, Hermansky-Pudlak syndrome, Wiskott-Aldrich syndrome, severe combined immunodeficiency, lysinuric protein intolerance as well as X-linked lymphoproliferative syndromes. To date HLH is widely accepted as a life threatening disorder secondary to uncontrolled hypercytokine surfing from hyperinflammatory response to various kinds of reactive or neoplastic state.

2. EPIDEMOLOGY

HLH is an extremely rare disorder with variable incidence rates (1 out of every 3000-800,000) depending on region and age [4]. According to prior two studies in pediatric patients, the incidence of HLH were reportedly 1 to 225 per 300 000 live births [5, 6]. Of note, 25% of pediatric cases are familial HLH whereas most of the adult onset HLH belong to secondary HLH [7]. In familial HLH, approximately 75-80% of cases present at younger age (<1 year old) [7]. The incidence of acquired HLH is difficult to be estimated given its rarity. Regardless of familial or acquired HLH, there is no predilection for race or gender [7, 8].

3. PATHOGENESIS

The exact mechanisms of HLH are still illusive. However, a defect of NK-cells has been proved in a subset of pediatric patients with familiar HLH who have genetic syndromes resulting in immune dysfunction. NK-cell malfunction has been documented in many types of malignancies, immune deficiency or compromised status, certain metabolic diseases [9-11]. Whether there is a direct link between dysfunctional NK-cells and susceptibility to develop acquired HLH is unclear. Also, the underlying mechanism for the frequent association of acquired HLH with certain T-/NK-cell lymphomas e.g., primary cutaneous γδ T-cell lymphoma and aggressive NK-cell leukemia is currently under investigation.

3.1. NK-Cell Dysfunction

NK-cell plays an essential role in the elimination of infected or tumor cells by secretion of perforin, granzymes and cytokine [9-12]. Activated NK-cells form immunological synapse with targets cells. Once granules are released, perforin permeabilizes the target cell membrane and induces caspase dependent cell death [12, 13]. Any defect in the cytolytic pathway in the NK-cell can lead to compromise of host defense system and immune surveillance escape of infected or malignant cells. In the preclinical models, cytotoxic deficient mice (*PRF1*, *STX11*, *Rab27a*, *LYST*, and *UNC13D*) were shown to develop a HLH like syndrome when they were infected with lymphocytic choriomeningitis virus (LCMV) [14-20]. Experimental studies have shown that the aberrant interaction of NK-cells with cytotoxic T-cells and histiocytes play an important role in HLH pathogenesis [21-23]. Growing evidence suggest that NK-cells regulates the differentiation and activation of cytotoxic CD8 T-cell response in perforin dependent mechanisms [24]. Cytotoic T-cells were shown to escape NK-cell surveillance by overexpression of MHC-I inhibitory NK ligands and downregulation of activating NK receptor ligands [25, 26]. In a recent study, *in vivo* depletion of cytotoxic proficient NK-cells was shown to be sufficient to induce HLH like syndrome, re-emphasizing the role of NK-cells cytotoxicity to prevent HLH development [27]. Abnormally active T-cells release proinflammatory cytokines such as tumor necrosis factor alpha (TNFα), interferon gamma (IFNγ), interleukin (IL)-1b, IL-2, IL-6, IL-8, IL-10, IL-12, and IL-18, further activating cytotoxic T-cells and histiocytes [28, 29]. Once the cytokine storm occurs, it is difficult to stop it without therapeutic intervention or even with appropriate treatment. The release of the cytokines as inflammatory mediators leads to systemic inflammatory response syndrome or HLH which can be complicated with adult reparatory distress syndrome, sepsis, or multi-organ failure, etc.

3.1.A. Primary HLH

13.3.1A-a Familial HLH: Familial HLH is defined as disease with obvious genetic causes or familial inheritance. Familial HLH patients typically present in their younger age although cases of late onset had been reported [7]. NK-cell dysfunction is observed in the particular settings. Typically, perforin gene mutation or mutations in genes that are involved in the biogenesis or transport of vesicles in NK-cells causes familial HLH [30-33]. There are five subtypes in familial HLH (Table 1). Approximately 10% familial HLH is subgrouped as type 1 and *HPLH1* (Hemophagocytic Lymphohistiocytosis 1) genes located at chromosome 9q [34]. However, specific genes and their mutations causing type 1 familial HLH are unknown. In type 2, about 20-40% of cases have *PRF1* mutation, which encodes a soluble pore-forming protein (perforin) that is normally stored in the cytotoxic T-lymphocytes (CTLs) and NK-cells. After stimulation, degranulation occurs in CTLs and NK-cells, which allows perforin to be released into cellular synapse to bind on targeted cells and form pores through oligomerization of calcium channel. Perforin, together with granzyme B, a serine protease, results in apoptosis of target cells [35]. In addition, *PRF2* mutation can cause impairment of perforin, preventing granzymes from getting into target cells (Figure 1). Approximately 10-20% of type 3 familial HLH patients harbor *UNC13D* gene mutations, which encodes unc-13 homolog D or Munc13-4 proteins (Figure 1) [16, 36-38]. This protein was shown to play a pivotal role in cytotoxic granule exocytosis [37]. There was no defect in lytic granule polarization or formation of immunological synapse in the type 3 familial HLH patients, however the cytokine release including IFN-γ was decreased, suggesting that Munc13-4 regulate the exocytosis of the granule (Figure 1) [37]. Complementation of Munc13-4 fully restored the cytotoxic activity of HLH patients' cells, further supporting the role of Munc13-4 in granular exocytosis [37].

In type 4, *STX11* gene mutations are found in 10-20% of cases. *STX11* protein binds to SNAP23 in NK-cells, facilitating endocytosis and excocytosis (Figure 1). Therefore, mutations in *STX11* gene impair NK-cell function. In type 5, *STXBP2* mutation has been described. *STXBP2* encodes Munc18-2 protein that is involved in intracellular trafficking and release of cytotoxic granules from NK-cells. In most of the primary HLH cases, there are concurrent medical conditions that seem to trigger HLH such as viral infection, autoimmune disorder, or underlying neoplastic disorders (discussed in the later sections). Thus, it is clinically difficult to make a diagnosis of primary vs. secondary HLH at the initial presentation, and extensive search for the underlying triggers should be performed [39].

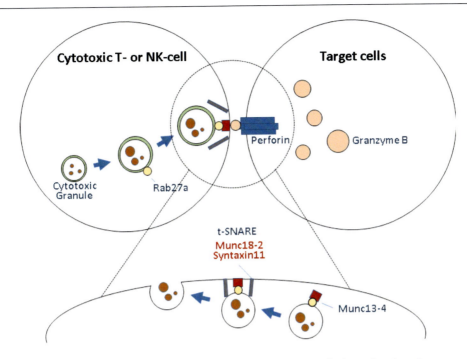

Figure 1. HLH-associated genetic abnormalities are involved in granule dependent lympho-cytotoxicity, impairing membranous fusion of granules, docking of effector cells to target cells, and trafficking of granules.

Table 1. Subtypes of primary or genetic HLH

Subtype	Gene and Locus
Familial HLH	
Type 1:	*HPLH1*, 9q21.3-q22
Type 2	*PRF1*, 10q21-22
Type3:	*Munc13-4/UNC13D*, 17q25
Type 4:	*STX11*, 6q24.1
Type 5	*STXBP2*, 19p13.3-13.2
Immune deficiency syndrome	
Chediak-Higashi syndrome	*LYST*, 1q42.1-q42.2
Griscelli syndrome	15q21
Hermansky-Pudiak syndrome	*HPS6*, 10q24.32
X-linked lymphoproliferative syndrome Type 1	*SH2D1A (SAP)*, Xq25
X-linked lymphoproliferative syndrome Type 2	*BIRC4 (XIAP)*, Xq25
Wiskott-Aldrich syndrome	*WAS*, Xp11.4-p11.21
Severe combined immunodeficiency	*IL2RG*, Xq13.1
Lysinuric protein intolerance:	*SLC7A7*, 14q1.2

13.3.1A-b Immune deficiency syndrome: Number of immune deficiency syndromes including Chediak-Higashi syndrome, Griscelli syndrome, X-linked lymphoproliferative syndrome, Wiskott-Aldrich syndrome, severe combined immunodeficiency, lysinuric protein intolerance, and Hermansky-Pudlak syndrome predispose patients to HLH [40] (Table 2). Griscelli syndrome [41-44], Chediak-Higash syndrome [45, 46], and Hermansky-Pudlak syndrome [47-50] are inherited in an autosomal recessive manner. The common clinical and laboratory findings of these syndromes include oculocutaneous albinism and impaired cytotoxic T- and NK-cells, leading to immune deficiency and susceptibility to infection [40].

Griscellin syndrome (GS): GS is an autosomal recessive disordered characterized by albinism, silvery gray hair, neurologic abnormality, and immunodeficiency. Two genetic deficiencies have been identified; *Rab27a* and myosin VA (*MYO-VA*). Since these proteins are colocalized in the melanosome, their genetic defects result in abnormal distribution of melanosome observed in GS patients [51]. Consistently, expression of Rab27a in the GS melanocytes restored the normal phenotype including melanosome transport to the dendritic tips [51]. Of importance, Rab27a protein binds to Munc13-4 proteins when perforin containing granules to interact with target cell membrane [41-44, 52, 53]. Thus, *RAB27A* mutation associated GS is characterized by defective cytotoxic T- and NK-cell activity, leading to lymphoproliferative syndrome including HLH and macrophage activation syndrome [41-44, 52].

Chediak–Higashi syndrome (CHS): CHS is an autosomal recessive disease that is clinically characterized by oculocutaneous albinism and frequent development of HLH in approximately 80% of such patients [45, 46]. Per clinical observation, a subset of CHS patients does not develop HLH. *LYST*, also named CHS1, gene, is located at 1q42.1-q42.2 and functions as the lysosomal trafficking regulator, transporting or trafficking materials into cytoplasmic lysosomes [54]. Studies have shown that the risk of HLH in the group of CHS patients depends upon the presence of *LYST* gene mutation [54]. Biallelic mutation in *LYST* geneimpairs degranulation, leading to hypergranulated cells including NK-cells with enlarged lysosomesin the patients with CHS [54]. Site and pattern of *LYST* mutations will determine whether HLH is developed. In an animal model, a splice-site frameshift mutation in intron 27 of *LYST* in souris mice resulted in HLH induced by LCMV (lymphocytic choriomeningitis virus) infection [19]. In a different model using beige mice, a 3-nucleotide in-frame deletion at the C-terminal encoding region of *LYST* was created. However, HLH did not occur upon similar infection [55]. Jessen's study also proved that T-/NK-cell cytotoxic function was more severely and uniformly compromised in the mouse model while only subtle changes were noted in patients who later or never have HLH [19]. Although that study did not find clear genotype-phenotype correlations, other clinical studies have suggested genotype-phenotype correlations that may explain CHS severity [56] and presumably also related to the onset of HLH as well.

Hermansky-Pudlak syndrome (HPS) type 2: HPS is a rare autosomal recessive disease associated with neutropenia, thrombocytopenia, hypopigmentation, granulomatous colitis, splenomegaly, bleeding disorder, and developmental delay [57, 58]. Mutations in the β3A subunit of adaptor protein 3 complex (AP3) was shown to cause lysosomal trafficking dysregulation [59, 60] and homozygous exon 15 deletion in *AP3B1* gene had been identified in HPS patients as well [57]. Preclinical and clinical studies showed that AP3 deficiency results in defect of T- and NK-cell cytotoxicity secondary to degranulation of perforin containing lytic granules [61-63], and cases of HLH in HPS type 2 patients had been reported [19, 59, 60, 62-66]. In a recent study using *Pearl* mouse model carrying a tandem duplication in the *AP3B1* gene resulting in truncation mutation, AP3B1 deficiency was shown to mimic the phenotypes of HPS patients and to induce degranulation defect in the cytotoxic T- and NK-cell leading to impaired cytotoxicity [66]. In an additional experiment, *Pearl* mice developed HLH when infected with LCMV although the mice spontaneously recovered from HLH without any treatment [66] of uncertain mechanism. Collectively, preclinical and clinical evidences suggest that defect in cytotoxic T- and NK-cell can predispose HPS patients to HLH.

X-linked lymphoproliferative syndrome: Hemizygous mutations in *SH2D1A (SAP)* and *BIRC4 (XIAP)* are associated with type 1 and type 2 X-linked lymphoproliferative syndrome, respectively, causing lymphocytic activation and inhibition of apoptosis, which collectively induces dysregulation of cytotoxic T- and NK-cells leading to vulnerability to EBV infection and development of HLH [28, 67, 68].

Wiskott-Aldrich syndrome (WAS): WAS is a rare X-linked hereditary disorder characterized by hemorrhagic diathesis, thrombocytopenia, recurrent infection, eczema, and immunodeficiency [69]. The gene for WAS is located on Xp11.22-p11.23 and familial WAS cases with nucleotides 73-74 deletion had been reported [70]. WAS protein is exclusively expressed in hematopoietic cells and lack of functional WAS results in thrombocytopenia, lymphopenia, or dysregulation of myeloid and lymphoid cells [69]. Laboratory findings in WAS patients typically show decrease number and function of cytotoxic T-cells and normal-to-increased number of NK-cells, but with reduced cytotoxicity [69]. Cases of HLH associated with WAS have sporadically been reported [71, 72].

Severe combined immunodeficiency (SCID): SCID is a syndrome characterized by T-cell deficiency and it is caused by a variety of mutations in *IL2RG, JAK3, IL7RA, PTPRC, CD3D, cD3E, CD3Z, CORO1A, RAG1/RAG2, DCLRE1C, PRKDC, AK2, ADA, LIG4,* and *NHEJ1*. SCID patients usually present with recurrent severe infection, failure to thrive, chronic diarrhea and typical laboratory findings include lymphopenia, lack of T-cell mitogen response, and hypogammaglobulinemia. HLH cases associated with SCID have been reported although the underlying mechanisms remain to be unclear [73-75].

Lysinuric protein intolerance (LPI): LPI is a genetic disorder caused by mutations in *SLC7A7* gene encoding y+LAT1 protein that plays an essential role in cationic amino acid (ornithine, arginine, lysine) transport [76-78]. Clinical manifestation of LPI includes vomiting, diarrhea, coma, and failure to thrive [79]. Also, it may cause multi-organ abnormalities including bone marrow, brain, kidney, spleen, liver, and kidney. HLH cases associated with LPI had been reported [71, 80], and it has been hypothesized that intracellular arginine accumulation due to y+LAT1 defect may induce nitric oxide (NO) overproduction and subsequent immune dysfunction as well as macrophage activation [81]. In addition to lysinuric protein intolerance, there are also associations between HLH and other inborn errors of metabolism such as Gaucher disease, Pearson syndrome, multiple sulfatase deficiency, galactosemia, and galactosialidosis [82]. The role of NK and TCL in development of HLH in these metabolic disease is unknown and worthy of exploration.

3.1.B. Secondary or Reactive HLH

13.3.1B-a. HLH associated with infection: The most common types of infection associated HLH are viral (41%), mycobacterial (23%), bacterial (23%), and fungal (13%). Among viral infection, Epstein-Bar Virsus (EBV) is the most commonly associated with secondary HLH. The majority of EBV infection in HLH occurs in younger age and its incidence is highest in the East Asia. Also, concurrent histoplasma and cytomegalorivus (CMV) infection are commonly found in HLH, representing 19% and 14% of HLH patients per reported study [83]. Additionally, human immunodeficiency virus (HIV), Human Herpesvirus-8 (HHV8), parvovirus B19, hepatitis, flavivirus, influenza virus, enterovirus infections were also reported in secondary HLH cases [83].

13.3.1B-b. Macrophage activation syndrome (MAS): MAS is a life-threatening complication associated with rheumatoid disease, and MAS is caused by pathologic activation of macrophages and T-cells, leading to systemic inflammation. Among many of rheumatoid disorder associated with MAS, Juvenile Rheumatoid Arthritis (JRA) is the most common (50.2%) followed by systemic lupus erythematosus (22.3%), Still disease (8.8%), and Kawasaki disease (5.9%). Previous reports showed that NK-cell function is substantially depressed in the majority of MAS patients based on the assay with coincubation of mononuclear cells with NK-cell sensitive K562 cells [84]. MAS can be triggered by infections, flares of underlying rheumatoid disease, or changes in medications, specifically administration of gold, methotrexate, sulfasalazine, or TNF inhibitors [71]. Although the exact mechanisms how cytotoxic T-cell and NK-cell dysfunction lead to MAS remain to be unclear, it has been hypothesized that dysfunctional T- and NK-cell fail to eradicate infected cells, leading to persistent antigenic stimulation and MAS [71]. In addition, dysfunctional T-cell may fail to trigger apoptotic signal for the removal of antigen presenting cells, causing persistent cytokine release exacerbating macrophage activation [71].

13.3.1B-c. HLH associated with malignancy: Although HLH cases associated with myeloid leukemia, germ cell tumors, anaplastic large cell lymphoma, classical Hodgkin lymphoma, and B-cell lymphoblastic leukemia have been reported, the majority of HLH cases are observed in T- or NK-cell lymphoma or leukemia for unknown reason [85, 86]. Of note, T- or NK-cell lymphoma is frequently associated with active EBV infection, and it is unclear if underlying EBV infection triggers HLH in these specific cancer types or T- or NK-cell dysfunction caused by EBV infection triggers cascade of inflammation. although cytokines released from malignant cells, immune dysregulation secondary to chemotherapy, persistent antigen stimulation from the cancer cells, and concurrent bacterial, fungal, or viral infection seem to collectively serve as trigger for HLH in cancer patients [85].

4. CLINICAL MANIFESTATIONS

The most common presentations of early stage HLH include unexplained fevers, splenomegaly, cytopenia, maculopapular or nodular rash and neurologic complications such as encephalopathy, meningismus, seizures, and nerve palsies [39, 83]. Given frequent association with infections such as EBV and CMV, acute viral infection related symptoms and signs are common. Fever of unknown origin (FUO) is frequent in general population and it is often difficult to differentiate HLH from other etiologies causing FUO. However, in patients with FUO associated with cytopenieas, elevated ferritin or serum CD25 levels, further work up for HLH should be promptly initiated [39]. The degree of liver function tests abnormalities is variable in HLH and acute liver failure has commonly been reported [39]. Neonates can present with hydrops fetalis and veno-occlusive disease [87, 88]. Of note, approximately 95% of HLH patients have disseminated intravascular coagulopathy (DIC) features with high risk of acute bleeding. More than 80% of HLH patients have cytopenia at the time of presentation. Despite the association of hemophagocytosis and HLH, absence of hemophagocytosis on bone marrow biopsy is common in HLH. Neurologic symptoms such as altered mental status, ataxia, hypotonia, seizure, and cranial nerve palsy can be present HLH patients and more than 50% of patients may have positive CSF findings [87, 88]. Cutaneous manifestation in HLH includes maculopapular erythematous rashes, petechiae, purpura, panniculitis, morbilliform erythema, conjunctivitis, and erythematous rash on the lips [87, 88]. Rarely, HLH can cause acute respiratory failure with high mortality up to 90%. In contrast to early stage, later stage HLH is complicated by multi-organ failure with poor survival [87, 88].

Table 2. Diagnostic criteria of HLH according to HLH-2004 protocol [88]

Clinical and Laboratory Parameters	Laboratory Value (Unit)
Fever	
Splenomegaly	
Cytopenia: affecting at least 2 lineages in the peripheral blood	Hemoglobin < 90 (g/L) (< 100 (g/L) for infants) Platelet < 100 x 10^9 (/L) Neutrophils < 1.0 x 10^9(/L)
Hypertriglyceridemia and/or hypofibrinogenemia	Fasting triglyceride ≥ 265 (mg/dL) Fibrinogen ≤ 1.5 (g/L)
Hemophagocytosis: found in the bone marrow, spleen, or lymph node biopsy	
Decreased or absent NK-cell activity	
Elevated ferritin	Ferritin ≥ 500 (ng/mL)
Elevated serum CD25	sCD25 ≥ 2400 (U/ml)

Presence of at least 5 of the 8 clinical or laboratory criteria.

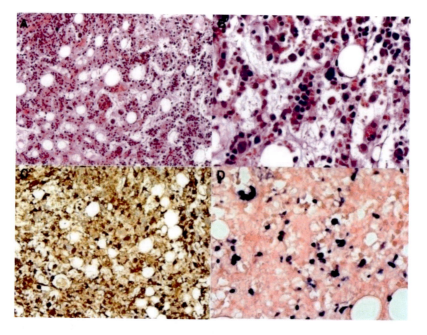

Figure 2. Bone marrow involvement by HLH secondary to an aggressive T-cell lymphoma. A. the bone marrow core biopsy (H&E, x 200) shows dilated sinusoidal space with accumulation of many histiocytes, which engulfed varied kinds of hematopoietic cells (hemophagocytosis). B. The higher magnification of review demonstrates a number of significantly enlarged histiocytes containing numerous hematopoietic cells and abundant clear cytoplasm (H&E, x 600). C. Histiocytes are stained positive for CD68 while normal erythroid and, granulocytic precursors as well as platelets in the cytoplasm of histiocytes are negative for the staining (Immunoperoxidase, x 200). D. in situ hybridization (ISH) with EBV encoded RNA probe (EBER) shows EBV infection or reactivation in the patient with HLH (ISH, x 600).

5. DIAGNOSIS

5.1. Diagnostic Criteria

HLH remains to be a syndromic disorder and the diagnosis is based on a constellation of clinical and laboratory findings. The Histiocyte Society proposed a definition of HLH and diagnostic criteria as part of HLH-2004 trials after update of its original guideline in HLH-1994 trial [88]. Although familial HLH usually presents in younger age, there are reports of adult onset familial HLH cases, and same diagnostic criteria should be applied to both pediatric and adult HLH patients. The diagnostic criteria from HLH-2004 trial are described in the Table 2. Briefly, HLH can be diagnosed when the patient has one of the pathologic mutations (*PRF1, UNC13D, Munc18-2, Rab27a, STX11, SH2D1A,* or *BIRC4*) or has at least five of the eight clinical criteria as follows; 1) fever ≥ 38.5°C, 2) splenomegaly, 3) cytopenia in at least two lineages (Hemoglobin <9.0 g/dL, platelets <100x10^9/L, neutrophils<1x10^9/L), 4) hypertriglyceridemia (>265 mg/dL fasting) and/or hypofibrinogenemia (<150 g/dL), 5) hemophagocytosis in bone marrow, spleen, lymph nodes, or liver, 6) low or absent NK-cell activity, 7) ferritin >500ng/mL, 8) elevated serum CD25 (α-chain of serum IL-2 receptor). Given dismal outcomes, diagnostic work up should be initiated immediately when HLH is clinically suspected, especially in critically ill patients. Among laboratory exam, serum soluble IL-2 receptor level (CD25) is the most specific diagnostic test with a good correlation with disease activity [39, 83]. Alternatively, ferritin could be a useful marker given high sensitivity and specificity when it is elevated (>10,000 ng/mL) [39, 83]. Importantly, hemophagocytosis is neither sensitive nor specific for the diagnosis of HLH, and not all patients have hemophagocytosis at the time of diagnosis [39, 83]. Therefore, diagnosis should not be delayed based on the absence of hemophagocytosis. Although not included in the HLH-2004 diagnostic criteria, newer laboratory studies including the measurement of the expression levels of perforin, XIAP, and surface CD107a are now available, which further helps the diagnosis of HLH [39].

5.2. Histologic Findings

Bone marrow or lymph node biopsy typically show reactive lymphocytosis, increased histiocytes, with or without marked left-shift myeloid maturation [83]. Also, enlarged histiocytes engulfing red blood cells, lymphocytes, and granulocytes are frequently observed in the bone marrow aspirate. When there is composite neoplasm e.g., lymphoma or leukemia found in the bone marrow, lymph node, spleen or other sites, the organ or tissue could be partially or diffusely replaced by neoplastic cells. Hemophagocytic phenomenon may not be striking. As it is also not uncommon for HLH to accompany with virus, bacteria, histoplasmosis, and flares of autoimmune disorder, a tunnel vision of the diseases may miss an early diagnosis of hemophagnocytosis [89]. Immunohistochemistry staining with histiocyte specific antibodies including anti-CD14, CD68, and CD163 are typically positive highlighting hemophagocytes (Figure 2). When acute liver failure occurs, a biopsy of liver often shows dense small lymphoid infiltrate [83].

5.3. Novel Diagnostic Markers

Several markers have been identified to help the diagnosis of HLH, especially the measurement of NK-cell function that is one of diagnostic criteria. Mutation analysis of known genes that are associated with familial HLH can be helpful to diagnose the inheritated immune difficiency syndrome and HLH. NK-cell degranulation assay may provide diagnostic value based on a large cohort study of 494 HLH patients [90]. Also, resting NK-cell degranulation activity less than 5% was shown to have sensitivity of 96% and specificity of 88% [90]. Serum ceramide and Secretory SMase (S-SMAse)/ceramide activity was also shown to be elevated in HLH cases and their clinical implication needs further validation [91]. Testing NK-cell perforin expression in combination with CD107a upregulation test have more sensitivity and specificity, that is superior to NK-cell cytotoxicity test for screening of genetic HLH [92].

6. TREATMENT

6.1. Front-Line Treatment

The survival of familial HLH patients without treatment was shown to be ~2 months, and the clinical course of untreated HLH is detrimental [39, 87, 88]. The prognosis significantly depends on early diagnosis and treatment. The goals of HLH treatment are 1) controlling the hyperinflammatory and hypercytokine status, 2) controlling underlying disorders (autoimmune disease, infection, and malignancy), and 3) eradicating hyperactive macrophages [39, 87, 88]. The HLH-2004 protocol that is composed of 2 weeks of induction treatment and 6 weeks of tapering phase is the most common regimen used for HLH as a front-line setting. The regimen includes dexamethasone, etoposide, intrathecal mtethotrexate and hydrocortisone (in the presence of CNS manifestations) [88]. Treatment lasts up to 8 weeks for secondary HLH wherease treatment should be continued until hematopoietic stem cell transplantation in case of familial HLH [88].

Meanwhile supportive care including antibiotics for concurrent infection and transfusion should be continued. Also, chemotherapy for the underlying malignancy can be incorporated into HLH-2004 regimen if the patient can tolerate treatment [88].

6.2. Salvage Treatments

Based on HLH-94 study, approximately 50% of HLH patients achieve complete remission, but 20% of patient die before stem cell transplant or 30% of patients experienced only partial response [87]. In refractory or relapsed HLH patients after initial chemotherapy, several alternative therapies have been shown to be active. High dose steroid and alemtuzumb could be an option since they suppress cytotoxic T-cells and histiocytes [39, 93]. Also, targeting IL-1, IL-6, and CD25 had been shown to be effective in MAS patients [39]. Recently, tocilizumab (an immunesuppressor drug used for rheumatoid arthirsis) is under investigation for treatment of HLH. Of note, in patients with recurrent disease during tapering treatment, re-intensification of standard agents could be attempted [39].

6.3. Allogeneic Stem Cell Transplantation

At this moment, allogeneic stem cell transplantation (SCT) is the only curative treatment for familial HLH. Due to chance of early relapse after initial chemotherapy, process for allogeneic SCT including donor identification should be promptly initiated after diagnosis of familial HLH. A nationwide retrospective study showed 65.4% of overall survival rate after reduced intensity conditioning (RIC) regimen followed by cord blood transplantation. A meta-analysis of total 342 patients from 11 studies have demonstrated 20% of treatment related mortality with no significant difference in survival outcomes in EBV associated HLH [94]. Allogeneic SCT should be considered in relapsed or refractory disease as long as the patient has good performance status without major comorbidities [95]. Primary graft loss is common in HLH patients. Therefore, donor engraftment should be monitored weekly for the first several months following transplant [39]. When engraftment declines down to 50-60% levels during the early post-transplant phase, tapering immunosuppressants or donor lymphocytes infusion can be tried to stabilize the donor chimerism. At this moment, the safe level of donor chimerism is not determined although healthy long-term survivors with very low donor chimerism levels had been reported [39]. For HLH patients with CNS disease, close post-transplant monitoring is required. CSF study within 100 days of transplant is recommended even in the asymptomatic patients. When CSF study turns out positive, the CNS disease can be effectively treated with intrathecal chemotherapy [39].

CONCLUSION

HLH is a heterogeneous disease regarding etiopathogenesis and comprehensive clinical and laboratory work up is required for early diagnosis. Inherited or acquired NK-cell dysfunction plays an important role in the pathobiology of both primary and secondary HLH. Despite advances in the diagnostics, therapeutics and supportive care, HLH remains to be difficult to treat. The role of cytotoxic T-cells and NK-cells in the development of HLH needs further investigation for the development of novel therapeutic strategies.

REFERENCES

[1] Scott R, Robb-Smith A. Histiocytic medullary reticulosis. *Lancet.* 1939;(2):194-198.

[2] Farquhar JW, Claireaux AE. Familial Haemophagocytic Reticulosis. *Archives of Disease in Childhood.* 1952;27(136):519-525.

[3] Boake WC, Card WH, Kimmey JF. Histiocytic Medullary Reticulosis; Concurrence In Father And Son. *Arch Intern Med.* 1965;116:245-252.

[4] Jordan MB, Allen CE, Weitzman S, Filipovich AH, McClain KL. How I treat hemophagocytic lymphohistiocytosis. *Blood.* 2011;118(15):4041-4052.

[5] Henter JI, Elinder G, Söder O, Ost A. Incidence in Sweden and clinical features of familial hemophagocytic lymphohistiocytosis. *Acta Paediatr Scand.* 1991;80(4):428-435.

[6] Ishii E, Ohga S, Tanimura M, et al. Clinical and epidemiologic studies of familial hemophagocytic lymphohistiocytosis in Japan. Japan LCH Study Group. *Med Pediatr Oncol.* 1998;30(5):276-283.

[7] Janka GE. Familial and Acquired Hemophagocytic Lymphohistiocytosis. *Annual Review of Medicine.* 2012;63(1):233-246.

[8] Rosado FGN, Kim AS. Hemophagocytic LymphohistiocytosisAn Update on Diagnosis and Pathogenesis. *American journal of clinical pathology.* 2013;139(6):713-727.

[9] Morvan MG, Lanier LL. NK cells and cancer: you can teach innate cells new tricks. *Nat Rev Cancer.* 2016;16(1):7-19.

[10] Vivier E, Tomasello E, Baratin M, Walzer T, Ugolini S. Functions of natural killer cells. *Nat Immunol.* 2008;9(5):503-510.

[11] Cerwenka A, Lanier LL. Natural killer cell memory in infection, inflammation and cancer. *Nat Rev Immunol.* 2016;16(2):112-123.

[12] de Saint Basile G, Menasche G, Fischer A. Molecular mechanisms of biogenesis and exocytosis of cytotoxic granules. *Nat Rev Immunol.* 2010;10.

[13] Caligiuri MA. Human natural killer cells. *Blood.* 2008;112(3):461-469.

[14] Jordan MB, Hildeman D, Kappler J, Marrack P. An animal model of hemophagocytic lymphohistiocytosis (HLH): $CD8^{+}$ T cells and interferon gamma are essential for the disorder. *Blood.* 2004;104(3):735-743.

[15] Pachlopnik Schmid J, Ho C-H, Diana J, et al. A Griscelli syndrome type 2 murine model of hemophagocytic lymphohistiocytosis (HLH). *European Journal of Immunology.* 2008;38(11):3219-3225.

[16] Crozat K, Hoebe K, Ugolini S, et al. *Jinx*, an MCMV susceptibility phenotype caused by disruption of *Unc13d*: a mouse model of type 3 familial hemophagocytic lymphohistiocytosis. *The Journal of Experimental Medicine.* 2007;204(4):853-863.

[17] Sepulveda FE, Debeurme F, Ménasché G, et al. Distinct severity of HLH in both human and murine mutants with complete loss of cytotoxic effector PRF1, RAB27A, and STX11. *Blood.* 2013;121(4):595-603.

[18] Kögl T, Müller J, Jessen B, et al. Hemophagocytic lymphohistiocytosis in syntaxin-11–deficient mice: T-cell exhaustion limits fatal disease. *Blood.* 2013;121(4):604-613.

[19] Jessen B, Maul-Pavicic A, Ufheil H, et al. Subtle differences in CTL cytotoxicity determine susceptibility to hemophagocytic lymphohistiocytosis in mice and humans with Chediak-Higashi syndrome. *Blood.* 2011;118(17):4620-4629.

[20] de Saint Basile G, Fischer A. Defective cytotoxic granule-mediated cell death pathway impairs T lymphocyte homeostasis. *Curr Opin Rheumatol.* 2003;15.

[21] Créput C, Galicier L, Buyse S, Azoulay E. Understanding organ dysfunction in hemophagocytic lymphohistiocytosis. *Intensive Care Medicine.* 2008;34(7):1177-1187.

[22] Ménasché G, Feldmann J, Fischer A, de Saint Basile G. Primary hemophagocytic syndromes point to a direct link between lymphocyte cytotoxicity and homeostasis. *Immunol Rev.* 2005;203:165-179.

[23] Bode SF, Lehmberg K, Maul-Pavicic A, et al. Recent advances in the diagnosis and treatment of hemophagocytic lymphohistiocytosis. *Arthritis Research & Therapy.* 2012;14(3):213.

[24] Long EO, Kim HS, Liu D, Peterson ME, Rajagopalan S. Controlling Natural Killer Cell Responses: Integration of Signals for Activation and Inhibition. *Annual Review of Immunology.* 2013;31(1):227-258.

[25] Waggoner SN, Cornberg M, Selin LK, Welsh RM. Natural killer cells act as rheostats modulating antiviral T cells. *Nature.* 2012;481(7381):394-398.

[26] Lang PA, Lang KS, Xu HC, et al. Natural killer cell activation enhances immune pathology and promotes chronic infection by limiting CD8+ T-cell immunity. *Proceedings of the National Academy of Sciences.* 2012;109(4):1210-1215.

[27] Sepulveda FE, Maschalidi S, Vosshenrich CAJ, et al. A novel immunoregulatory role for NK-cell cytotoxicity in protection from HLH-like immunopathology in mice. *Blood.* 2015;125(9):1427-1434.

[28] Yang X, Miyawaki T, Kanegane H. SAP and XIAP deficiency in hemophagocytic lymphohistiocytosis. *Pediatrics International.* 2012;54(4):447-454.

[29] Jordan MB, Hildeman D, Kappler J, Marrack P. An animal model of hemophagocytic lymphohistiocytosis (HLH): CD8+ T cells and interferon gamma are essential for the disorder. *Blood.* 2004;104.

[30] de Saint Basile G, Ménasché G, Fischer A. Molecular mechanisms of biogenesis and exocytosis of cytotoxic granules. *Nat Rev Immunol.* 2010;10(8):568-579.

[31] Stepp SE, Dufourcq-Lagelouse R, Deist FL, et al. Perforin Gene Defects in Familial Hemophagocytic Lymphohistiocytosis. *Science.* 1999;286(5446):1957-1959.

[32] Feldmann J, Callebaut I, Raposo G, et al. Munc13-4 Is Essential for Cytolytic Granules Fusion and Is Mutated in a Form of Familial Hemophagocytic Lymphohistiocytosis (FHL3). *Cell.*115(4):461-473.

[33] xF, te M, xE, et al. Munc18-2 deficiency causes familial hemophagocytic lymphohistiocytosis type 5 and impairs cytotoxic granule exocytosis in patient NK cells. *The Journal of Clinical Investigation.* 2009;119(12):3765-3773.

[34] Ohadi M, Lalloz MRA, Sham P, et al. Localization of a Gene for Familial Hemophagocytic Lymphohistiocytosis at Chromosome 9q21.3-22 by Homozygosity Mapping. *The American Journal of Human Genetics.* 64(1):165-171.

[35] Trapani JA. Target cell apoptosis induced by cytotoxic T cells and natural killer cells involves synergy between the pore-forming protein, perforin, and the serine protease, granzyme B. *Aust N Z J Med.* 1995;25(6):793-799.

[36] Hazen MM, Woodward AL, Hofmann I, et al. Mutations of the hemophagocytic lymphohistiocytosis–associated gene UNC13D in a patient with systemic juvenile idiopathic arthritis. *Arthritis & Rheumatism.* 2008;58(2):567-570.

[37] Feldmann J, Callebaut I, Raposo G, et al. Munc13-4 is essential for cytolytic granules fusion and is mutated in a form of familial hemophagocytic lymphohistiocytosis (FHL3). *Cell.* 2003;115.

[38] Marcenaro S, Gallo F, Martini S, et al. Analysis of natural killer-cell function in familial hemophagocytic lymphohistiocytosis (FHL): defective CD107a surface expression heralds Munc13-4 defect and discriminates between genetic subtypes of the disease. *Blood.* 2006;108.

[39] Jordan MB, Allen CE, Weitzman S, Filipovich AH, McClain KL. How I treat hemophagocytic lymphohistiocytosis. *Blood.* 2011;118(15):4041-4052.

[40] Bode SF, Ammann S, Al-Herz W, et al. The syndrome of hemophagocytic lymphohistiocytosis in primary immunodeficiencies: implications for differential diagnosis and pathogenesis. *Haematologica.* 2015;100(7):978-988.

[41] Mancini AJ, Chan LS, Paller AS. Partial albinism with immunodeficiency: Griscelli syndrome: Report of a case and review of the literature. *J Am Acad Dermatol.* 1998;38(2):295-300.

[42] Barral DC, Ramalho JS, Anders R, et al. Functional redundancy of Rab27 proteins and the pathogenesis of Griscelli syndrome. *The Journal of Clinical Investigation.* 2002;110(2):247-257.

[43] Mahalingashetti PB, Krishnappa MH, Kalyan PSP, Subramanian RA, Padhy S. Griscelli Syndrome: Hemophagocytic Lymphohistiocytosis with Silvery Hair. *Journal of Laboratory Physicians.* 2012;4(2):129-130.

[44] Nouriel A, Zisquit J, Helfand AM, Anikster Y, Greenberger S. Griscelli Syndrome Type 3: Two New Cases and Review of the Literature. *Pediatric Dermatology.* 2015;32(6):e245-e248.

[45] Blume RS, Wolff SM. The Chediak-Higashi Syndrome: Studies in Four Patients and a Review of the Literature. *Medicine.* 1972;51(4):247-280.

[46] Kaplan J, De Domenico I, Ward DM. Chediak-Higashi syndrome. *Curr Opin Hematol.* 2008;15(1):22-29.

[47] Seward SL, Gahl WA. Hermansky-Pudlak Syndrome: Health Care Throughout Life. *Pediatrics.* 2013;132(1):153-160.

[48] Krisp A, Hoffman R, Happle R, König A, Freyschmidt-Paul P. Hermansky-Pudlak syndrome. *Eur J Dermatol.* 2001;11(4):372-373.

[49] Dell'Angelica EC, Shotelersuk V, Aguilar RC, Gahl WA, Bonifacino JS. Altered Trafficking of Lysosomal Proteins in Hermansky-Pudlak Syndrome Due to Mutations in the β3A Subunit of the AP-3 Adaptor. *Molecular Cell.* 1999;3(1):11-21.

[50] Li W, Zhang Q, Oiso N, et al. Hermansky-Pudlak syndrome type 7 (HPS-7) results from mutant dysbindin, a member of the biogenesis of lysosome-related organelles complex 1 (BLOC-1). *Nat Genet.* 2003;35(1):84-89.

[51] Bahadoran P, Aberdam E, Mantoux F, et al. Rab27a: A key to melanosome transport in human melanocytes. *J Cell Biol.* 2001;152(4):843-850.

[52] Stepp SE, Dufourcq-Lagelouse R, Le Deist F, et al. Perforin gene defects in familial hemophagocytic lymphohistiocytosis. *Science.* 1999;286.

[53] Elstak ED, Neeft M, Nehme NT, et al. The munc13-4–rab27 complex is specifically required for tethering secretory lysosomes at the plasma membrane. *Blood.* 2011;118(6):1570-1578.

[54] Al-Tamemi S, Al-Zadjali S, Al-Ghafri F, Dennison D. Chediak-Higashi Syndrome: Novel Mutation of the CHS1/LYST Gene in 3 Omani Patients. *Journal of pediatric hematology/oncology.* 2014;36(4):e248-e250.

[55] Chiang SCC, Wood SM, Tesi B, et al. Differences in Granule Morphology yet Equally Impaired Exocytosis among Cytotoxic T Cells and NK Cells from Chediak–Higashi Syndrome Patients. *Frontiers in Immunology.* 2017;8:426.

[56] Karim MA, Suzuki K, Fukai K, et al. Apparent genotype-phenotype correlation in childhood, adolescent, and adult Chediak-Higashi syndrome. *Am J Med Genet.* 2002;108(1):16-22.

[57] Jung J, Bohn G, Allroth A, et al. Identification of a homozygous deletion in the AP3B1 gene causing Hermansky-Pudlak syndrome, type 2. *Blood.* 2006;108(1):362-369.

[58] Hermansky F, Pudlak P. Albinism associated with hemorrhagic diathesis and unusual pigmented reticular cells in the bone marrow: report of two cases with histochemical studies. *Blood.* 1959;14(2):162-169.

[59] Shotelersuk V, Dell'Angelica EC, Hartnell L, Bonifacino JS, Gahl WA. A new variant of Hermansky-Pudlak syndrome due to mutations in a gene responsible for vesicle formation. *Am J Med.* 2000;108(5):423-427.

[60] Clark RH, Stinchcombe JC, Day A, et al. Adaptor protein 3-dependent microtubule-mediated movement of lytic granules to the immunological synapse. *Nat Immunol.* 2003;4(11):1111-1120.

[61] Enders A, Zieger B, Schwarz K, et al. Lethal hemophagocytic lymphohistiocytosis in Hermansky-Pudlak syndrome type II. *Blood.* 2006;108(1):81-87.

[62] Wenham M, Grieve S, Cummins M, et al. Two patients with Hermansky Pudlak syndrome type 2 and novel mutations in AP3B1. *Haematologica.* 2010;95(2):333-337.

[63] Fontana S, Parolini S, Vermi W, et al. Innate immunity defects in Hermansky-Pudlak type 2 syndrome. *Blood.* 2006;107(12):4857-4864.

[64] Enders A, Zieger B, Schwarz K, et al. Lethal hemophagocytic lymphohistiocytosis in Hermansky-Pudlak syndrome type II. *Blood.* 2006;108.

[65] Chiang PW, Spector E, Thomas M, Frei-Jones M. Novel mutation causing Hermansky-Pudlak Syndrome Type 2. *Pediatr Blood Cancer.* 2010;55(7):1438.

[66] Jessen B, Bode SF, Ammann S, et al. The risk of hemophagocytic lymphohistiocytosis in Hermansky-Pudlak syndrome type 2. *Blood.* 2013;121(15):2943-2951.

[67] Marsh RA, Madden L, Kitchen BJ, et al. XIAP deficiency: a unique primary immunodeficiency best classified as X-linked familial hemophagocytic lymphohistiocytosis and not as X-linked lymphoproliferative disease. *Blood.* 2010;116(7):1079-1082.

[68] Arico M, Imashuku S, Clementi R, et al. Hemophagocytic lymphohistiocytosis due to germline mutations inSH2D1A, the X-linked lymphoproliferative disease gene. *Blood.* 2001;97(4):1131-1133.

[69] Massaad MJ, Ramesh N, Geha RS. Wiskott-Aldrich syndrome: a comprehensive review. *Annals of the New York Academy of Sciences*. 2013;1285(1):26-43.

[70] Binder V, Albert MH, Kabus M, Bertone M, Meindl A, Belohradsky BH. The Genotype of the Original Wiskott Phenotype. *New England Journal of Medicine*. 2006;355(17):1790-1793.

[71] Grom AA. Natural killer cell dysfunction: A common pathway in systemic-onset juvenile rheumatoid arthritis, macrophage activation syndrome, and hemophagocytic lymphohistiocytosis? *Arthritis & Rheumatism*. 2004;50(3):689-698.

[72] Pasic S, Micic D, Kuzmanovic M. Epstein-Barr virus-associated haemophagocytic lymphohistiocytosis in Wiskott-Aldrich syndrome. *Acta Pædiatrica*. 2003;92(7):859-861.

[73] Dvorak CC, Sandford A, Fong A, Cowan MJ, George TI, Lewis DB. Maternal T-cell Engraftment Associated With Severe Hemophagocytosis of the Bone Marrow in Untreated X-linked Severe Combined Immunodeficiency. *Journal of pediatric hematology/oncology*. 2008;30(5):396-400.

[74] Patiroglu T, Haluk Akar H, van den Burg M, et al. X-linked severe combined immunodeficiency due to a novel mutation complicated with hemophagocytic lymphohistiocytosis and presented with invagination: A case report. *European Journal of Microbiology & Immunology*. 2014;4(3):174-176.

[75] Grunebaum E, Zhang J, Dadi H, Roifman CM. Haemophagocytic lymphohistiocytosis in X-linked severe combined immunodeficiency. *British Journal of Haematology*. 2000;108(4):834-837.

[76] Torrents D, Mykkanen J, Pineda M, et al. Identification of SLC7A7, encoding y+LAT-1, as the lysinuric protein intolerance gene. *Nat Genet*. 1999;21(3):293-296.

[77] Yanagida O, Kanai Y, Chairoungdua A, et al. Human L-type amino acid transporter 1 (LAT1): characterization of function and expression in tumor cell lines. *Biochimica et Biophysica Acta (BBA) - Biomembranes*. 2001;1514(2):291-302.

[78] Palacín M, Bertran J, Chillarón J, Estévez R, Zorzano A. Lysinuric protein intolerance: mechanisms of pathophysiology. *Molecular Genetics and Metabolism*. 81:27-37.

[79] Simell O, Perheentupa J, Rapola J, Visakorpi JK, Eskelin L-E. Lysinuric protein intolerance. *The American Journal of Medicine*. 59(2):229-240.

[80] Mauhin W, Habarou F, Gobin S, et al. Update on Lysinuric Protein Intolerance, a Multi-faceted Disease Retrospective cohort analysis from birth to adulthood. *Orphanet Journal of Rare Diseases*. 2017;12(1):3.

[81] Mendes Ribeiro AC, Brunini TMC, Ellory JC, Mann GE. Abnormalities in l-arginine transport and nitric oxide biosynthesis in chronic renal and heart failure. *Cardiovascular Research*. 2001;49(4):697-712.

[82] Gokce M, Unal O, Hismi B, et al. Secondary hemophagocytosis in 3 patients with organic acidemia involving propionate metabolism. *Pediatr Hematol Oncol.* 2011;29.

[83] Filipovich AH. Hemophagocytic lymphohistiocytosis (HLH) and related disorders. *ASH Education Program Book.* 2009;2009(1):127-131.

[84] Grom AA, Villanueva J, Lee S, Goldmuntz EA, Passo MH, Filipovich A. Natural killer cell dysfunction in patients with systemic-onset juvenile rheumatoid arthritis and macrophage activation syndrome. *The Journal of Pediatrics.* 142(3):292-296.

[85] Tamamyan GN, Kantarjian HM, Ning J, et al. Malignancy-associated hemophagocytic lymphohistiocytosis in adults: Relation to hemophagocytosis, characteristics, and outcomes. *Cancer.* 2016;122(18):2857-2866.

[86] Han A-R, Lee HR, Park B-B, et al. Lymphoma-associated hemophagocytic syndrome: clinical features and treatment outcome. *Annals of Hematology.* 2007;86(7):493.

[87] Henter JI, Samuelsson-Horne A, Aricò M, et al. Treatment of hemophagocytic lymphohistiocytosis with HLH-94 immunochemotherapy and bone marrow transplantation. *Blood.* 2002;100.

[88] Henter JI, Horne A, Aricó M, et al. HLH-2004: Diagnostic and therapeutic guidelines for hemophagocytic lymphohistiocytosis. *Pediatr Blood Cancer.* 2007;48(2):124-131.

[89] Akenroye AT, Madan N, Mohammadi F, Leider J. Hemophagocytic Lymphohistiocytosis mimics many common conditions: case series and review of literature. *Eur Ann Allergy Clin Immunol.* 2017;49(1):31-41.

[90] Jenkins RW, Clarke CJ, Lucas JT, et al. Evaluation of the Role of Secretory Sphingomyelinase and Bioactive Sphingolipids as Biomarkers in Hemophagocytic Lymphohistiocytosis. *American journal of hematology.* 2013;88(11):E265-E272.

[91] Bryceson YT, Pende D, Maul-Pavicic A, et al. A prospective evaluation of degranulation assays in the rapid diagnosis of familial hemophagocytic syndromes. *Blood.* 2012;119(12):2754-2763.

[92] Rubin TS, Zhang K, Gifford C, et al. Perforin and CD107a testing is superior to NK cell function testing for screening patients for genetic HLH. *Blood.* 2017;129(22):2993-2999.

[93] Marsh RA, Allen CE, McClain KL, et al. Salvage Therapy of Refractory Hemophagocytic Lymphohistiocytosis with Alemtuzumab. *Pediatric blood & cancer.* 2013;60(1):101-109.

[94] Qin Q, Xie Z, Shen Y, et al. Assessment of immunochemotherapy and stem cell transplantation on EBV-associated hemophagocytic lymphohistiocytosis in children: a systematic review and meta analysis. *Eur Rev Med Pharmacol Sci.* 2012;16(5):672-678.

[95] Seo JJ. Hematopoietic cell transplantation for hemophagocytic lymphohistiocytosis: recent advances and controversies. *Blood res.* 2015;50(3):131-139.

EDITORS' CONTACT INFORMATION

Dr. Ling Zhang, MD
Program Director
Hematopathology Fellowship Program
Associate Member/Associate Professor
Department of Hematopathology and Laboratory Medicine
H Lee Moffitt Cancer Center and Research Institute
University of South Florida
Email: Ling.zhang@moffitt.org

Dr. Lubomir Sokol, MD, PhD
Head, Lymphoma Section
Senior Member/Professor
Department of Malignant Hematology
H Lee Moffitt Cancer Center and Research Institute
University of South Florida
Email: Lubomir.sokol@moffitt.org

INDEX

A

A20, 12, 13, 23
abnormal function, v, 25
activated NK-cells, 183, 189, 281
activating natural killer receptors (NKRs), 30, 31, 34
activation-induced cell death (AICD), 5, 33, 166
acute lymphoblastic leukemia (ALL), 13, 14, 23, 44, 51, 54, 55, 56, 57, 58, 59, 63, 65, 66, 69, 70, 101, 106, 107, 112, 257, 263, 265, 266
acute myeloid leukemia (AML), 9, 13, 51, 52, 54, 55, 56, 58, 59, 64, 65, 67, 68, 73, 75, 78, 84, 85, 90, 91, 95, 159, 161, 168
adaptive immune systems, v, 25, 26
adhesion molecules, 27, 97
aggressive natural killer (NK) cell leukemia (ANKL), vii, 2, 115, 116, 117, 118, 128, 130, 131, 132, 136, 145, 152, 153, 157, 192, 216, 222, 228, 249, 250, 251, 252, 253, 254, 255, 256, 257, 258, 259, 260, 261, 262, 263, 265, 266, 267, 268, 269, 270, 271, 272, 273, 274, 275, 276, 277
aggressive variants of T-LGLL, 122, 124
alemtuzumab, 24, 83, 159, 170, 171, 173, 177, 179, 180, 298
allogeneic hematopoietic stem cell transplantation (alloHSCT), 43, 44, 49, 51, 53, 54, 55, 61, 62, 65, 68, 85, 271, 275, 276
anemia, 7, 11, 17, 18, 26, 64, 75, 76, 78, 79, 81, 84, 85, 86, 87, 88, 89, 92, 93, 94, 95, 97, 98, 99, 103, 117, 122, 131, 138, 156, 157, 165, 166, 168, 169, 171, 172, 176, 187, 251, 266
angiocentric, 183, 184, 188, 189, 191, 192, 194, 195, 196, 197, 198, 204, 213, 222, 226
angiocentric lymphoma, 184, 213
angiodestruction, 184, 192, 195, 197, 229, 253
angiodestructive, 183, 188, 189, 192, 194, 195, 196, 198
angioinvasion, 184, 192, 195, 197, 229, 253, 254
antibody-dependent cell-mediated cytotoxicity (ADCC), 27, 151
antigen, 1, 2, 3, 7, 8, 15, 17, 21, 25, 26, 27, 28, 29, 32, 33, 38, 40, 44, 45, 46, 47, 48, 54, 58, 61, 62, 64, 66, 71, 73, 76, 79, 88, 98, 101, 102, 108, 110, 113, 115, 116, 139, 140, 149, 150, 153, 162, 172, 178, 187, 189, 192, 199, 208, 223, 226, 242, 264, 268, 270, 275, 287
anti-thymocyte globulin (ATG), 51, 56, 84, 85, 86, 87, 97, 98
aplastic anemia (AA), 11, 17, 18, 38, 67, 75, 76, 79, 81, 84, 85, 86, 87, 92, 93, 94, 95, 97, 98, 99, 122, 146, 166, 171, 172, 243, 245, 297, 298
atypical lymphocytes, 192, 251
autoimmune, 3, 18, 26, 28, 30, 31, 33, 34, 35, 37, 81, 83, 88, 89, 103, 104, 108, 115, 116, 118, 135, 138, 149, 152, 156, 165, 166, 280, 282, 290
autoimmune cytopenias, 156, 166
autoimmune disease/disorders, 3, 26, 28, 30, 31, 33, 34, 35, 37, 81, 83, 88, 108, 115, 116, 118, 149, 152, 156, 165, 166, 280, 290
autoimmunity, 1, 25, 26, 28, 34, 36, 75, 76, 88, 118, 129, 136, 138, 149, 153, 279
autosomal-dominant hyper-IgE syndrome (AD-HIES), 81

B

BCL11B, 12, 13, 23
bendamustine, 270, 272, 276
benign inflammatory dermatosis, 194, 228
benign LGL Proliferation, 129
BIRC4, 279, 283, 285, 289
blastic plasmacytoid dendritic cell neoplasm, 136, 147, 195, 228
bone marrow infiltrate, 116, 121, 259
bone marrow involvement, 122, 127, 130, 188, 202, 226, 227, 231, 251, 252, 253, 288
boolean model, 5
bortezomib, 174
brentuximab vedotin, 242, 265, 270, 272, 276

C

CD16, 27, 45, 46, 48, 69, 102, 103, 105, 106, 107, 109, 115, 123, 125, 126, 129, 130, 131, 132, 134, 135, 140, 149, 150, 151, 152, 154, 155, 157, 160, 189, 192, 195, 226, 228, 243, 250, 254, 256, 258, 259, 260, 268
CD3ε, 115, 183, 189, 192, 195, 196, 197, 202, 254, 268
CD4, 12, 17, 23, 34, 72, 82, 86, 87, 90, 96, 98, 100, 103, 104, 107, 108, 109, 113, 123, 125, 126, 130, 131, 132, 133, 134, 135, 136, 137, 140, 146, 155, 157, 187, 189, 191, 194, 195, 215, 250, 254, 260
CD4 positive LGLL, 133
CD45RA, 3, 88, 123
CD56, 12, 23, 27, 38, 45, 102, 103, 106, 107, 108, 109, 112, 115, 123, 125, 126, 128, 129, 130, 131, 132, 134, 135, 136, 140, 142, 143, 144, 149, 150, 151, 152, 154, 155, 156, 157, 160, 183, 184, 189, 191, 192, 193, 194, 195, 196, 197, 202, 203, 207, 210, 211, 214, 215, 226, 228, 243, 249, 250, 253, 254, 255, 256, 258, 260, 262, 264, 268, 269, 275
CD57, 102, 103, 104, 105, 108, 110, 111, 115, 119, 123, 125, 126, 127, 130, 131, 132, 133, 134, 135, 143, 150, 151, 154, 155, 160, 189, 254, 256, 258, 259, 260, 268
CD62L, 3, 123
CD8, 2, 6, 13, 17, 33, 34, 35, 37, 38, 78, 79, 81, 82, 86, 87, 89, 91, 94, 96, 102, 103, 104, 105, 107, 108, 109, 110, 111, 113, 114, 115, 119, 123, 125, 126, 127, 129, 130, 131, 132, 133, 134, 135, 137, 139, 140, 141, 143, 146, 150, 154, 155, 157, 160, 162, 189, 191, 194, 196, 228, 229, 250, 254, 258, 259, 260, 268, 281, 293, 294
CD94, 30, 47, 123, 129, 131, 132, 149, 150, 151, 154, 157, 160, 189, 202, 215, 223
CD94-NKG2 families, 30
Chediak-Higashi syndrome, 280, 283, 284, 293, 295, 296
chemokines, 27, 45, 198, 200
chemotherapy, 54, 59, 101, 102, 106, 109, 110, 113, 131, 145, 171, 183, 187, 200, 201, 202, 212, 221, 223, 225, 230, 231, 233, 235, 236, 237, 238, 239, 240, 242, 246, 247, 248, 260, 265, 266, 269, 270, 271, 272, 273, 276, 287, 291
chimeric antigen receptor T cells (CAR-T), 44, 63, 64, 66
chromosome 7 anomalies, 134
chronic active EBV infection, 185, 192, 207, 250, 263
chronic lymphoproliferative disorder, v, vii, 2, 18, 21, 93, 111, 115, 116, 129, 143, 149, 163, 250, 258, 260, 264, 266
chronic lymphoproliferative disorder of natural killer (NK) cells (CLPD-NK), vii, 2, 7, 18, 115, 116, 117, 122, 128, 129, 131, 132, 149, 152, 153, 154, 155, 156, 157, 158, 159, 163, 250, 258, 260, 266
circulating large granular lymphocytes, 1, 115, 120, 133
clonal episomal EBV, 130
clonal expansion, 7, 14, 15, 33, 75, 76, 78, 80, 81, 83, 84, 87, 88, 105, 112, 159, 165, 261
clonality, 7, 20, 36, 76, 79, 109, 124, 127, 140, 141, 144, 154, 163, 217, 254
clone(s), 2, 3, 7, 8, 11, 13, 15, 18, 21, 30, 69, 75, 78, 81, 83, 87, 89, 94, 107, 109, 122, 127, 158, 167, 171, 176
coagulation necrosis, 188
comparative genomic hybridization (CGH), 131, 145, 197, 213, 217, 244, 249, 257, 259, 263, 276
corticosteroids, 167
cyclophosphamide (Cy), 35, 57, 83, 135, 159, 165, 167, 168, 170, 177, 179, 200, 235, 269
cyclosporine (CsA), 18, 83, 84, 86, 92, 97, 98, 99, 135, 139, 159, 165, 167, 168, 170, 177, 181
cyclosporine A (CSA), 99, 159, 165, 167, 168, 170, 177, 181
cytokine(s), 1, 13, 16, 27, 28, 31, 34, 38, 39, 45, 48, 50, 61, 64, 79, 80, 81, 82, 83, 88, 94, 95, 96, 100,

115, 116, 118, 151, 154, 159, 160, 198, 200, 281, 282, 287
cytopenias, 36, 78, 79, 117, 134, 139, 149, 152, 156, 158, 159, 165, 166, 167, 169, 177, 251, 258, 265, 266, 267, 279
cytotoxic markers, 124, 157, 183, 189, 191, 192, 194, 195, 196, 197, 202, 254, 268
cytotoxic T cells, 30, 33, 71, 83, 93, 105, 106, 115, 158, 196, 294

D

D661H, 10, 12
D661V, 10, 12
ddPCR, 11
death-inducing signaling complex (DISC), 4, 17, 33, 40, 178
deletion of 6q, 131, 257
dendritic cells, 14, 27, 28, 61, 72, 83, 85, 136, 242
diffuse large B-cell lymphoma, 113, 193, 200, 245
DNA methylation, 12, 82
DNMT3A, 12, 13, 14, 23, 77, 82, 91
dysphagia, 187

E

Eastern cooperative oncology group (ECOG), 11, 83, 142, 167, 178, 233
EBV DNA fragments, 130
EBV DNA titer, 130, 227, 228
EBV encoded RNA probe (EBER), 130, 183, 185, 191, 192, 193, 194, 195, 196, 197, 202, 231, 255, 268, 269, 288
EBV nuclear antigen-2 (EBNA-2) proteins, 257
EBV-associated lymphoid neoplasms, 228
EBV-negative aggressive NK cell leukemia, 254, 257, 263
effector memory cytotoxic T cells, 115
enteropathy-associated T-cell lymphoma type II, 196
epigenetic modifier, 13, 199
epistaxis, 187, 192, 193, 227
Epstein-Barr virus (EBV), 3, 16, 81, 115, 118, 129, 130, 131, 145, 152, 153, 156, 162, 172, 175, 180, 183, 184, 185, 187, 189, 191, 192, 193, 194, 195, 196, 198, 199, 200, 201, 202, 204, 205, 206, 207, 208, 209, 210, 215, 216, 217, 221, 223, 224, 225, 226, 227, 228, 229, 231, 232, 233, 239, 242, 243,
244, 245, 248, 249, 250, 254, 256, 257, 258, 259, 260, 261, 262, 263, 265, 266, 267, 268, 269, 270, 273, 274, 277, 285, 286, 287, 288, 291, 297, 299
erythropoietin (EPO), 169
extracellular matrix, 27, 198
extracellular signal-regulated kinase, 31, 40
extranodal NK/T cell lymphoma, nasal type (ENKTL), 115, 116, 117, 118, 128, 130, 131, 132, 136, 142, 145, 183, 184, 185, 186, 187, 188, 189, 191, 192, 193, 194, 195, 196, 197, 198, 199, 200, 201, 202, 210, 222, 225, 226, 227, 228, 229, 230, 231, 232, 233, 234, 243, 244, 246, 247, 248, 257, 260, 264, 270, 272, 274
extra-upper aerodigestive tract NK/T-cell (EUNKTL), 201, 230

F

farnesyltransferase Inhibitor, 173
Fas, 4, 5, 17, 18, 27, 29, 37, 40, 84, 93, 118, 178, 189, 197, 215, 220, 251
Fas Ligand (FasL), 1, 27, 118, 199, 251
Fas-associated death domain protein (FADD), 27, 33, 197
FAS–FASL-mediated apoptosis, 25
FasL, 1, 27, 118, 199, 251
fludarabine, 51, 165, 171, 179
FOXO3, 198, 218, 249, 257, 263
French-American-British (FAB) system, 78

G

gamma-delta (γδ) variant of T-LGLL, 124
G-CSF, 29, 169, 237
gene expression profiling, 197, 218
generalized lymphadenopathy, 133, 251
genetic defect(s), 280, 284
germinal configuration, 152
graft- versus- host disease (GVHD), 43, 44, 49, 51, 54, 55, 57, 58, 59, 60, 61, 62, 63, 65, 67, 72, 103, 104
graft- versus- leukemia effect (GvL), 44, 49, 54, 62, 66
granulocyte colony-stimulating factor (G-CSF), 29, 169, 237
granulocyte-macrophage colony -stimulating factor (GM-CSF), 28, 29
granuloma gangrenescens, 184

granulomatosis with polyangiitis, 192
granzyme, 27, 30, 31, 39, 40, 105, 124, 127, 135, 152, 157, 162, 189, 191, 202, 223, 226, 231, 246, 260, 282, 294
Griscelli syndrome, 280, 283, 284, 293, 295

H

HACE1 hypermethylation, 249, 257
hematopoietic stem cell transplant (SCT), v, 43, 44, 53, 67, 68, 69, 73, 85, 110, 111, 116, 129, 170, 172, 173, 180, 239, 241, 248, 265, 273, 275, 276, 290, 291
hemolytic anemia, 89, 103, 117, 138, 172
hemophagocytic lymphohistiocytosis (HLH), 119, 131, 139, 187, 249, 251, 253, 259, 260, 262, 265, 266, 267, 279, 280, 281, 282, 283, 284, 285, 286, 287, 288, 289, 290, 291, 292, 293, 294, 295, 296, 297, 298, 299
hemophagocytic syndrome, 135, 187, 212, 262, 274, 293, 298
hemophagocytosis, 131, 132, 134, 279, 280, 287, 288, 289, 297, 298
hepatosplenic T-cell lymphoma, 134, 141
hepatosplenomegaly, 131, 134, 192, 195, 196, 251, 259, 266
Hermansky-Pudlak syndrome, 280, 284, 285, 295, 296
herpes simplex virus, 191
HLA class I molecules, 150
HLA-B7, 4
HLA-DR, 4, 18, 58, 86, 87, 97, 99, 118, 123, 125, 126, 132, 135, 139, 154, 181
HLA-DR15, 4, 87, 97
HLA-DR4, 4, 18, 118, 139, 181
HTLV, 3, 16, 30, 80, 83, 94, 118, 138, 153, 162
human immunodeficiency virus, 118, 186, 208, 286
human T cell lymphotropic virus (HTLV), 3, 16, 30, 80, 83, 94, 118, 138, 153, 162
Hu-MiK-Beta 1, 172
hydroa vacciniforme-like lymphoma, 195, 196
hypercytokinemia, 280
hypoplastic myelodysplastic syndrome (MDS), 11, 54, 55, 56, 64, 65, 73, 75, 76, 77, 78, 79, 80, 81, 82, 83, 84, 85, 86, 87, 89, 93, 95, 98, 99, 100, 122, 168, 171, 172

I

idiopathic midline destructive disease, 184, 226
IFN-γ, 28, 58, 61, 79, 282
IL-15, 1, 5, 20, 26, 61, 62, 63, 72, 81, 82, 83, 88, 95, 96, 159, 166, 172, 180
IL-3, 28, 198
immunoreceptor tyrosine-based activation motifs (ITAMs), 30, 31
immunosuppressive therapy, 22, 78, 87, 93, 97, 99, 142, 150, 159, 165, 166, 169, 176, 177, 178, 181
immunosurveillance, 25, 118
indolent chronic lymphoproliferative disorder of NK cells (CLPD-NK), 2, 7, 115, 116, 117, 122, 128, 129, 131, 132, 149, 152, 153, 154, 155, 156, 157, 158, 159, 258, 260, 266
innate and adaptive immune systems, v, 25, 26
innate immune systems, 35
interferon (IFN)-gamma, 92
interferon gamma (INF gamma), 151
interferon-gamma (IFN-γ), 28, 58, 61, 79, 282
interleukin 1 (IL-1), 1, 5, 16, 20, 26, 28, 61, 62, 63, 72, 81, 82, 83, 88, 95, 96, 100, 159, 166, 172, 180, 200, 221, 281, 291
international prognostic index (IPI), 144, 184, 188, 200, 201, 202, 222, 229, 230, 232, 245

J

JAK/STAT, 4, 5, 12, 13, 14, 22, 23, 24, 115, 116, 128, 142, 158, 162, 199, 220, 248, 257
JAK3-specific inhibitor, 174
JAK3-Specific Inhibitor, 173

K

killer, v, vi, vii, 2, 3, 7, 16, 17, 18, 20, 27, 30, 36, 37, 38, 39, 40, 43, 44, 46, 47, 48, 53, 66, 67, 68, 69, 70, 71, 72, 73, 76, 84, 85, 91, 94, 96, 102, 110, 112, 113, 138, 139, 141, 142, 143, 144, 145, 146, 149, 150, 160, 161, 162, 163, 166, 181, 183, 184, 189, 201, 203, 204, 205, 207, 208, 209, 210, 211, 212, 213, 214, 215, 216, 217, 218, 219, 220, 221, 222, 223, 225, 232, 243, 244, 245, 246, 247, 248, 249, 250, 254, 260, 261, 262, 263, 264, 265, 266, 274, 275, 276, 277, 279, 292, 293, 294, 297, 298
killer T-cell, 144, 210, 222, 246

Index

killer-cell immunoglobulin-like receptor(s) (KIRs), 3, 7, 18, 30, 31, 43, 46, 47, 49, 50, 51, 52, 53, 54, 55, 56, 57, 58, 59, 65, 66, 67, 68, 69, 70, 72, 124, 129, 132, 149, 150, 151, 153, 154, 155, 157, 158, 159, 160, 163, 189, 215, 254, 258, 264
Korean prognostic index, 184, 200, 201, 202
Korean Prognostic Index, 232

L

latent membrane protein (LMP-1), 199, 204, 208, 227, 257
lethal midline granuloma, 184, 203, 205, 206, 207, 226, 262
leukemia-free survival (LFS), 59
LGL expansion, 3, 102, 103, 104, 105, 106, 107, 108, 110, 116, 128
LGL leukemia (large granular lymphocytic leukemia), v, vi, vii, 1, 2, 3, 16, 17, 18, 19, 20, 21, 22, 23, 24, 25, 26, 35, 36, 37, 39, 40, 41, 45, 71, 76, 89, 91, 93, 94, 95, 96, 101, 102, 104, 110, 111, 112, 113, 114, 115, 116, 117, 118, 120, 133, 137, 138, 139, 140, 141, 142, 143, 144, 146, 147, 152, 153,158, 159, 161, 162, 163, 164, 165, 166, 168, 173, 178, 179, 180, 181, 184, 203, 250, 251, 252, 256, 258, 259, 261, 262, 264, 266, 274, 275, 276
LGL lymphocytosis, 17, 103, 106, 107, 108, 109, 152
ligand-receptor interaction, 150
lymphoglobulin, 84, 85, 86
lymphomatoid granulomatosis, 193, 226, 228, 245
lysinuric protein intolerance, 280, 283, 284, 286, 297

M

macrophage activation, 280, 284, 286, 287, 297, 298
major histocompatibility complex (MHC), 20, 27, 28, 29, 30, 38, 45, 46, 47, 48, 49, 66, 68, 69, 76, 124, 140, 150, 154, 160, 161, 162, 187, 199, 281
MAPK, 31, 35, 115, 116
matrix metalloproteinase, 33, 261
metastatic neuroendocrine tumor, 193
methotrexate (MTX), 1, 11, 14, 24, 35, 83, 108, 113, 128, 135, 159, 165, 167, 168, 169, 177, 179, 237, 238, 239, 247, 248, 265, 269, 270, 276, 286
microthrombi, 189

midline malignant reticulosis, 184, 207, 226
monoclonal, 3, 8, 17, 18, 44, 47, 62, 108, 109, 116, 118, 122, 124, 129, 137, 141, 143, 156, 158, 159, 163, 166, 171, 172, 180, 227, 264
monoclonal antibody(ies), 44, 47, 62, 108, 116, 124, 141, 156, 159, 171, 172, 180
monoclonal gammopathy (MGUS), 116, 118, 137, 166
monomorphic epitheliotropic intestinal T-cell lymphoma, 196, 228
mosquito bite allergy, 250
mosquito-bite hypersensitivity, 196
Munc18-2, 279, 282, 289, 294
mutation(s), 1, 2, 4, 9, 10, 11, 12, 13, 14, 15, 18, 21, 22, 23, 33, 60, 64, 76, 77, 80, 81, 82, 89, 90, 91, 93, 94, 95, 96, 104, 111, 115, 128, 135, 142, 149, 157, 158, 159, 163, 166, 168, 171, 173, 180, 197, 199, 209, 215, 219, 220, 227, 241, 249, 257, 279, 282, 284, 285, 286, 289, 290, 294, 295, 296, 297
mycosis fungiodes, 195
myelodysplastic syndromes (MDS), 11, 54, 55, 56, 64, 65, 73, 75, 76, 77, 78, 79, 80, 81, 82, 83, 84, 85, 86, 87, 89, 90, 91, 92, 93, 95, 97, 98, 99, 100, 122, 139, 159, 166, 168, 171, 172

N

nasal cavity, 130, 183, 184, 187, 206, 221, 226, 227, 229, 230
nasal congestion, 130, 187
nasal NK/T cell lymphoma, 204, 219, 220, 237, 250
nasal type, 142, 144, 145, 183, 184, 191, 201, 202, 203, 204, 209, 210, 211, 212, 213, 214, 215, 217, 218, 220, 222, 223, 225, 226, 232, 233, 234, 238, 242, 243, 244, 245, 246, 247, 248, 257, 259, 263, 270, 276
nasopharyngeal carcinoma, 193, 221, 228
nasopharynx, 184, 187, 191, 226, 230, 235
natural cytotoxicity receptors (NCR), 18, 46, 151, 264
natural killer (NK) cell(s), vi, vii, 2, 3, 7, 9, 11, 16, 18, 19, 21, 25, 26, 27, 28, 29, 30, 31, 32, 34, 35, 36, 37, 38, 39, 40, 43, 44, 45, 46, 47, 48, 49, 50, 51, 53, 54, 56, 57, 58, 59, 60, 61, 62, 63, 64, 65, 66, 67, 68, 69, 70, 71, 72, 73, 75, 76, 81, 91, 93, 94, 96, 101, 102,106, 107, 110, 111, 112, 113, 115, 116, 117, 118, 119, 128, 129, 130, 131, 132, 133, 136, 138, 142, 143, 144, 145, 146, 149, 150,

151, 152, 153, 154, 155, 156, 157, 158, 159, 160, 161, 162, 163, 181, 184, 192, 195, 196, 198, 203, 204, 205, 207, 208, 209, 211, 212, 213, 214, 215, 216, 217, 218, 220, 221, 222, 223, 226, 228, 243, 244, 246, 249, 250, 251, 252, 253, 254, 255, 256, 257, 258, 259, 260, 261, 262, 263, 264, 265, 266, 267, 268, 270, 271, 274, 275, 276, 277, 279, 292, 293, 294, 297, 298
NCCN guidelines for NHL, 159
network model, 5, 6, 19, 40, 178
neutropenia, 7, 11, 18, 26, 28, 35, 36, 78, 85, 89, 103, 105, 108, 109, 113, 114, 117, 118, 138, 156, 157, 162, 165, 166, 167, 168, 169, 172, 176, 179, 181, 237, 251, 266, 270, 285
next generation sequencing (NGS), 7, 9, 15, 128, 199, 227
NF-κB, 6, 12, 13, 26, 115, 198
NK cell-associated receptors (NKR), 25, 31, 34, 60, 64, 65, 154, 189
NK prognostic index, 184, 200, 202
NK/T cell lymphoma prognostic index (NKPI), 232
NK-cell dysfunction, 280, 282, 286, 287, 292
NK-cell enteropathy, 197, 217, 228
NKG2D, 30, 31, 40, 48, 61, 64, 72, 73, 150, 154, 160, 161
NKR-DAP10/DAP12 signaling pathways, 25, 34
non-Hodgkin lymphoma, 144, 225
NOS, 81, 133, 229
NRP1, 12, 14

P

palate, 184, 187, 227, 235
panniculitis, 189, 194, 214, 228, 287
paranasal sinuses, 184, 187, 193, 206, 216, 221, 226
paroxysmal nocturnal hemoglobinuria (PNH), 17, 75, 76, 87, 91, 99, 122, 166
pembrolizumab, 242, 265, 270, 272, 276
pentostatin, 165, 171, 179
perforin, 27, 30, 31, 37, 40, 45, 66, 124, 127, 131, 135, 141, 150, 151, 157, 189, 192, 215, 226, 268, 279, 281, 282, 284, 285, 289, 290, 294, 295, 298
peripheral T-cell lymphoma, 133, 146, 195, 204, 244
perisinasoidal arrangement, 123
pesticides, 186, 209, 226
phosphatidylinositol 3-kinase (PI3K)-AKT, 115

phosphoinositide 3-kinase (PI3K), 1, 4, 5, 19, 26, 31, 34, 35, 113, 115, 116
PINK-E, 201, 232
platelet drived growth factor (PDGF), 1, 4, 5, 26, 166
polymorphic reticulosis, 184, 203, 205, 206, 207, 210, 226
PRCA, 11, 181
PRDM1, 183, 197, 218, 227, 244, 249, 257, 263
PRDMI, 183, 197, 218, 227, 244, 249, 257, 263
PRF1, 279, 281, 282, 283, 289, 293
primary cutaneous CD56-positive peripheral T cell lymphoma, 195
primary cutaneous CD8 positive aggressive epidermotropic cytotoxic T-cell lymphoma, 196, 228
prognostic index of natural killer lymphoma, 201, 232
programmed cell death ligand-1 (PD-L1), 227, 242, 244
proteasome inhibitor, 174
pseudoepitheliomatous hyperplasia, 189, 193
PTPN2 (G224V) mutations, 249
PTPRT, 12, 23
pulmonary artery hypertension, 29, 116
pure red cell aplasia (PRCA), 11, 22, 122, 139, 166, 168, 181
purine analog(s), 165, 170, 173, 177
purine nucleoside analogs, 171

R

Rab27a, 279, 281, 284, 289, 295
RAS-RAF, 115, 116
red pulps, 123
regulators, 13, 27
regulators of the extracellular matrix, 27
rheumatoid arthritis (RA), 11, 26, 28, 34, 40, 78, 83, 86, 90, 108, 110, 113, 116, 118, 135, 139, 165, 166, 174, 180, 295, 296, 297, 298
rhinorrhea, 187, 192, 227

S

S1P, 4
serum lactate dehydrogenase, 200, 232, 251
severe combined immunodeficiency, 61, 62, 96, 280, 283, 284, 285, 297

Index

Sezary Syndrome, 134, 146
SH2 domain, 10, 11, 94, 149, 279
SH2D1A, 279, 283, 285, 289, 296
siplizumab, 172, 175, 180
SLIT2, 12, 13, 24
SOCS3, 13
sphingosine, 4, 6, 19, 20
splenectomy, 134, 135, 152, 170, 172, 173, 177
splenomegaly, 26, 115, 116, 118, 132, 139, 149, 156, 166, 167, 169, 171, 172, 258, 280, 285, 287, 288, 289
squamous cell carcinoma, 193
STAT3, 1, 4, 5, 6, 9, 10, 11, 12, 13, 14, 15, 18, 21, 22, 23, 80, 81, 82, 93, 94, 95, 104, 109, 111, 115, 128, 135, 142, 149, 158, 163, 166, 168, 171, 173, 174, 177, 178, 198, 199, 219, 220, 241, 249, 257
STAT3 (Y640F), 10, 11, 12, 13, 80, 168, 249, 257
STAT3 mutations, 9, 11, 12, 13, 15, 18, 21, 22, 23, 80, 81, 93, 94, 111, 128, 142, 163, 171
STAT5, 6, 10, 12, 80, 81, 82, 174
STAT5b, 10, 11, 12, 22, 23, 94, 95, 142, 166, 173, 176, 177, 180
STAT5B, 23, 115, 128, 142, 199, 220, 249, 257
stem cell transplant (SCT), 44, 53, 67, 68, 69, 70, 72, 73, 110, 111, 112, 116, 129, 135, 143, 170, 172, 173, 180, 239, 241, 248, 260, 265, 266, 270, 273, 276, 290, 291, 299
steroids, 159, 169, 177, 270, 271
STX11, 279, 281, 282, 283, 289, 293
subcutaneous panniculitis-like T-cell lymphoma, 194
surface CD3, 45, 102, 115, 118, 123, 125, 126, 129, 130, 131, 132, 134, 135, 152, 153, 154, 155, 189, 196, 250, 254, 256, 258, 259, 260, 268
Syk protein tyrosine kinase, 31
systemic EBV related T/NK cell lymphoproliferative disorders, 250
systemic EBV-positive T-cell lymphoma of childhood, 259, 260

T

T cell lymphoma, 115, 116, 130, 133, 142, 145, 146, 147, 154, 163, 183, 184, 186, 195, 204, 207, 210, 214, 215, 219, 220, 222, 225, 226, 228, 230, 232, 233, 234, 235, 236, 237, 239, 243, 244, 247, 248, 250, 257, 260, 264, 266, 270, 274, 276

T cell receptor (TCR), 3, 7, 8, 15, 17, 20, 40, 45, 76, 78, 79, 86, 88, 90, 98, 102, 103, 104, 105, 106, 107, 108, 109, 115, 124, 125, 126, 127, 128, 129, 130, 132, 134, 135, 140, 141, 146, 152, 154, 155, 176, 189, 195, 196, 200, 226, 249, 250, 254, 256, 259, 260, 268
T-cell clonality, 127
T-cell large granular lymphocytic leukemia (T-LGLL), vi, vii, 2, 3, 5, 6, 7, 8, 9, 10, 11, 12, 13, 14, 21, 22, 23, 25, 30, 31, 34, 78, 83, 115, 116, 117, 118, 119, 121, 122, 123, 125, 126, 127, 128, 129, 130, 131, 132, 133, 134, 135, 137, 139, 140, 146, 152, 153, 156, 158, 159, 165, 171, 173, 178, 179, 180, 258, 259
TCRαβ, 17, 125, 126, 131, 132, 135, 254, 256
TCRγδ, 21, 131, 135, 254
TET2, 12, 13, 14, 23, 77, 83, 90
TFNAIP3, 12
thrombocytopenia, 18, 26, 78, 85, 89, 131, 138, 156, 166, 187, 251, 266, 285
thymoglobulin, 84, 85, 86, 104
TIA1, 124, 135, 152, 189, 191
tipifarnib (zarnestra), 159, 173, 175
TNFA-IP3, 115, 128
Tofacitinib, 173, 174, 180
tumor necrosis factor (TNF), 13, 28, 32, 61, 79, 81, 92, 95, 108, 113, 115, 151, 198, 281, 286
tumor necrosis factor beta (TNF β), 151
tumor necrosis factor-alpha (TNF-α), 61, 79, 81

U

UCB transplant (UCBT), 59
umbilical, 58, 70
umbilical cord blood (UCB), 58, 59, 70
UNC13D, 279, 281, 282, 283, 289, 294
upper aerodigestive tract NK/T cell lymphoma (UNKTL), 201, 230

V

variable β-chain repertoire, 124

W

whole exome sequencing (WES), 9
whole genome sequencing (WGS), 9, 14
Wilms-tumor 1 (WT1), 79

Wiskott-Aldrich syndrome, 280, 283, 284, 285, 297
world health organization (WHO), vii, 2, 16, 76, 78, 90, 91, 92, 117, 129, 136, 137, 141, 144, 149, 152, 158, 161, 184, 204, 206, 214, 216, 229, 242, 243, 245, 250, 258, 261, 264, 274

X

x-linked lymphoproliferative syndromes, 280

Α

αβ T-LGLL, 8, 124

Γ

γδ T-cells, 27, 134